50% OFF

Online HESI A^2 Prep Course!

By Mometrix

FREE Study Skills Videos/DVD Offer

Dear Customer,

Thank you for your purchase from Mometrix! We consider it an honor and a privilege that you have purchased our product and we want to ensure your satisfaction.

As part of our ongoing effort to meet the needs of test takers, we have developed a set of Study Skills Videos that we would like to give you for FREE. These videos cover our *best practices* for getting ready for your exam, from how to use our study materials to how to best prepare for the day of the test.

All that we ask is that you email us with feedback that would describe your experience so far with our product. Good, bad, or indifferent, we want to know what you think!

To get your FREE Study Skills Videos, you can use the **QR code** below, or send us an **email** at studyvideos@mometrix.com with *FREE VIDEOS* in the subject line and the following information in the body of the email:

- The name of the product you purchased.
- Your product rating on a scale of 1-5, with 5 being the highest rating.
- Your feedback. It can be long, short, or anything in between. We just want to know your impressions and experience so far with our product. (Good feedback might include how our study material met your needs and ways we might be able to make it even better. You could highlight features that you found helpful or features that you think we should add.)

If you have any questions or concerns, please don't hesitate to contact me directly.

Thanks again!

Sincerely,

Jay Willis
Vice President
jay.willis@mometrix.com
1-800-673-8175

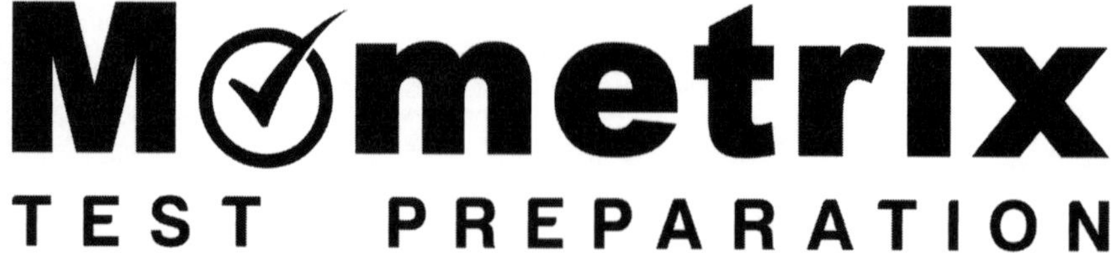

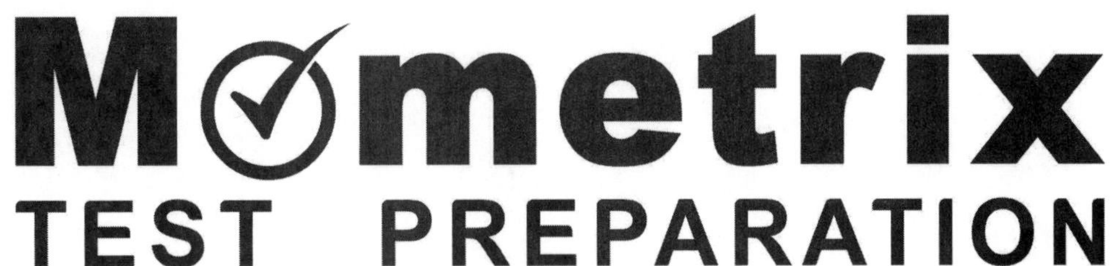

HESI® A^2

Secrets Study Guide 2024-2025

1000+ Practice Test Questions

Comprehensive Review Prep
with 200+ Online Videos
for the HESI Admission
Assessment Exam

5th Edition

Written and edited by Mometrix Test Prep

Printed in the United States of America

This paper meets the requirements of ANSI/NISO Z39.48-1992 (Permanence of Paper).

Mometrix offers volume discount pricing to institutions. For more information or a price quote, please contact our sales department at sales@mometrix.com or 888-248-1219.

Paperback
ISBN 13: 978-1-5167-2607-3
ISBN 10: 1-5167-2607-3

Dear Future HESI A^2 Success Story

First of all, **THANK YOU** for purchasing Mometrix study materials!

Second, congratulations! You are one of the few determined test-takers who are committed to doing whatever it takes to excel on your exam. **You have come to the right place.** We developed these study materials with one goal in mind: to deliver you the information you need in a format that's concise and easy to use.

In addition to optimizing your guide for the content of the test, we've outlined our recommended steps for breaking down the preparation process into small, attainable goals so you can make sure you stay on track.

We've also analyzed the entire test-taking process, identifying the most common pitfalls and showing how you can overcome them and be ready for any curveball the test throws you.

Standardized testing is one of the biggest obstacles on your road to success, which only increases the importance of doing well in the high-pressure, high-stakes environment of test day. Your results on this test could have a significant impact on your future, and this guide provides the information and practical advice to help you achieve your full potential on test day.

Your success is our success

We would love to hear from you! If you would like to share the story of your exam success or if you have any questions or comments in regard to our products, please contact us at support@mometrix.com.

Thanks again for your business and we wish you continued success!

Sincerely,
The Mometrix Test Preparation Team

Need more help? Check out our flashcards at:
http://mometrixflashcards.com/HESI

Table of Contents

Introduction

Thank you for purchasing this resource! You have made the choice to prepare yourself for a test that could have a huge impact on your future, and this guide is designed to help you be fully ready for test day. Obviously, it's important to have a solid understanding of the test material, but you also need to be prepared for the unique environment and stressors of the test, so that you can perform to the best of your abilities.

For this purpose, the first section that appears in this guide is the **Secret Keys**. We've devoted countless hours to meticulously researching what works and what doesn't, and we've boiled down our findings to the four most impactful steps you can take to improve your performance on the test. We start at the beginning with study planning and move through the preparation process, all the way to the testing strategies that will help you get the most out of what you know when you're finally sitting in front of the test.

We recommend that you start preparing for your test as far in advance as possible. However, if you've bought this guide as a last-minute study resource and only have a few days before your test, we recommend that you skip over the first two Secret Keys since they address a long-term study plan.

If you struggle with **test anxiety**, we strongly encourage you to check out our recommendations for how you can overcome it. Test anxiety is a formidable foe, but it can be beaten, and we want to make sure you have the tools you need to defeat it.

Secret Key #1 – Plan Big, Study Small

There's a lot riding on your performance. If you want to ace this test, you're going to need to keep your skills sharp and the material fresh in your mind. You need a plan that lets you review everything you need to know while still fitting in your schedule. We'll break this strategy down into three categories.

Information Organization

Start with the information you already have: the official test outline. From this, you can make a complete list of all the concepts you need to cover before the test. Organize these concepts into groups that can be studied together, and create a list of any related vocabulary you need to learn so you can brush up on any difficult terms. You'll want to keep this vocabulary list handy once you actually start studying since you may need to add to it along the way.

Time Management

Once you have your set of study concepts, decide how to spread them out over the time you have left before the test. Break your study plan into small, clear goals so you have a manageable task for each day and know exactly what you're doing. Then just focus on one small step at a time. When you manage your time this way, you don't need to spend hours at a time studying. Studying a small block of content for a short period each day helps you retain information better and avoid stressing over how much you have left to do. You can relax knowing that you have a plan to cover everything in time. In order for this strategy to be effective though, you have to start studying early and stick to your schedule. Avoid the exhaustion and futility that comes from last-minute cramming!

Study Environment

The environment you study in has a big impact on your learning. Studying in a coffee shop, while probably more enjoyable, is not likely to be as fruitful as studying in a quiet room. It's important to keep distractions to a minimum. You're only planning to study for a short block of time, so make the most of it. Don't pause to check your phone or get up to find a snack. It's also important to **avoid multitasking**. Research has consistently shown that multitasking will make your studying dramatically less effective. Your study area should also be comfortable and well-lit so you don't have the distraction of straining your eyes or sitting on an uncomfortable chair.

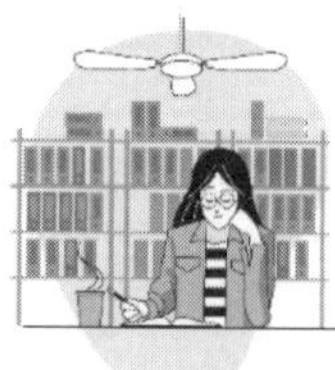

The time of day you study is also important. You want to be rested and alert. Don't wait until just before bedtime. Study when you'll be most likely to comprehend and remember. Even better, if you know what time of day your test will be, set that time aside for study. That way your brain will be used to working on that subject at that specific time and you'll have a better chance of recalling information.

Finally, it can be helpful to team up with others who are studying for the same test. Your actual studying should be done in as isolated an environment as possible, but the work of organizing the information and setting up the study plan can be divided up. In between study sessions, you can discuss with your teammates the concepts that you're all studying and quiz each other on the details. Just be sure that your teammates are as serious about the test as you are. If you find that your study time is being replaced with social time, you might need to find a new team.

Secret Key #2 – Make Your Studying Count

You're devoting a lot of time and effort to preparing for this test, so you want to be absolutely certain it will pay off. This means doing more than just reading the content and hoping you can remember it on test day. It's important to make every minute of study count. There are two main areas you can focus on to make your studying count.

Retention

It doesn't matter how much time you study if you can't remember the material. You need to make sure you are retaining the concepts. To check your retention of the information you're learning, try recalling it at later times with minimal prompting. Try carrying around flashcards and glance at one or two from time to time or ask a friend who's also studying for the test to quiz you.

To enhance your retention, look for ways to put the information into practice so that you can apply it rather than simply recalling it. If you're using the information in practical ways, it will be much easier to remember. Similarly, it helps to solidify a concept in your mind if you're not only reading it to yourself but also explaining it to someone else. Ask a friend to let you teach them about a concept you're a little shaky on (or speak aloud to an imaginary audience if necessary). As you try to summarize, define, give examples, and answer your friend's questions, you'll understand the concepts better and they will stay with you longer. Finally, step back for a big picture view and ask yourself how each piece of information fits with the whole subject. When you link the different concepts together and see them working together as a whole, it's easier to remember the individual components.

Finally, practice showing your work on any multi-step problems, even if you're just studying. Writing out each step you take to solve a problem will help solidify the process in your mind, and you'll be more likely to remember it during the test.

Modality

Modality simply refers to the means or method by which you study. Choosing a study modality that fits your own individual learning style is crucial. No two people learn best in exactly the same way, so it's important to know your strengths and use them to your advantage.

For example, if you learn best by visualization, focus on visualizing a concept in your mind and draw an image or a diagram. Try color-coding your notes, illustrating them, or creating symbols that will trigger your mind to recall a learned concept. If you learn best by hearing or discussing information, find a study partner who learns the same way or read aloud to yourself. Think about how to put the information in your own words. Imagine that you are giving a lecture on the topic and record yourself so you can listen to it later.

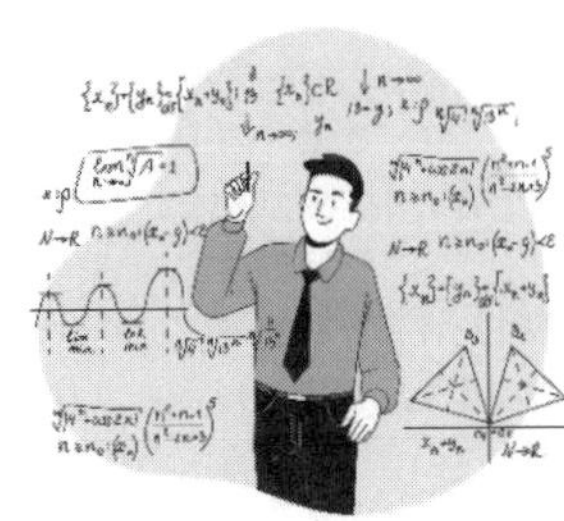

For any learning style, flashcards can be helpful. Organize the information so you can take advantage of spare moments to review. Underline key words or phrases. Use different colors for different categories. Mnemonic devices (such as creating a short list in which every item starts with the same letter) can also help with retention. Find what works best for you and use it to store the information in your mind most effectively and easily.

Secret Key #3 – Practice the Right Way

Your success on test day depends not only on how many hours you put into preparing, but also on whether you prepared the right way. It's good to check along the way to see if your studying is paying off. One of the most effective ways to do this is by taking practice tests to evaluate your progress. Practice tests are useful because they show exactly where you need to improve. Every time you take a practice test, pay special attention to these three groups of questions:

- The questions you got wrong
- The questions you had to guess on, even if you guessed right
- The questions you found difficult or slow to work through

This will show you exactly what your weak areas are, and where you need to devote more study time. Ask yourself why each of these questions gave you trouble. Was it because you didn't understand the material? Was it because you didn't remember the vocabulary? Do you need more repetitions on this type of question to build speed and confidence? Dig into those questions and figure out how you can strengthen your weak areas as you go back to review the material.

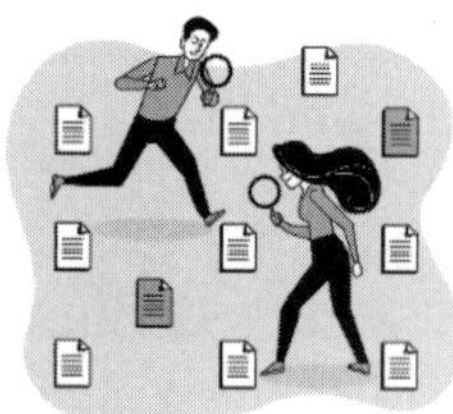

Additionally, many practice tests have a section explaining the answer choices. It can be tempting to read the explanation and think that you now have a good understanding of the concept. However, an explanation likely only covers part of the question's broader context. Even if the explanation makes perfect sense, **go back and investigate** every concept related to the question until you're positive you have a thorough understanding.

As you go along, keep in mind that the practice test is just that: practice. Memorizing these questions and answers will not be very helpful on the actual test because it is unlikely to have any of the same exact questions. If you only know the right answers to the sample questions, you won't be prepared for the real thing. **Study the concepts** until you understand them fully, and then you'll be able to answer any question that shows up on the test.

It's important to wait on the practice tests until you're ready. If you take a test on your first day of study, you may be overwhelmed by the amount of material covered and how much you need to learn. Work up to it gradually.

On test day, you'll need to be prepared for answering questions, managing your time, and using the test-taking strategies you've learned. It's a lot to balance, like a mental marathon that will have a big impact on your future. Like training for a marathon, you'll need to start slowly and work your way up. When test day arrives, you'll be ready.

Start with the strategies you've read in the first two Secret Keys—plan your course and study in the way that works best for you. If you have time, consider using multiple study resources to get different approaches to the same concepts. It can be helpful to see difficult concepts from more than one angle. Then find a good source for practice tests. Many times, the test website will suggest potential study resources or provide sample tests.

Secret Key #4 – Have a Plan for Guessing

When you're taking the test, you may find yourself stuck on a question. Some of the answer choices seem better than others, but you don't see the one answer choice that is obviously correct. What do you do?

The scenario described above is very common, yet most test takers have not effectively prepared for it. Developing and practicing a plan for guessing may be one of the single most effective uses of your time as you get ready for the exam.

In developing your plan for guessing, there are three questions to address:

- When should you start the guessing process?
- How should you narrow down the choices?
- Which answer should you choose?

When to Start the Guessing Process

Unless your plan for guessing is to select C every time (which, despite its merits, is not what we recommend), you need to leave yourself enough time to apply your answer elimination strategies. Since you have a limited amount of time for each question, that means that if you're going to give yourself the best shot at guessing correctly, you have to decide quickly whether or not you will guess.

Of course, the best-case scenario is that you don't have to guess at all, so first, see if you can answer the question based on your knowledge of the subject and basic reasoning skills. Focus on the key words in the question and try to jog your memory of related topics. Give yourself a chance to bring the knowledge to mind, but once you realize that you don't have (or you can't access) the knowledge you need to answer the question, it's time to start the guessing process.

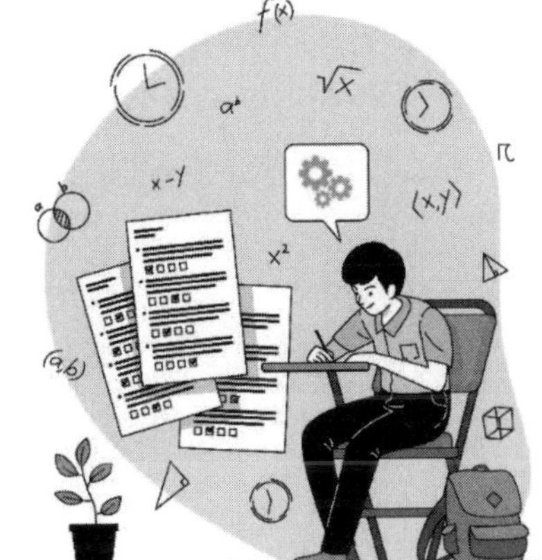

It's almost always better to start the guessing process too early than too late. It only takes a few seconds to remember something and answer the question from knowledge. Carefully eliminating wrong answer choices takes longer. Plus, going through the process of eliminating answer choices can actually help jog your memory.

Summary: Start the guessing process as soon as you decide that you can't answer the question based on your knowledge.

How to Narrow Down the Choices

The next chapter in this book (**Test-Taking Strategies**) includes a wide range of strategies for how to approach questions and how to look for answer choices to eliminate. You will definitely want to read those carefully, practice them, and figure out which ones work best for you. Here though, we're going to address a mindset rather than a particular strategy.

Your odds of guessing an answer correctly depend on how many options you are choosing from.

Number of options left	5	4	3	2	1
Odds of guessing correctly	20%	25%	33%	50%	100%

You can see from this chart just how valuable it is to be able to eliminate incorrect answers and make an educated guess, but there are two things that many test takers do that cause them to miss out on the benefits of guessing:

- Accidentally eliminating the correct answer
- Selecting an answer based on an impression

We'll look at the first one here, and the second one in the next section.

To avoid accidentally eliminating the correct answer, we recommend a thought exercise called **the $5 challenge**. In this challenge, you only eliminate an answer choice from contention if you are willing to bet $5 on it being wrong. Why $5? Five dollars is a small but not insignificant amount of money. It's an amount you could afford to lose but wouldn't want to throw away. And while losing $5 once might not hurt too much, doing it twenty times will set you back $100. In the same way, each small decision you make—eliminating a choice here, guessing on a question there—won't by itself impact your score very much, but when you put them all together, they can make a big difference. By holding each answer choice elimination decision to a higher standard, you can reduce the risk of accidentally eliminating the correct answer.

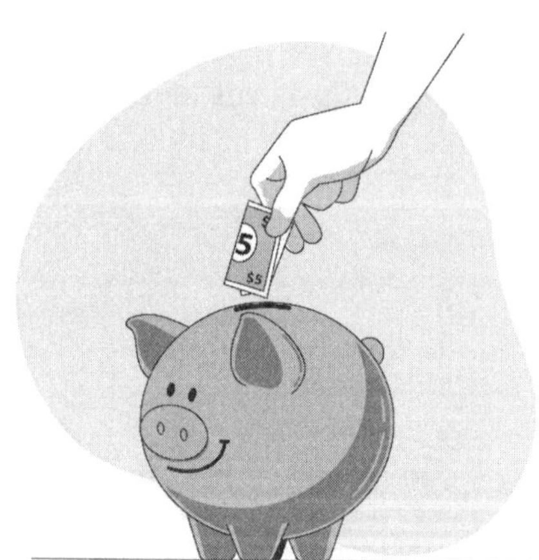

The $5 challenge can also be applied in a positive sense: If you are willing to bet $5 that an answer choice *is* correct, go ahead and mark it as correct.

Summary: Only eliminate an answer choice if you are willing to bet $5 that it is wrong.

Which Answer to Choose

You're taking the test. You've run into a hard question and decided you'll have to guess. You've eliminated all the answer choices you're willing to bet $5 on. Now you have to pick an answer. Why do we even need to talk about this? Why can't you just pick whichever one you feel like when the time comes?

The answer to these questions is that if you don't come into the test with a plan, you'll rely on your impression to select an answer choice, and if you do that, you risk falling into a trap. The test writers know that everyone who takes their test will be guessing on some of the questions, so they intentionally write wrong answer choices to seem plausible. You still have to pick an answer though, and if the wrong answer choices are designed to look right, how can you ever be sure that you're not falling for their trap? The best solution we've found to this dilemma is to take the decision out of your hands entirely. Here is the process we recommend:

Once you've eliminated any choices that you are confident (willing to bet $5) are wrong, select the first remaining choice as your answer.

Whether you choose to select the first remaining choice, the second, or the last, the important thing is that you use some preselected standard. Using this approach guarantees that you will not be enticed into selecting an answer choice that looks right, because you are not basing your decision on how the answer choices look.

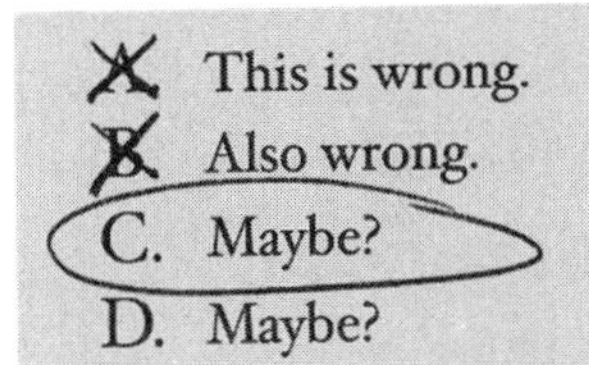

This is not meant to make you question your knowledge. Instead, it is to help you recognize the difference between your knowledge and your impressions. There's a huge difference between thinking an answer is right because of what you know, and thinking an answer is right because it looks or sounds like it should be right.

Summary: To ensure that your selection is appropriately random, make a predetermined selection from among all answer choices you have not eliminated.

Test-Taking Strategies

This section contains a list of test-taking strategies that you may find helpful as you work through the test. By taking what you know and applying logical thought, you can maximize your chances of answering any question correctly!

It is very important to realize that every question is different and every person is different: no single strategy will work on every question, and no single strategy will work for every person. That's why we've included all of them here, so you can try them out and determine which ones work best for different types of questions and which ones work best for you.

Question Strategies

READ CAREFULLY

Read the question and the answer choices carefully. Don't miss the question because you misread the terms. You have plenty of time to read each question thoroughly and make sure you understand what is being asked. Yet a happy medium must be attained, so don't waste too much time. You must read carefully and efficiently.

CONTEXTUAL CLUES

Look for contextual clues. If the question includes a word you are not familiar with, look at the immediate context for some indication of what the word might mean. Contextual clues can often give you all the information you need to decipher the meaning of an unfamiliar word. Even if you can't determine the meaning, you may be able to narrow down the possibilities enough to make a solid guess at the answer to the question.

PREFIXES

If you're having trouble with a word in the question or answer choices, try dissecting it. Take advantage of every clue that the word might include. Prefixes can be a huge help. Usually, they allow you to determine a basic meaning. *Pre-* means before, *post-* means after, *pro-* is positive, *de-* is negative. From prefixes, you can get an idea of the general meaning of the word and try to put it into context.

HEDGE WORDS

Watch out for critical hedge words, such as *likely, may, can, sometimes, often, almost, mostly, usually, generally, rarely,* and *sometimes*. Question writers insert these hedge phrases to cover every possibility. Often an answer choice will be wrong simply because it leaves no room for exception. Be on guard for answer choices that have definitive words such as *exactly* and *always*.

SWITCHBACK WORDS

Stay alert for *switchbacks*. These are the words and phrases frequently used to alert you to shifts in thought. The most common switchback words are *but, although*, and *however*. Others include *nevertheless, on the other hand, even though, while, in spite of, despite*, and *regardless of*. Switchback words are important to catch because they can change the direction of the question or an answer choice.

✓ FACE VALUE

When in doubt, use common sense. Accept the situation in the problem at face value. Don't read too much into it. These problems will not require you to make wild assumptions. If you have to go beyond creativity and warp time or space in order to have an answer choice fit the question, then you should move on and consider the other answer choices. These are normal problems rooted in reality. The applicable relationship or explanation may not be readily apparent, but it is there for you to figure out. Use your common sense to interpret anything that isn't clear.

Answer Choice Strategies

✓ ANSWER SELECTION

The most thorough way to pick an answer choice is to identify and eliminate wrong answers until only one is left, then confirm it is the correct answer. Sometimes an answer choice may immediately seem right, but be careful. The test writers will usually put more than one reasonable answer choice on each question, so take a second to read all of them and make sure that the other choices are not equally obvious. As long as you have time left, it is better to read every answer choice than to pick the first one that looks right without checking the others.

✓ ANSWER CHOICE FAMILIES

An answer choice family consists of two (in rare cases, three) answer choices that are very similar in construction and cannot all be true at the same time. If you see two answer choices that are direct opposites or parallels, one of them is usually the correct answer. For instance, if one answer choice says that quantity x increases and another either says that quantity x decreases (opposite) or says that quantity y increases (parallel), then those answer choices would fall into the same family. An answer choice that doesn't match the construction of the answer choice family is more likely to be incorrect. Most questions will not have answer choice families, but when they do appear, you should be prepared to recognize them.

✓ ELIMINATE ANSWERS

Eliminate answer choices as soon as you realize they are wrong, but make sure you consider all possibilities. If you are eliminating answer choices and realize that the last one you are left with is also wrong, don't panic. Start over and consider each choice again. There may be something you missed the first time that you will realize on the second pass.

✓ AVOID FACT TRAPS

Don't be distracted by an answer choice that is factually true but doesn't answer the question. You are looking for the choice that answers the question. Stay focused on what the question is asking for so you don't accidentally pick an answer that is true but incorrect. Always go back to the question and make sure the answer choice you've selected actually answers the question and is not merely a true statement.

✓ EXTREME STATEMENTS

In general, you should avoid answers that put forth extreme actions as standard practice or proclaim controversial ideas as established fact. An answer choice that states the "process should be used in certain situations, if..." is much more likely to be correct than one that states the "process should be discontinued completely." The first is a calm rational statement and doesn't even make a definitive, uncompromising stance, using a hedge word *if* to provide wiggle room, whereas the second choice is far more extreme.

☑ Benchmark

As you read through the answer choices and you come across one that seems to answer the question well, mentally select that answer choice. This is not your final answer, but it's the one that will help you evaluate the other answer choices. The one that you selected is your benchmark or standard for judging each of the other answer choices. Every other answer choice must be compared to your benchmark. That choice is correct until proven otherwise by another answer choice beating it. If you find a better answer, then that one becomes your new benchmark. Once you've decided that no other choice answers the question as well as your benchmark, you have your final answer.

☑ Predict the Answer

Before you even start looking at the answer choices, it is often best to try to predict the answer. When you come up with the answer on your own, it is easier to avoid distractions and traps because you will know exactly what to look for. The right answer choice is unlikely to be word-for-word what you came up with, but it should be a close match. Even if you are confident that you have the right answer, you should still take the time to read each option before moving on.

General Strategies

☑ Tough Questions

If you are stumped on a problem or it appears too hard or too difficult, don't waste time. Move on! Remember though, if you can quickly check for obviously incorrect answer choices, your chances of guessing correctly are greatly improved. Before you completely give up, at least try to knock out a couple of possible answers. Eliminate what you can and then guess at the remaining answer choices before moving on.

☑ Check Your Work

Since you will probably not know every term listed and the answer to every question, it is important that you get credit for the ones that you do know. Don't miss any questions through careless mistakes. If at all possible, try to take a second to look back over your answer selection and make sure you've selected the correct answer choice and haven't made a costly careless mistake (such as marking an answer choice that you didn't mean to mark). This quick double check should more than pay for itself in caught mistakes for the time it costs.

☑ Don't Rush

It is very easy to make errors when you are in a hurry. Maintaining a fast pace in answering questions is pointless if it makes you miss questions that you would have gotten right otherwise. Test writers like to include distracting information and wrong answers that seem right. Taking a little extra time to avoid careless mistakes can make all the difference in your test score. Find a pace that allows you to be confident in the answers that you select.

☑ Keep Moving

Panicking will not help you pass the test, so do your best to stay calm and keep moving. Taking deep breaths and going through the answer elimination steps you practiced can help to break through a stress barrier and keep your pace.

Final Notes

The combination of a solid foundation of content knowledge and the confidence that comes from practicing your plan for applying that knowledge is the key to maximizing your performance on test day. As your foundation of content knowledge is built up and strengthened, you'll find that the strategies included in this chapter become more and more effective in helping you quickly sift through the distractions and traps of the test to isolate the correct answer.

Now that you're preparing to move forward into the test content chapters of this book, be sure to keep your goal in mind. As you read, think about how you will be able to apply this information on the test. If you've already seen sample questions for the test and you have an idea of the question format and style, try to come up with questions of your own that you can answer based on what you're reading. This will give you valuable practice applying your knowledge in the same ways you can expect to on test day.

Good luck and good studying!

About the HESI Test

Thank you for your purchase of *HESI A^2 Secrets* by Mometrix Test Preparation. This study manual includes comprehensive review sections for each of the eight* HESI Admission Assessment subtests: Reading Comprehension, Vocabulary and General Knowledge, Grammar, Basic Math Skills, Biology, Chemistry, Anatomy and Physiology, and Physics. Following those review sections is a full-length practice test for each subtest. The answer key also includes detailed answer explanations.

***Note: You probably will not have to take all eight subtests. Check with each of the schools where you are applying to see which subtests they require.**

In the table below is a breakdown of the exam subtests, including the number and categories of questions found in each subtest. Two additional subtests, Personality Profile and Learning Style, are not scored but are used as supplemental assessments. Both of these assessments are designed to help the student by providing useful feedback as to how the student can maximize their odds of succeeding academically based on their personality and learning style.

None of the subtests are individually timed, but your full test session has a limit of 4 hours. If there are some subtest you are required to take and others that are optional, you should work on the required subtests first so you don't feel rushed. Once those are out of the way, you can use any leftover time to work on the optional subtests.

SUBTEST	NUMBER OF TEST ITEMS
Mathematics	**50**
Basic Operations	
Fractions, Percentages, and Related Concepts	
Algebra	
Reading Comprehension	**47**
Main Ideas, Supporting Details, and Context	
Purpose and Tone	
Fact and Opinion, Logical Inferences, and Summarizing	
Vocabulary and General Knowledge	**50**
Grammar	**50**
The Eight Parts of Speech	
Agreement and Sentence Structure	
Word Confusion	
Biology	**25**
Macromolecules	
DNA	
RNA	
Mendel's Laws	
Non-Mendelian Concepts	

Chemistry	**25**
Metric System and Scientific Reasoning	
Atomic Structure	
Bonding	
The Periodic Table	
Properties of Substances	
States of Matter	
Chemical Reactions	
Acids, Bases, and Salts	
Biochemistry	
Anatomy and Physiology	**25**
General Anatomy and Physiology	
Respiratory System	
Cardiovascular System	
Gastrointestinal System	
Nervous System	
Muscular System	
Reproductive System	
Integumentary System	
Endocrine System	
Urinary System	
Immune System	
Skeletal System	
Physics	**25**
Kinematics	
Acceleration	
Projectile Motion	
Newton's Laws of Motion	
Friction	
Rotation	
Kinetic and Potential Energy	
Linear Momentum and Impulse	
Nature of Electricity	
Magnetism and Electricity	
Personality Profile	**15**
Learning Style	**14**
Total	**Up to 326**

Mathematics

Transform passive reading into active learning! After immersing yourself in this chapter, put your comprehension to the test by taking a quiz. The insights you gained will stay with you longer this way. Scan the QR code to go directly to the chapter quiz interface for this study guide. If you're using a computer, simply visit the bonus page at **mometrix.com/bonus948/hesia2** and click the Chapter Quizzes link.

The Mathematics Test section of the HESI A^2 exam consists of 50 questions. All numbers used are real numbers.

Number Basics

Classifications of Numbers

Numbers are the basic building blocks of mathematics. Specific features of numbers are identified by the following terms:

Integer – any positive or negative whole number, including zero. Integers do not include fractions $\left(\frac{1}{3}\right)$, decimals (0.56), or mixed numbers $\left(7\frac{3}{4}\right)$.

Prime number – any whole number greater than 1 that has only two factors, itself and 1; that is, a number that can be divided evenly only by 1 and itself.

Composite number – any whole number greater than 1 that has more than two different factors; in other words, any whole number that is not a prime number. For example: The composite number 8 has the factors of 1, 2, 4, and 8.

Even number – any integer that can be divided by 2 without leaving a remainder. For example: 2, 4, 6, 8, and so on.

Odd number – any integer that cannot be divided evenly by 2. For example: 3, 5, 7, 9, and so on.

Decimal number – any number that uses a decimal point to show the part of the number that is less than one. Example: 1.234.

Decimal point – a symbol used to separate the ones place from the tenths place in decimals or dollars from cents in currency.

Decimal place – the position of a number to the right of the decimal point. In the decimal 0.123, the 1 is in the first place to the right of the decimal point, indicating tenths; the 2 is in the second place, indicating hundredths; and the 3 is in the third place, indicating thousandths.

The **decimal**, or base 10, system is a number system that uses ten different digits (0, 1, 2, 3, 4, 5, 6, 7, 8, 9). An example of a number system that uses something other than ten digits is the **binary**, or base 2, number system, used by computers, which uses only the numbers 0 and 1. It is thought that the decimal system originated because people had only their 10 fingers for counting.

Rational numbers include all integers, decimals, and fractions. Any terminating or repeating decimal number is a rational number.

Irrational numbers cannot be written as fractions or decimals because the number of decimal places is infinite and there is no recurring pattern of digits within the number. For example, pi (π) begins with 3.141592 and continues without terminating or repeating, so pi is an irrational number.

Real numbers are the set of all rational and irrational numbers.

Review Video: Classification of Numbers
Visit mometrix.com/academy and enter code: 461071

Review Video: Prime and Composite Numbers
Visit mometrix.com/academy and enter code: 565581

Numbers in Word Form and Place Value

When writing numbers out in word form or translating word form to numbers, it is essential to understand how a place value system works. In the decimal or base-10 system, each digit of a number represents how many of the corresponding place value—a specific factor of 10—are contained in the number being represented. To make reading numbers easier, every three digits to the left of the decimal place is preceded by a comma. The following table demonstrates some of the place values:

Power of 10	10^3	10^2	10^1	10^0	10^{-1}	10^{-2}	10^{-3}
Value	1,000	100	10	1	0.1	0.01	0.001
Place	thousands	hundreds	tens	ones	tenths	hundredths	thousandths

For example, consider the number 4,546.09, which can be separated into each place value like this:

4: thousands
5: hundreds
4: tens
6: ones
0: tenths
9: hundredths

This number in word form would be *four thousand five hundred forty-six and nine hundredths.*

Review Video: Place Value
Visit mometrix.com/academy and enter code: 205433

Rounding and Estimation

Rounding and Estimation

Rounding is reducing the digits in a number while still trying to keep the value similar. The result will be less accurate but in a simpler form and easier to use. Whole numbers can be rounded to the nearest ten, hundred, or thousand.

When you are asked to estimate the solution to a problem, you will need to provide only an approximate figure or **estimation** for your answer. In this situation, you will need to round each number in the calculation to the level indicated (nearest hundred, nearest thousand, etc.) or to a level that makes sense for the numbers involved. When estimating a sum **all numbers must be rounded to the same level**. You cannot round one number to the nearest thousand while rounding another to the nearest hundred.

Review Video: Rounding and Estimation
Visit mometrix.com/academy and enter code: 126243

Absolute Value

Absolute Value

A precursor to working with negative numbers is understanding what **absolute values** are. A number's absolute value is simply the distance away from zero a number is on the number line. The absolute value of a number is always positive and is written $|x|$. For example, the absolute value of 3, written as $|3|$, is 3 because the distance between 0 and 3 on a number line is three units. Likewise, the absolute value of –3, written as $|-3|$, is 3 because the distance between 0 and –3 on a number line is three units. So $|3| = |-3|$.

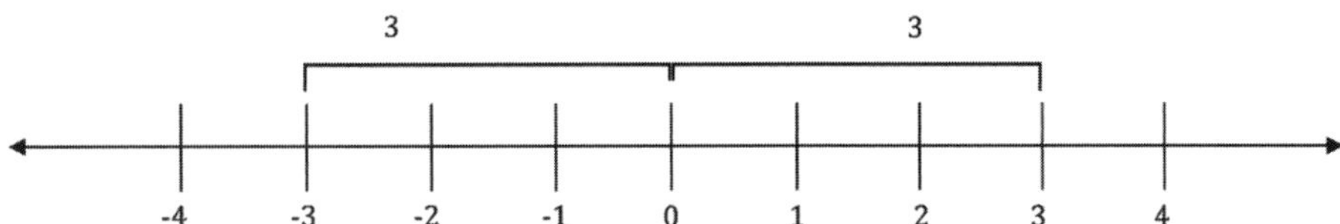

Review Video: Absolute Value
Visit mometrix.com/academy and enter code: 314669

Operations

Operations

An **operation** is simply a mathematical process that takes some value(s) as input(s) and produces an output. Elementary operations are often written in the following form: *value operation value*. For instance, in the expression $1 + 2$ the values are 1 and 2 and the operation is addition. Performing the operation gives the output of 3. In this way we can say that $1 + 2$ and 3 are equal, or $1 + 2 = 3$.

Addition

Addition increases the value of one quantity by the value of another quantity (both called **addends**). Example: $2 + 4 = 6$ or $8 + 9 = 17$. The result is called the **sum**. With addition, the order does not matter, $4 + 2 = 2 + 4$.

When adding signed numbers, if the signs are the same simply add the absolute values of the addends and apply the original sign to the sum. For example, $(+4) + (+8) = +12$ and $(-4) + (-8) = -12$. When the original signs are different, take the absolute values of the addends and subtract the smaller value from the larger value, then apply the original sign of the larger value to the difference. Example: $(+4) + (-8) = -4$ and $(-4) + (+8) = +4$.

Subtraction

Subtraction is the opposite operation to addition; it decreases the value of one quantity (the **minuend**) by the value of another quantity (the **subtrahend**). For example, $6 - 4 = 2$ or $17 - 8 = 9$. The result is called the **difference**. Note that with subtraction, the order does matter, $6 - 4 \neq 4 - 6$.

For subtracting signed numbers, change the sign of the subtrahend and then follow the same rules used for addition. Example: $(+4) - (+8) = (+4) + (-8) = -4$

Multiplication

Multiplication can be thought of as repeated addition. One number (the **multiplier**) indicates how many times to add the other number (the **multiplicand**) to itself. Example: $3 \times 2 = 2 + 2 + 2 = 6$. With multiplication, the order does not matter, $2 \times 3 = 3 \times 2$ or $3 + 3 = 2 + 2 + 2$, either way the result (the **product**) is the same.

If the signs are the same, the product is positive when multiplying signed numbers. Example: $(+4) \times (+8) = +32$ and $(-4) \times (-8) = +32$. If the signs are opposite, the product is negative. Example: $(+4) \times (-8) = -32$ and $(-4) \times (+8) = -32$. When more than two factors are multiplied together, the sign of the product is determined by how many negative factors are present. If there are an odd number of negative factors then the product is negative, whereas an even number of negative factors indicates a positive product. Example: $(+4) \times (-8) \times (-2) = +64$ and $(-4) \times (-8) \times (-2) = -64$.

Division

Division is the opposite operation to multiplication; one number (the **divisor**) tells us how many parts to divide the other number (the **dividend**) into. The result of division is called the **quotient**. Example: $20 \div 4 = 5$. If 20 is split into 4 equal parts, each part is 5. With division, the order of the numbers does matter, $20 \div 4 \neq 4 \div 20$.

The rules for dividing signed numbers are similar to multiplying signed numbers. If the dividend and divisor have the same sign, the quotient is positive. If the dividend and divisor have opposite signs, the quotient is negative. Example: $(-4) \div (+8) = -0.5$.

Review Video: Mathematical Operations
Visit mometrix.com/academy and enter code: 208095

Parentheses

Parentheses are used to designate which operations should be done first when there are multiple operations. Example: $4 - (2 + 1) = 1$; the parentheses tell us that we must add 2 and 1, and then subtract the sum from 4, rather than subtracting 2 from 4 and then adding 1 (this would give us an answer of 3).

Review Video: Mathematical Parentheses
Visit mometrix.com/academy and enter code: 978600

Exponents

An **exponent** is a superscript number placed next to another number at the top right. It indicates how many times the base number is to be multiplied by itself. Exponents provide a shorthand way to write what would be a longer mathematical expression, Example: $2^4 = 2 \times 2 \times 2 \times 2$. A number with an exponent of 2 is said to be "squared," while a number with an exponent of 3 is said to be "cubed." The value of a number raised to an exponent is called its power. So 8^4 is read as "8 to the 4th power," or "8 raised to the power of 4."

Review Video: What is an Exponent?
Visit mometrix.com/academy and enter code: 600998

Roots

A **root**, such as a square root, is another way of writing a fractional exponent. Instead of using a superscript, roots use the radical symbol ($\sqrt{\ }$) to indicate the operation. A radical will have a number underneath the bar, and may sometimes have a number in the upper left: $\sqrt[n]{a}$, read as "the nth root of a." The relationship between radical notation and exponent notation can be described by this equation:

$$\sqrt[n]{a} = a^{\frac{1}{n}}$$

The two special cases of $n = 2$ and $n = 3$ are called square roots and cube roots. If there is no number to the upper left, the radical is understood to be a square root ($n = 2$). Nearly all of the roots you encounter will be square roots. A square root is the same as a number raised to the one-half power. When we say that a is the square root of b ($a = \sqrt{b}$), we mean that a multiplied by itself equals b: ($a \times a = b$).

A **perfect square** is a number that has an integer for its square root. There are 10 perfect squares from 1 to 100: 1, 4, 9, 16, 25, 36, 49, 64, 81, 100 (the squares of integers 1 through 10).

Review Video: Roots
Visit mometrix.com/academy and enter code: 795655

Review Video: Perfect Squares and Square Roots
Visit mometrix.com/academy and enter code: 648063

WORD PROBLEMS AND MATHEMATICAL SYMBOLS

When working on word problems, you must be able to translate verbal expressions or "math words" into math symbols. This chart contains several "math words" and their appropriate symbols:

Phrase	Symbol
equal, is, was, will be, has, costs, gets to, is the same as, becomes	$=$
times, of, multiplied by, product of, twice, doubles, halves, triples	$\times$
divided by, per, ratio of/to, out of	$\div$
plus, added to, sum, combined, and, more than, totals of	$+$
subtracted from, less than, decreased by, minus, difference between	$-$
what, how much, original value, how many, a number, a variable	x, n, etc.

EXAMPLES OF TRANSLATED MATHEMATICAL PHRASES

- The phrase four more than twice a number can be written algebraically as $2x + 4$.
- The phrase half a number decreased by six can be written algebraically as $\frac{1}{2}x - 6$.
- The phrase the sum of a number and the product of five and that number can be written algebraically as $x + 5x$.
- You may see a test question that says, "Olivia is constructing a bookcase from seven boards. Two of them are for vertical supports and five are for shelves. The height of the bookcase is twice the width of the bookcase. If the seven boards total 36 feet in length, what will be the height of Olivia's bookcase?" You would need to make a sketch and then create the equation to determine the width of the shelves. The height can be represented as double the width. (If x represents the width of the shelves in feet, then the height of the bookcase is $2x$. Since the seven boards total 36 feet, $2x + 2x + x + x + x + x + x = 36$ or $9x = 36$; $x = 4$. The height is twice the width, or 8 feet.)

Subtraction with Regrouping

Subtraction with Regrouping

A great way to make use of some of the features built into the decimal system would be regrouping when attempting longform subtraction operations. When subtracting within a place value, sometimes the minuend is smaller than the subtrahend, **regrouping** enables you to 'borrow' a unit from a place value to the left in order to get a positive difference. For example, consider subtracting 189 from 525 with regrouping.

First, set up the subtraction problem in vertical form:

$$\begin{array}{r} 525 \\ -\ 189 \\ \hline \end{array}$$

Notice that the numbers in the ones and tens columns of 525 are smaller than the numbers in the ones and tens columns of 189. This means you will need to use regrouping to perform subtraction:

$$\begin{array}{rrrr} & 5 & 2 & 5 \\ - & 1 & 8 & 9 \\ \hline \end{array}$$

To subtract 9 from 5 in the ones column you will need to borrow from the 2 in the tens columns:

$$\begin{array}{rrrr} & 5 & 1 & 15 \\ - & 1 & 8 & 9 \\ \hline & & & 6 \end{array}$$

Next, to subtract 8 from 1 in the tens column you will need to borrow from the 5 in the hundreds column:

$$\begin{array}{rrrr} & 4 & 11 & 15 \\ - & 1 & 8 & 9 \\ \hline & & 3 & 6 \end{array}$$

Last, subtract the 1 from the 4 in the hundreds column:

$$\begin{array}{rrrr} & 4 & 11 & 15 \\ - & 1 & 8 & 9 \\ \hline & 3 & 3 & 6 \end{array}$$

Review Video: Subtracting Large Numbers
Visit mometrix.com/academy and enter code: 603350

Order of Operations

ORDER OF OPERATIONS

The **order of operations** is a set of rules that dictates the order in which we must perform each operation in an expression so that we will evaluate it accurately. If we have an expression that includes multiple different operations, the order of operations tells us which operations to do first. The most common mnemonic for the order of operations is **PEMDAS**, or "Please Excuse My Dear Aunt Sally." PEMDAS stands for parentheses, exponents, multiplication, division, addition, and subtraction. It is important to understand that multiplication and division have equal precedence, as do addition and subtraction, so those pairs of operations are simply worked from left to right in order.

For example, evaluating the expression $5 + 20 \div 4 \times (2 + 3)^2 - 6$ using the correct order of operations would be done like this:

- **P:** Perform the operations inside the parentheses: $(2 + 3) = 5$
- **E:** Simplify the exponents: $(5)^2 = 5 \times 5 = 25$
  - The expression now looks like this: $5 + 20 \div 4 \times 25 - 6$
- **MD:** Perform multiplication and division from left to right: $20 \div 4 = 5$; then $5 \times 25 = 125$
  - The expression now looks like this: $5 + 125 - 6$
- **AS:** Perform addition and subtraction from left to right: $5 + 125 = 130$; then $130 - 6 = 124$

Review Video: Order of Operations
Visit mometrix.com/academy and enter code: 259675

Properties of Exponents

The properties of exponents are as follows:

Property	Description
$a^1 = a$	Any number to the power of 1 is equal to itself
$1^n = 1$	The number 1 raised to any power is equal to 1
$a^0 = 1$	Any number raised to the power of 0 is equal to 1
$a^n \times a^m = a^{n+m}$	Add exponents to multiply powers of the same base number
$a^n \div a^m = a^{n-m}$	Subtract exponents to divide powers of the same base number
$(a^n)^m = a^{n \times m}$	When a power is raised to a power, the exponents are multiplied
$(a \times b)^n = a^n \times b^n$ $(a \div b)^n = a^n \div b^n$	Multiplication and division operations inside parentheses can be raised to a power. This is the same as each term being raised to that power.
$a^{-n} = \frac{1}{a^n}$	A negative exponent is the same as the reciprocal of a positive exponent

Note that exponents do not have to be integers. Fractional or decimal exponents follow all the rules above as well. Example: $5^{\frac{1}{4}} \times 5^{\frac{3}{4}} = 5^{\frac{1}{4}+\frac{3}{4}} = 5^1 = 5$.

Review Video: Properties of Exponents
Visit mometrix.com/academy and enter code: 532558

Scientific Notation

Scientific Notation

Scientific notation is a way of writing large numbers in a shorter form. The form $a \times 10^n$ is used in scientific notation, where a is greater than or equal to 1 but less than 10, and n is the number of places the decimal must move to get from the original number to a. Example: The number 230,400,000 is cumbersome to write. To write the value in scientific notation, place a decimal point between the first and second numbers, and include all digits through the last non-zero digit ($a = 2.304$). To find the appropriate power of 10, count the number of places the decimal point had to move ($n = 8$). The number is positive if the decimal moved to the left, and negative if it moved to the right. We can then write 230,400,000 as 2.304×10^8. If we look instead at the number 0.00002304, we have the same value for a, but this time the decimal moved 5 places to the right ($n = -5$). Thus, 0.00002304 can be written as 2.304×10^{-5}. Using this notation makes it simple to compare very large or very small numbers. By comparing exponents, it is easy to see that 3.28×10^4 is smaller than 1.51×10^5, because 4 is less than 5.

Review Video: Scientific Notation
Visit mometrix.com/academy and enter code: 976454

Factors and Multiples

Factors and Greatest Common Factor

Factors are numbers that are multiplied together to obtain a **product**. For example, in the equation $2 \times 3 = 6$, the numbers 2 and 3 are factors. A **prime number** has only two factors (1 and itself), but other numbers can have many factors.

A **common factor** is a number that divides exactly into two or more other numbers. For example, the factors of 12 are 1, 2, 3, 4, 6, and 12, while the factors of 15 are 1, 3, 5, and 15. The common factors of 12 and 15 are 1 and 3.

A **prime factor** is also a prime number. Therefore, the prime factors of 12 are 2 and 3. For 15, the prime factors are 3 and 5.

The **greatest common factor** (**GCF**) is the largest number that is a factor of two or more numbers. For example, the factors of 15 are 1, 3, 5, and 15; the factors of 35 are 1, 5, 7, and 35. Therefore, the greatest common factor of 15 and 35 is 5.

Review Video: Factors
Visit mometrix.com/academy and enter code: 920086

Review Video: Prime Numbers and Factorization
Visit mometrix.com/academy and enter code: 760669

Review Video: Greatest Common Factor and Least Common Multiple
Visit mometrix.com/academy and enter code: 838699

Multiples and Least Common Multiple

Often listed out in multiplication tables, **multiples** are integer increments of a given factor. In other words, dividing a multiple by the factor will result in an integer. For example, the multiples of 7 include: $1 \times 7 = 7, 2 \times 7 = 14, 3 \times 7 = 21, 4 \times 7 = 28, 5 \times 7 = 35$. Dividing 7, 14, 21, 28, or 35 by 7 will result in the integers 1, 2, 3, 4, and 5, respectively.

The least common multiple (**LCM**) is the smallest number that is a multiple of two or more numbers. For example, the multiples of 3 include 3, 6, 9, 12, 15, etc.; the multiples of 5 include 5, 10, 15, 20, etc. Therefore, the least common multiple of 3 and 5 is 15.

Review Video: Multiples
Visit mometrix.com/academy and enter code: 626738

Fractions, Decimals, and Percentages

Fractions

A **fraction** is a number that is expressed as one integer written above another integer, with a dividing line between them $\left(\frac{x}{y}\right)$. It represents the **quotient** of the two numbers "x divided by y." It can also be thought of as x out of y equal parts.

The top number of a fraction is called the **numerator**, and it represents the number of parts under consideration. The 1 in $\frac{1}{4}$ means that 1 part out of the whole is being considered in the calculation. The bottom number of a fraction is called the **denominator**, and it represents the total number of equal parts. The 4 in $\frac{1}{4}$ means that the whole consists of 4 equal parts. A fraction cannot have a denominator of zero; this is referred to as "*undefined*."

Fractions can be manipulated, without changing the value of the fraction, by multiplying or dividing (but not adding or subtracting) both the numerator and denominator by the same number. If you divide both numbers by a common factor, you are **reducing** or simplifying the fraction. Two fractions that have the same value but are expressed differently are known as **equivalent fractions**. For example, $\frac{2}{10}, \frac{3}{15}, \frac{4}{20}$, and $\frac{5}{25}$ are all equivalent fractions. They can also all be reduced or simplified to $\frac{1}{5}$.

When two fractions are manipulated so that they have the same denominator, this is known as finding a **common denominator**. The number chosen to be that common denominator should be the least common multiple of the two original denominators. Example: $\frac{3}{4}$ and $\frac{5}{6}$; the least common multiple of 4 and 6 is 12. Manipulating to achieve the common denominator: $\frac{3}{4} = \frac{9}{12}; \frac{5}{6} = \frac{10}{12}$.

Review Video: Overview of Fractions
Visit mometrix.com/academy and enter code: 262335

Proper Fractions and Mixed Numbers

A fraction whose denominator is greater than its numerator is known as a **proper fraction**, while a fraction whose numerator is greater than its denominator is known as an **improper fraction**. Proper fractions have values *less than one* and improper fractions have values *greater than one*.

A **mixed number** is a number that contains both an integer and a fraction. Any improper fraction can be rewritten as a mixed number. Example: $\frac{8}{3} = \frac{6}{3} + \frac{2}{3} = 2 + \frac{2}{3} = 2\frac{2}{3}$. Similarly, any mixed number can be rewritten as an improper fraction. Example: $1\frac{3}{5} = 1 + \frac{3}{5} = \frac{5}{5} + \frac{3}{5} = \frac{8}{5}$.

Review Video: Proper and Improper Fractions and Mixed Numbers
Visit mometrix.com/academy and enter code: 211077

Adding and Subtracting Fractions

If two fractions have a common denominator, they can be added or subtracted simply by adding or subtracting the two numerators and retaining the same denominator. If the two fractions do not already have the same denominator, one or both of them must be manipulated to achieve a common denominator before they can be added or subtracted. Example: $\frac{1}{2} + \frac{1}{4} = \frac{2}{4} + \frac{1}{4} = \frac{3}{4}$.

Review Video: Adding and Subtracting Fractions
Visit mometrix.com/academy and enter code: 378080

Multiplying Fractions

Two fractions can be multiplied by multiplying the two numerators to find the new numerator and the two denominators to find the new denominator. Example: $\frac{1}{3} \times \frac{2}{3} = \frac{1 \times 2}{3 \times 3} = \frac{2}{9}$.

Dividing Fractions

Two fractions can be divided by flipping the numerator and denominator of the second fraction and then proceeding as though it were a multiplication problem. Example: $\frac{2}{3} \div \frac{3}{4} = \frac{2}{3} \times \frac{4}{3} = \frac{8}{9}$.

Review Video: Multiplying and Dividing Fractions
Visit mometrix.com/academy and enter code: 473632

Multiplying a Mixed Number by a Whole Number or a Decimal

When multiplying a mixed number by something, it is usually best to convert it to an improper fraction first. Additionally, if the multiplicand is a decimal, it is most often simplest to convert it to a fraction. For instance, to multiply $4\frac{3}{8}$ by 3.5, begin by rewriting each quantity as a whole number plus a proper fraction. Remember, a mixed number is a fraction added to a whole number and a decimal is a representation of the sum of fractions, specifically tenths, hundredths, thousandths, and so on:

$$4\frac{3}{8} \times 3.5 = \left(4 + \frac{3}{8}\right) \times \left(3 + \frac{1}{2}\right)$$

Next, the quantities being added need to be expressed with the same denominator. This is achieved by multiplying and dividing the whole number by the denominator of the fraction. Recall that a whole number is equivalent to that number divided by 1:

$$= \left(\frac{4}{1} \times \frac{8}{8} + \frac{3}{8}\right) \times \left(\frac{3}{1} \times \frac{2}{2} + \frac{1}{2}\right)$$

When multiplying fractions, remember to multiply the numerators and denominators separately:

$$= \left(\frac{4 \times 8}{1 \times 8} + \frac{3}{8}\right) \times \left(\frac{3 \times 2}{1 \times 2} + \frac{1}{2}\right)$$
$$= \left(\frac{32}{8} + \frac{3}{8}\right) \times \left(\frac{6}{2} + \frac{1}{2}\right)$$

Now that the fractions have the same denominators, they can be added:

$$= \frac{35}{8} \times \frac{7}{2}$$

Finally, perform the last multiplication and then simplify:

$$= \frac{35 \times 7}{8 \times 2} = \frac{245}{16} = \frac{240}{16} + \frac{5}{16} = 15\frac{5}{16}$$

Comparing Fractions

It is important to master the ability to compare and order fractions. This skill is relevant to many real-world scenarios. For example, carpenters often compare fractional construction nail lengths when preparing for a project, and bakers often compare fractional measurements to have the correct ratio of ingredients. There are three commonly used strategies when comparing fractions. These strategies are referred to as the common denominator approach, the decimal approach, and the cross-multiplication approach.

Using a Common Denominator to Compare Fractions

The fractions $\frac{2}{3}$ and $\frac{4}{7}$ have different denominators. $\frac{2}{3}$ has a denominator of 3, and $\frac{4}{7}$ has a denominator of 7. In order to precisely compare these two fractions, it is necessary to use a common denominator. A common denominator is a common multiple that is shared by both denominators. In this case, the denominators 3 and 7 share a multiple of 21. In general, it is most efficient to select the least common multiple for the two denominators.

Rewrite each fraction with the common denominator of 21. Then, calculate the new numerators as illustrated below.

$$\frac{2}{3} \overset{\times 7}{=} \frac{\mathbf{14}}{21} \qquad \frac{4}{7} \overset{\times 3}{=} \frac{\mathbf{12}}{21}$$

For $\frac{2}{3}$, multiply the numerator and denominator by 7. The result is $\frac{14}{21}$.

For $\frac{4}{7}$, multiply the numerator and denominator by 3. The result is $\frac{12}{21}$.

Now that both fractions have a denominator of 21, the fractions can accurately be compared by comparing the numerators. Since 14 is greater than 12, the fraction $\frac{14}{21}$ is greater than $\frac{12}{21}$. This means that $\frac{2}{3}$ is greater than $\frac{4}{7}$.

Using Decimals to Compare Fractions

Sometimes decimal values are easier to compare than fraction values. For example, $\frac{5}{8}$ is equivalent to 0.625 and $\frac{3}{5}$ is equivalent to 0.6. This means that the comparison of $\frac{5}{8}$ and $\frac{3}{5}$ can be determined by comparing the decimals 0.625 and 0.6. When both decimal values are extended to the thousandths place, they become 0.625 and 0.600, respectively. It becomes clear that 0.625 is greater than 0.600 because 625 thousandths is greater than 600 thousandths. In other words, $\frac{5}{8}$ is greater than $\frac{3}{5}$ because 0.625 is greater than 0.6.

Using Cross-Multiplication to Compare Fractions

Cross-multiplication is an efficient strategy for comparing fractions. This is a shortcut for the common denominator strategy. Start by writing each fraction next to one another. Multiply the numerator of the fraction on the left by the denominator of the fraction on the right. Write down the result next to the fraction on the left. Now multiply the numerator of the fraction on the right by the denominator of the fraction on the left. Write down the result next to the fraction on the right. Compare both products. The fraction with the larger result is the larger fraction.

Consider the fractions $\frac{4}{7}$ and $\frac{5}{9}$.

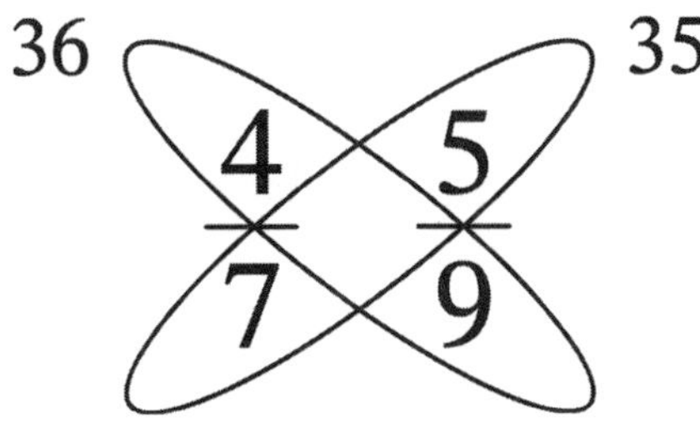

36 is greater than 35. Therefore, $\frac{4}{7}$ is greater than $\frac{5}{9}$.

Decimals

Decimals are one way to represent parts of a whole. Using the place value system, each digit to the right of a decimal point denotes the number of units of a corresponding *negative* power of ten. For example, consider the decimal 0.24. We can use a model to represent the decimal. Since a dime is worth one-tenth of a dollar and a penny is worth one-hundredth of a dollar, one possible model to represent this fraction is to have 2 dimes representing the 2 in the tenths place and 4 pennies representing the 4 in the hundredths place:

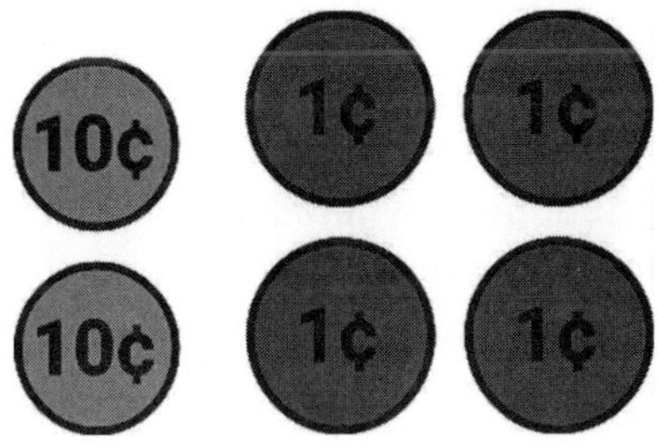

To write the decimal as a fraction, put the decimal in the numerator with 1 in the denominator. Multiply the numerator and denominator by tens until there are no more decimal places. Then simplify the fraction to lowest terms. For example, converting 0.24 to a fraction:

$$0.24 = \frac{0.24}{1} = \frac{0.24 \times 100}{1 \times 100} = \frac{24}{100} = \frac{6}{25}$$

Review Video: Decimals
Visit mometrix.com/academy and enter code: 837268

Operations with Decimals

Adding and Subtracting Decimals

When adding and subtracting decimals, the decimal points must always be aligned. Adding decimals is just like adding regular whole numbers. Example: $4.5 + 2.0 = 6.5$.

If the problem-solver does not properly align the decimal points, an incorrect answer of 4.7 may result. An easy way to add decimals is to align all of the decimal points in a vertical column visually. This will allow you to see exactly where the decimal should be placed in the final answer. Begin adding from right to left. Add each column in turn, making sure to carry the number to the left if a column adds up to more than 9. The same rules apply to the subtraction of decimals.

Review Video: Adding and Subtracting Decimals
Visit mometrix.com/academy and enter code: 381101

Multiplying Decimals

A simple multiplication problem has two components: a **multiplicand** and a **multiplier**. When multiplying decimals, work as though the numbers were whole rather than decimals. Once the final product is calculated, count the number of places to the right of the decimal in both the multiplicand and the multiplier. Then, count that number of places from the right of the product and place the decimal in that position.

For example, 12.3×2.56 has a total of three places to the right of the respective decimals. Multiply 123×256 to get 31,488. Now, beginning on the right, count three places to the left and insert the decimal. The final product will be 31.488.

Review Video: How to Multiply Decimals
Visit mometrix.com/academy and enter code: 731574

Dividing Decimals

Every division problem has a **divisor** and a **dividend**. The dividend is the number that is being divided. In the problem $14 \div 7$, 14 is the dividend and 7 is the divisor. In a division problem with decimals, the divisor must be converted into a whole number. Begin by moving the decimal in the divisor to the right until a whole number is created. Next, move the decimal in the dividend the same number of spaces to the right. For example, 4.9 into 24.5 would become 49 into 245. The decimal was moved one space to the right to create a whole number in the divisor, and then the same was done for the dividend. Once the whole numbers are created, the problem is carried out normally: $245 \div 49 = 5$.

Review Video: Dividing Decimals
Visit mometrix.com/academy and enter code: 560690

Review Video: Dividing Decimals by Whole Numbers
Visit mometrix.com/academy and enter code: 535669

PERCENTAGES

Percentages can be thought of as fractions that are based on a whole of 100; that is, one whole is equal to 100%. The word **percent** means "per hundred." Percentage problems are often presented in three main ways:

- Find what percentage of some number another number is.
  - Example: What percentage of 40 is 8?
- Find what number is some percentage of a given number.
  - Example: What number is 20% of 40?
- Find what number another number is a given percentage of.
  - Example: What number is 8 20% of?

There are three components in each of these cases: a **whole** (W), a **part** (P), and a **percentage** (%). These are related by the equation: $P = W \times \%$. This can easily be rearranged into other forms that may suit different questions better: $\% = \frac{P}{W}$ and $W = \frac{P}{\%}$. Percentage problems are often also word problems. As such, a large part of solving them is figuring out which quantities are what. For example, consider the following word problem:

In a school cafeteria, 7 students choose pizza, 9 choose hamburgers, and 4 choose tacos. What percentage of student choose tacos?

To find the whole, you must first add all of the parts: $7 + 9 + 4 = 20$. The percentage can then be found by dividing the part by the whole $\left(\% = \frac{P}{W}\right)$: $\frac{4}{20} = \frac{20}{100} = 20\%$.

Review Video: Computation with Percentages
Visit mometrix.com/academy and enter code: 693099

CONVERTING BETWEEN PERCENTAGES, FRACTIONS, AND DECIMALS

Converting decimals to percentages and percentages to decimals is as simple as moving the decimal point. To *convert from a decimal to a percentage*, move the decimal point **two places to the right.** To *convert from a percentage to a decimal*, move it **two places to the left**. It may be helpful to remember that the percentage number will always be larger than the equivalent decimal number. Example:

$$0.23 = 23\% \quad 5.34 = 534\% \quad 0.007 = 0.7\%$$
$$700\% = 7.00 \quad 86\% = 0.86 \quad 0.15\% = 0.0015$$

To convert a fraction to a decimal, simply divide the numerator by the denominator in the fraction. To convert a decimal to a fraction, put the decimal in the numerator with 1 in the denominator.

Multiply the numerator and denominator by tens until there are no more decimal places. Then simplify the fraction to lowest terms. For example, converting 0.24 to a fraction:

$$0.24 = \frac{0.24}{1} = \frac{0.24 \times 100}{1 \times 100} = \frac{24}{100} = \frac{6}{25}$$

Fractions can be converted to a percentage by finding equivalent fractions with a denominator of 100. Example:

$$\frac{7}{10} = \frac{70}{100} = 70\% \quad \frac{1}{4} = \frac{25}{100} = 25\%$$

To convert a percentage to a fraction, divide the percentage number by 100 and reduce the fraction to its simplest possible terms. Example:

$$60\% = \frac{60}{100} = \frac{3}{5} \quad 96\% = \frac{96}{100} = \frac{24}{25}$$

Review Video: Converting Fractions to Percentages and Decimals
Visit mometrix.com/academy and enter code: 306233

Review Video: Converting Percentages to Decimals and Fractions
Visit mometrix.com/academy and enter code: 287297

Review Video: Converting Decimals to Fractions and Percentages
Visit mometrix.com/academy and enter code: 986765

Review Video: Converting Decimals, Improper Fractions, and Mixed Numbers
Visit mometrix.com/academy and enter code: 696924

Proportions and Ratios

Proportions

A proportion is a relationship between two quantities that dictates how one changes when the other changes. A **direct proportion** describes a relationship in which a quantity increases by a set amount for every increase in the other quantity, or decreases by that same amount for every decrease in the other quantity. Example: Assuming a constant driving speed, the time required for a car trip increases as the distance of the trip increases. The distance to be traveled and the time required to travel are directly proportional.

An **inverse proportion** is a relationship in which an increase in one quantity is accompanied by a decrease in the other, or vice versa. Example: the time required for a car trip decreases as the speed increases and increases as the speed decreases, so the time required is inversely proportional to the speed of the car.

Review Video: Proportions
Visit mometrix.com/academy and enter code: 505355

Ratios

A **ratio** is a comparison of two quantities in a particular order. Example: If there are 14 computers in a lab, and the class has 20 students, there is a student to computer ratio of 20 to 14, commonly written as $20:14$. Ratios are normally reduced to their smallest whole number representation, so $20:14$ would be reduced to $10:7$ by dividing both sides by 2.

Review Video: Ratios
Visit mometrix.com/academy and enter code: 996914

Constant of Proportionality

When two quantities have a proportional relationship, there exists a **constant of proportionality** between the quantities. The product of this constant and one of the quantities is equal to the other quantity. For example, if one lemon costs $0.25, two lemons cost $0.50, and three lemons cost $0.75, there is a proportional relationship between the total cost of lemons and the number of lemons purchased. The constant of proportionality is the **unit price**, namely $0.25/lemon. Notice that the total price of lemons, t, can be found by multiplying the unit price of lemons, p, and the number of lemons, n: $t = pn$.

Work/Unit Rate

Unit rate expresses a quantity of one thing in terms of one unit of another. For example, if you travel 30 miles every two hours, a unit rate expresses this comparison in terms of one hour: in one hour you travel 15 miles, so your unit rate is 15 miles per hour. Other examples are how much one ounce of food costs (price per ounce) or figuring out how much one egg costs out of the dozen (price per 1 egg, instead of price per 12 eggs). The denominator of a unit rate is always 1. Unit rates are used to compare different situations to solve problems. For example, to make sure you get the best deal when deciding which kind of soda to buy, you can find the unit rate of each. If soda #1 costs $1.50 for a 1-liter bottle, and soda #2 costs $2.75 for a 2-liter bottle, it would be a better deal to buy soda #2, because its unit rate is only $1.375 per 1-liter, which is cheaper than soda #1. Unit rates can also help determine the length of time a given event will take. For example, if you can paint 2 rooms in 4.5 hours, you can determine how long it will take you to paint 5 rooms by solving for the unit rate per room and then multiplying that by 5.

Review Video: Rates and Unit Rates
Visit mometrix.com/academy and enter code: 185363

Linear Expressions

Terms and Coefficients

Mathematical expressions consist of a combination of one or more values arranged in terms that are added together. As such, an expression could be just a single number, including zero. A **variable term** is the product of a real number, also called a **coefficient**, and one or more variables, each of which may be raised to an exponent. Expressions may also include numbers without a variable, called **constants** or **constant terms**. The expression $6s^2$, for example, is a single term where the coefficient is the real number 6 and the variable term is s^2. Note that if a term is written as simply a variable to some exponent, like t^2, then the coefficient is 1, because $t^2 = 1t^2$.

Linear Expressions

A **single variable linear expression** is the sum of a single variable term, where the variable has no exponent, and a constant, which may be zero. For instance, the expression $2w + 7$ has $2w$ as the variable term and 7 as the constant term. It is important to realize that terms are separated by addition or subtraction. Since an expression is a sum of terms, expressions such as $5x - 3$ can be written as $5x + (-3)$ to emphasize that the constant term is negative. A real-world example of a single variable linear expression is the perimeter of a square, four times the side length, often expressed: $4s$.

In general, a **linear expression** is the sum of any number of variable terms so long as none of the variables have an exponent. For example, $3m + 8n - \frac{1}{4}p + 5.5q - 1$ is a linear expression, but $3y^3$ is not. In the same way, the expression for the perimeter of a general triangle, the sum of the side lengths $(a + b + c)$ is considered to be linear, but the expression for the area of a square, the side length squared $(s^2)$is not.

Slope

Slope

On a graph with two points, (x_1, y_1) and (x_2, y_2), the **slope** is found with the formula $m = \frac{y_2 - y_1}{x_2 - x_1}$; where $x_1 \neq x_2$ and m stands for slope. If the value of the slope is **positive**, the line has an *upward direction* from left to right. If the value of the slope is **negative**, the line has a *downward direction* from left to right. Consider the following example:

A new book goes on sale in bookstores and online stores. In the first month, 5,000 copies of the book are sold. Over time, the book continues to grow in popularity. The data for the number of copies sold is in the table below.

# of Months on Sale	1	2	3	4	5
# of Copies Sold (In Thousands)	5	10	15	20	25

So, the number of copies that are sold and the time that the book is on sale is a proportional relationship. In this example, an equation can be used to show the data: $y = 5x$, where x is the number of months that the book is on sale. Also, y is the number of copies sold. So, the slope of the corresponding line is $\frac{\text{rise}}{\text{run}} = \frac{5}{1} = 5$.

> **Review Video: Finding the Slope of a Line**
> Visit mometrix.com/academy and enter code: 766664

Linear Equations

Linear Equations

Equations that can be written as $ax + b = 0$, where $a \neq 0$, are referred to as **one variable linear equations.** A solution to such an equation is called a **root**. In the case where we have the equation $5x + 10 = 0$, if we solve for x we get a solution of $x = -2$. In other words, the root of the equation is -2. This is found by first subtracting 10 from both sides, which gives $5x = -10$. Next, simply divide both sides by the coefficient of the variable, in this case 5, to get $x = -2$. This can be checked by plugging -2 back into the original equation $(5)(-2) + 10 = -10 + 10 = 0$.

The **solution set** is the set of all solutions of an equation. In our example, the solution set would simply be -2. If there were more solutions (there usually are in multivariable equations) then they would also be included in the solution set. When an equation has no true solutions, it is referred to as an **empty set**. Equations with identical solution sets are **equivalent equations**. An **identity** is a term whose value or determinant is equal to 1.

Linear equations can be written many ways. Below is a list of some forms linear equations can take:

- **Standard Form**: $Ax + By = C$; the slope is $\frac{-A}{B}$ and the y-intercept is $\frac{C}{B}$
- **Slope Intercept Form**: $y = mx + b$, where m is the slope and b is the y-intercept
- **Point-Slope Form**: $y - y_1 = m(x - x_1)$, where m is the slope and (x_1, y_1) is a point on the line
- **Two-Point Form**: $\frac{y-y_1}{x-x_1} = \frac{y_2-y_1}{x_2-x_1}$, where (x_1, y_1) and (x_2, y_2) are two points on the given line
- **Intercept Form**: $\frac{x}{x_1} + \frac{y}{y_1} = 1$, where $(x_1, 0)$ is the point at which a line intersects the x-axis, and $(0, y_1)$ is the point at which the same line intersects the y-axis

> **Review Video: Slope-Intercept and Point-Slope Forms**
> Visit mometrix.com/academy and enter code: 113216
>
> **Review Video: Linear Equations Basics**
> Visit mometrix.com/academy and enter code: 793005

Solving Equations

Solving One-Variable Linear Equations

Multiply all terms by the lowest common denominator to eliminate any fractions. Look for addition or subtraction to undo so you can isolate the variable on one side of the equal sign. Divide both sides by the coefficient of the variable. When you have a value for the variable, substitute this value into the original equation to make sure you have a true equation. Consider the following example:

Kim's savings are represented by the table below. Represent her savings, using an equation.

X (Months)	Y (Total Savings)
2	$1,300
5	$2,050
9	$3,050
11	$3,550
16	$4,800

The table shows a function with a constant rate of change, or slope, of 250. Given the points on the table, the slopes can be calculated as $\frac{(2{,}050-1300)}{(5-2)}$, $\frac{(3{,}050-2{,}050)}{(9-5)}$, $\frac{(3{,}550-3{,}050)}{(11-9)}$, and $\frac{(4{,}800-3{,}550)}{(16-11)}$, each of which equals 250. Thus, the table shows a constant rate of change, indicating a linear function. The slope-intercept form of a linear equation is written as $y = mx + b$, where m represents the slope and b represents the y-intercept. Substituting the slope into this form gives $y = 250x + b$. Substituting corresponding x- and y-values from any point into this equation will give the y-intercept, or b. Using the point, (2, 1,300), gives $1{,}300 = 250(2) + b$, which simplifies as $b = 800$. Thus, her savings may be represented by the equation, $y = 250x + 800$.

Rules for Manipulating Equations

Like Terms

Like terms are terms in an equation that have the same variable, regardless of whether or not they also have the same coefficient. This includes terms that *lack* a variable; all constants (i.e., numbers without variables) are considered like terms. If the equation involves terms with a variable raised to different powers, the like terms are those that have the variable raised to the same power.

For example, consider the equation $x^2 + 3x + 2 = 2x^2 + x - 7 + 2x$. In this equation, 2 and -7 are like terms; they are both constants. $3x$, x, and $2x$ are like terms, they all include the variable x raised to the first power. x^2 and $2x^2$ are like terms, they both include the variable x, raised to the second power. $2x$ and $2x^2$ are not like terms; although they both involve the variable x, the variable is not raised to the same power in both terms. The fact that they have the same coefficient, 2, is not relevant.

Review Video: Rules for Manipulating Equations
Visit mometrix.com/academy and enter code: 838871

Carrying Out the Same Operation on Both Sides of an Equation

When solving an equation, the general procedure is to carry out a series of operations on both sides of an equation, choosing operations that will tend to simplify the equation when doing so. The reason why the same operation must be carried out on both sides of the equation is because that leaves the meaning of the equation unchanged, and yields a result that is equivalent to the original equation. This would not be the case if we carried out an operation on one side of an equation and not the other. Consider what an equation means: it is a statement that two values or expressions are equal. If we carry out the same operation on both sides of the equation—add 3 to both sides, for example—then the two sides of the equation are changed in the same way, and so remain equal. If we do that to only one side of the equation—add 3 to one side but not the other—then that wouldn't be true; if we change one side of the equation but not the other then the two sides are no longer equal.

Advantage of Combining Like Terms

Combining like terms refers to adding or subtracting like terms—terms with the same variable—and therefore reducing sets of like terms to a single term. The main advantage of doing this is that it simplifies the equation. Often, combining like terms can be done as the first step in solving an equation, though it can also be done later, such as after distributing terms in a product.

For example, consider the equation $2(x + 3) + 3(2 + x + 3) = -4$. The 2 and the 3 in the second set of parentheses are like terms, and we can combine them, yielding $2(x + 3) + 3(x + 5) = -4$. Now we can carry out the multiplications implied by the parentheses, distributing the outer 2 and 3 accordingly: $2x + 6 + 3x + 15 = -4$. The $2x$ and the $3x$ are like terms, and we can add them together: $5x + 6 + 15 = -4$. Now, the constants 6, 15, and -4 are also like terms, and we can combine them as well: subtracting 6 and 15 from both sides of the equation, we get $5x = -4 - 6 - 15$, or $5x = -25$, which simplifies further to $x = -5$.

Review Video: Solving Equations by Combining Like Terms
Visit mometrix.com/academy and enter code: 668506

Canceling Terms on Opposite Sides of an Equation

Two terms on opposite sides of an equation can be canceled if and only if they *exactly* match each other. They must have the same variable raised to the same power and the same coefficient. For example, in the equation $3x + 2x^2 + 6 = 2x^2 - 6$, $2x^2$ appears on both sides of the equation and can be canceled, leaving $3x + 6 = -6$. The 6 on each side of the equation *cannot* be canceled, because it is added on one side of the equation and subtracted on the other. While they cannot be canceled, however, the 6 and -6 are like terms and can be combined, yielding $3x = -12$, which simplifies further to $x = -4$.

It's also important to note that the terms to be canceled must be independent terms and cannot be part of a larger term. For example, consider the equation $2(x + 6) = 3(x + 4) + 1$. We cannot cancel the x's, because even though they match each other they are part of the larger terms $2(x + 6)$ and $3(x + 4)$. We must first distribute the 2 and 3, yielding $2x + 12 = 3x + 12 + 1$. Now we see that the terms with the x's do not match, but the 12s do, and can be canceled, leaving $2x = 3x + 1$, which simplifies to $x = -1$.

Process for Manipulating Equations

Isolating Variables

To **isolate a variable** means to manipulate the equation so that the variable appears by itself on one side of the equation, and does not appear at all on the other side. Generally, an equation or inequality is considered to be solved once the variable is isolated and the other side of the equation or inequality is simplified as much as possible. In the case of a two-variable equation or inequality, only one variable needs to be isolated; it will not usually be possible to simultaneously isolate both variables.

For a linear equation—an equation in which the variable only appears raised to the first power—isolating a variable can be done by first moving all the terms with the variable to one side of the equation and all other terms to the other side. (*Moving* a term really means adding the inverse of the term to both sides; when a term is *moved* to the other side of the equation its sign is flipped.)

Then combine like terms on each side. Finally, divide both sides by the coefficient of the variable, if applicable. The steps need not necessarily be done in this order, but this order will always work.

Review Video: Solving One-Step Equations
Visit mometrix.com/academy and enter code: 777004

Equations with More Than One Solution

Some types of non-linear equations, such as equations involving squares of variables, may have more than one solution. For example, the equation $x^2 = 4$ has two solutions: 2 and –2. Equations with absolute values can also have multiple solutions: $|x| = 1$ has the solutions $x = 1$ and $x = -1$.

It is also possible for a linear equation to have more than one solution, but only if the equation is true regardless of the value of the variable. In this case, the equation is considered to have infinitely many solutions, because any possible value of the variable is a solution. We know a linear equation has infinitely many solutions if when we combine like terms the variables cancel, leaving a true statement. For example, consider the equation $2(3x + 5) = x + 5(x + 2)$. Distributing, we get $6x + 10 = x + 5x + 10$; combining like terms gives $6x + 10 = 6x + 10$, and the $6x$-terms cancel to leave $10 = 10$. This is clearly true, so the original equation is true for any value of x. We could also have canceled the 10s leaving $0 = 0$, but again this is clearly true—in general if both sides of the equation match exactly, it has infinitely many solutions.

Equations with No Solution

Some types of non-linear equations, such as equations involving squares of variables, may have no solution. For example, the equation $x^2 = -2$ has no solutions in the real numbers, because the square of any real number must be positive. Similarly, $|x| = -1$ has no solution, because the absolute value of a number is always positive.

It is also possible for an equation to have no solution even if does not involve any powers greater than one, absolute values, or other special functions. For example, the equation $2(x + 3) + x = 3x$ has no solution. We can see that if we try to solve it: first we distribute, leaving $2x + 6 + x = 3x$. But now if we try to combine all the terms with the variable, we find that they cancel: we have $3x$ on the left and $3x$ on the right, canceling to leave us with $6 = 0$. This is clearly false. In general, whenever the variable terms in an equation cancel leaving different constants on both sides, it means that the equation has no solution. (If we are left with the *same* constant on both sides, the equation has infinitely many solutions instead.)

Features of Equations That Require Special Treatment

Linear Equations

A linear equation is an equation in which variables only appear by themselves: not multiplied together, not with exponents other than one, and not inside absolute value signs or any other functions. For example, the equation $x + 1 - 3x = 5 - x$ is a linear equation; while x appears multiple times, it never appears with an exponent other than one, or inside any function. The two-variable equation $2x - 3y = 5 + 2x$ is also a linear equation. In contrast, the equation $x^2 - 5 = 3x$ is *not* a linear equation, because it involves the term x^2. $\sqrt{x} = 5$ is not a linear equation, because it involves a square root. $(x - 1)^2 = 4$ is not a linear equation because even though there's no exponent on the x directly, it appears as part of an expression that is squared. The two-variable equation $x + xy - y = 5$ is not a linear equation because it includes the term xy, where two variables are multiplied together.

Linear equations can always be solved (or shown to have no solution) by combining like terms and performing simple operations on both sides of the equation. Some non-linear equations can be solved by similar methods, but others may require more advanced methods of solution, if they can be solved analytically at all.

Solving Equations Involving Roots

In an equation involving roots, the first step is to isolate the term with the root, if possible, and then raise both sides of the equation to the appropriate power to eliminate it. Consider an example equation, $2\sqrt{x+1}-1=3$. In this case, begin by adding 1 to both sides, yielding $2\sqrt{x+1}=4$, and then dividing both sides by 2, yielding $\sqrt{x+1}=2$. Now square both sides, yielding $x+1=4$. Finally, subtracting 1 from both sides yields $x=3$.

Squaring both sides of an equation may, however, yield a spurious solution—a solution to the squared equation that is *not* a solution of the original equation. It's therefore necessary to plug the solution back into the original equation to make sure it works. In this case, it does: $2\sqrt{3+1}-1=2\sqrt{4}-1=2(2)-1=4-1=3$.

The same procedure applies for other roots as well. For example, given the equation $3+\sqrt[3]{2x}=5$, we can first subtract 3 from both sides, yielding $\sqrt[3]{2x}=2$ and isolating the root. Raising both sides to the third power yields $2x=2^3$; i.e., $2x=8$. We can now divide both sides by 2 to get $x=4$.

Review Video: Solving Equations Involving Roots
Visit mometrix.com/academy and enter code: 297670

Solving Equations with Exponents

To solve an equation involving an exponent, the first step is to isolate the variable with the exponent. We can then take the appropriate root of both sides to eliminate the exponent. For instance, for the equation $2x^3+17=5x^3-7$, we can subtract $5x^3$ from both sides to get $-3x^3+17=-7$, and then subtract 17 from both sides to get $-3x^3=-24$. Finally, we can divide both sides by -3 to get $x^3=8$. Finally, we can take the cube root of both sides to get $x=\sqrt[3]{8}=2$.

One important but often overlooked point is that equations with an exponent greater than 1 may have more than one answer. The solution to $x^2=9$ isn't simply $x=3$; it's $x=\pm 3$ (that is, $x=3$ or $x=-3$). For a slightly more complicated example, consider the equation $(x-1)^2-1=3$. Adding 1 to both sides yields $(x-1)^2=4$; taking the square root of both sides yields $x-1=2$. We can then add 1 to both sides to get $x=3$. However, there's a second solution. We also have the possibility that $x-1=-2$, in which case $x=-1$. Both $x=3$ and $x=-1$ are valid solutions, as can be verified by substituting them both into the original equation.

Review Video: Solving Equations with Exponents
Visit mometrix.com/academy and enter code: 514557

Solving Equations with Absolute Values

When solving an equation with an absolute value, the first step is to isolate the absolute value term. We then consider two possibilities: when the expression inside the absolute value is positive or when it is negative. In the former case, the expression in the absolute value equals the expression on the other side of the equation; in the latter, it equals the additive inverse of that expression—the expression times negative one. We consider each case separately and finally check for spurious solutions.

For instance, consider solving $|2x - 1| + x = 5$ for x. We can first isolate the absolute value by moving the x to the other side: $|2x - 1| = -x + 5$. Now, we have two possibilities. First, that $2x - 1$ is positive, and hence $2x - 1 = -x + 5$. Rearranging and combining like terms yields $3x = 6$, and hence $x = 2$. The other possibility is that $2x - 1$ is negative, and hence $2x - 1 = -(-x + 5) = x - 5$. In this case, rearranging and combining like terms yields $x = -4$. Substituting $x = 2$ and $x = -4$ back into the original equation, we see that they are both valid solutions.

Note that the absolute value of a sum or difference applies to the sum or difference as a whole, not to the individual terms; in general, $|2x - 1|$ is not equal to $|2x + 1|$ or to $|2x| - 1$.

Spurious Solutions

A **spurious solution** may arise when we square both sides of an equation as a step in solving it or under certain other operations on the equation. It is a solution to the squared or otherwise modified equation that is *not* a solution of the original equation. To identify a spurious solution, it's useful when you solve an equation involving roots or absolute values to plug the solution back into the original equation to make sure it's valid.

Choosing Which Variable to Isolate in Two-Variable Equations

Similar to methods for a one-variable equation, solving a two-variable equation involves isolating a variable: manipulating the equation so that a variable appears by itself on one side of the equation, and not at all on the other side. However, in a two-variable equation, you will usually only be able to isolate one of the variables; the other variable may appear on the other side along with constant terms, or with exponents or other functions.

Often one variable will be much more easily isolated than the other, and therefore that's the variable you should choose. If one variable appears with various exponents, and the other is only raised to the first power, the latter variable is the one to isolate: given the equation $a^2 + 2b = a^3 + b + 3$, the b only appears to the first power, whereas a appears squared and cubed, so b is the variable that can be solved for: combining like terms and isolating the b on the left side of the equation, we get $b = a^3 - a^2 + 3$. If both variables are equally easy to isolate, then it's best to isolate the dependent variable, if one is defined; if the two variables are x and y, the convention is that y is the dependent variable.

Review Video: Solving Equations with Variables on Both Sides
Visit mometrix.com/academy and enter code: 402497

Cross Multiplication

Finding an Unknown in Equivalent Expressions

It is often necessary to apply information given about a rate or proportion to a new scenario. For example, if you know that Jedha can run a marathon (26.2 miles) in 3 hours, how long would it take her to run 10 miles at the same pace? Start by setting up equivalent expressions:

$$\frac{26.2\text{ mi}}{3\text{ hr}} = \frac{10\text{ mi}}{x\text{ hr}}$$

Now, cross multiply and solve for x:

$$26.2x = 30$$
$$x = \frac{30}{26.2} = \frac{15}{13.1}$$
$$x \approx 1.15 \text{ hrs } or \text{ } 1 \text{ hr } 9 \text{ min}$$

So, at this pace, Jedha could run 10 miles in about 1.15 hours or about 1 hour and 9 minutes.

Review Video: Cross Multiplying Fractions
Visit mometrix.com/academy and enter code: 893904

Graphing Equations

Graphical Solutions to Equations

When equations are shown graphically, they are usually shown on a **Cartesian coordinate plane**. The Cartesian coordinate plane consists of two number lines placed perpendicular to each other and intersecting at the zero point, also known as the origin. The horizontal number line is known as the x-axis, with positive values to the right of the origin, and negative values to the left of the origin. The vertical number line is known as the y-axis, with positive values above the origin, and negative values below the origin. Any point on the plane can be identified by an ordered pair in the form (x, y), called coordinates. The x-value of the coordinate is called the abscissa, and the y-value of the coordinate is called the ordinate. The two number lines divide the plane into **four quadrants**: I, II, III, and IV.

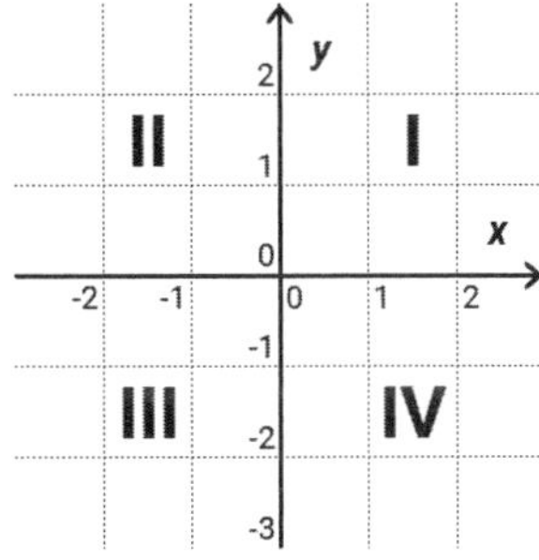

Note that in quadrant I $x > 0$ and $y > 0$, in quadrant II $x < 0$ and $y > 0$, in quadrant III $x < 0$ and $y < 0$, and in quadrant IV $x > 0$ and $y < 0$.

Recall that if the value of the slope of a line is positive, the line slopes upward from left to right. If the value of the slope is negative, the line slopes downward from left to right. If the y-coordinates are the same for two points on a line, the slope is 0 and the line is a **horizontal line**. If the x-coordinates are the same for two points on a line, there is no slope and the line is a **vertical line**. Two or more lines that have equivalent slopes are **parallel lines**. **Perpendicular lines** have slopes that are negative reciprocals of each other, such as $\frac{a}{b}$ and $\frac{-b}{a}$.

Review Video: Cartesian Coordinate Plane and Graphing
Visit mometrix.com/academy and enter code: 115173

Graphing Equations in Two Variables

One way of graphing an equation in two variables is to plot enough points to get an idea for its shape and then draw the appropriate curve through those points. A point can be plotted by substituting in a value for one variable and solving for the other. If the equation is linear, we only need two points and can then draw a straight line between them.

For example, consider the equation $y = 2x - 1$. This is a linear equation—both variables only appear raised to the first power—so we only need two points. When $x = 0$, $y = 2(0) - 1 = -1$. When $x = 2$, $y = 2(2) - 1 = 3$. We can therefore choose the points $(0, -1)$ and $(2, 3)$, and draw a line between them:

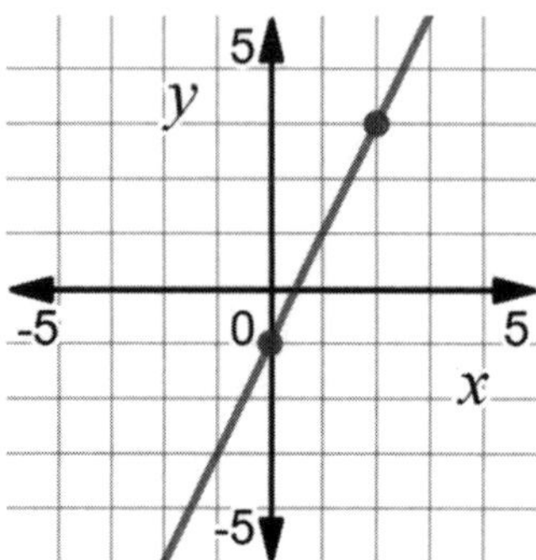

Inequalities

Working with Inequalities

Commonly in algebra and other upper-level fields of math you find yourself working with mathematical expressions that do not equal each other. The statement comparing such expressions with symbols such as $<$ (less than) or $>$ (greater than) is called an *inequality*. An example of an inequality is $7x > 5$. To solve for x, simply divide both sides by 7 and the solution is shown to be $x > \frac{5}{7}$. Graphs of the solution set of inequalities are represented on a number line. Open circles are used to show that an expression approaches a number but is never quite equal to that number.

> **Review Video: Solving Multi-Step Inequalities**
> Visit mometrix.com/academy and enter code: 347842
>
> **Review Video: Solving Inequalities Using All 4 Basic Operations**
> Visit mometrix.com/academy and enter code: 401111

Conditional inequalities are those with certain values for the variable that will make the condition true and other values for the variable where the condition will be false. **Absolute inequalities** can have any real number as the value for the variable to make the condition true, while there is no real number value for the variable that will make the condition false. Solving inequalities is done by following the same rules for solving equations with the exception that when multiplying or dividing by a negative number the direction of the inequality sign must be flipped or reversed. **Double inequalities** are situations where two inequality statements apply to the same variable expression. Example: $-c < ax + b < c$.

> **Review Video: Conditional and Absolute Inequalities**
> Visit mometrix.com/academy and enter code: 980164

Determining Solutions to Inequalities

To determine whether a coordinate is a solution of an inequality, you can substitute the values of the coordinate into the inequality, simplify, and check whether the resulting statement holds true. For instance, to determine whether $(-2,4)$ is a solution of the inequality $y \geq -2x + 3$, substitute the values into the inequality, $4 \geq -2(-2) + 3$. Simplify the right side of the inequality and the result is $4 \geq 7$, which is a false statement. Therefore, the coordinate is not a solution of the inequality. You can also use this method to determine which part of the graph of an inequality is shaded. The graph of $y \geq -2x + 3$ includes the solid line $y = -2x + 3$ and, since it excludes the point $(-2,4)$ to the left of the line, it is shaded to the right of the line.

> **Review Video: Graphing Linear Inequalities**
> Visit mometrix.com/academy and enter code: 439421

Flipping Inequality Signs

When given an inequality, we can always turn the entire inequality around, swapping the two sides of the inequality and changing the inequality sign. For instance, $x + 2 > 2x - 3$ is equivalent to $2x - 3 < x + 2$. Aside from that, normally the inequality does not change if we carry out the same operation on both sides of the inequality. There is, however, one principal exception: if we *multiply* or *divide* both sides of the inequality by a *negative number*, the inequality is flipped. For example, if we take the inequality $-2x < 6$ and divide both sides by -2, the inequality flips and we are left with

$x > -3$. This *only* applies to multiplication and division, and only with negative numbers. Multiplying or dividing both sides by a positive number, or adding or subtracting any number regardless of sign, does not flip the inequality. Another special case that flips the inequality sign is when reciprocals are used. For instance, $3 > 2$ but the relation of the reciprocals is $\frac{1}{2} < \frac{1}{3}$.

Compound Inequalities

A **compound inequality** is an equality that consists of two inequalities combined with *and* or *or*. The two components of a proper compound inequality must be of opposite type: that is, one must be greater than (or greater than or equal to), the other less than (or less than or equal to). For instance, "$x + 1 < 2$ or $x + 1 > 3$" is a compound inequality, as is "$2x \geq 4$ and $2x \leq 6$." An *and* inequality can be written more compactly by having one inequality on each side of the common part: "$2x \geq 1$ and $2x \leq 6$," can also be written as $1 \leq 2x \leq 6$.

In order for the compound inequality to be meaningful, the two parts of an *and* inequality must overlap; otherwise, no numbers satisfy the inequality. On the other hand, if the two parts of an *or* inequality overlap, then *all* numbers satisfy the inequality and as such the inequality is usually not meaningful.

Solving a compound inequality requires solving each part separately. For example, given the compound inequality "$x + 1 < 2$ or $x + 1 > 3$," the first inequality, $x + 1 < 2$, reduces to $x < 1$, and the second part, $x + 1 > 3$, reduces to $x > 2$, so the whole compound inequality can be written as "$x < 1$ or $x > 2$." Similarly, $1 \leq 2x \leq 6$ can be solved by dividing each term by 2, yielding $\frac{1}{2} \leq x \leq 3$.

Review Video: Compound Inequalities
Visit mometrix.com/academy and enter code: 786318

Solving Inequalities Involving Absolute Values

To solve an inequality involving an absolute value, first isolate the term with the absolute value. Then proceed to treat the two cases separately as with an absolute value equation, but flipping the inequality in the case where the expression in the absolute value is negative (since that essentially involves multiplying both sides by –1.) The two cases are then combined into a compound inequality; if the absolute value is on the greater side of the inequality, then it is an *or* compound inequality, if on the lesser side, then it's an *and*.

Consider the inequality $2 + |x - 1| \geq 3$. We can isolate the absolute value term by subtracting 2 from both sides: $|x - 1| \geq 1$. Now, we're left with the two cases $x - 1 \geq 1$ or $x - 1 \leq -1$: note that in the latter, negative case, the inequality is flipped. $x - 1 \geq 1$ reduces to $x \geq 2$, and $x - 1 \leq -1$ reduces to $x \leq 0$. Since in the inequality $|x - 1| \geq 1$ the absolute value is on the greater side, the two cases combine into an *or* compound inequality, so the final, solved inequality is "$x \leq 0$ or $x \geq 2$."

Review Video: Solving Absolute Value Inequalities
Visit mometrix.com/academy and enter code: 997008

Solving Inequalities Involving Square Roots

Solving an inequality with a square root involves two parts. First, we solve the inequality as if it were an equation, isolating the square root and then squaring both sides of the equation. Second, we restrict the solution to the set of values of x for which the value inside the square root sign is non-negative.

For example, in the inequality, $\sqrt{x-2}+1<5$, we can isolate the square root by subtracting 1 from both sides, yielding $\sqrt{x-2}<4$. Squaring both sides of the inequality yields $x-2<16$, so $x<18$. Since we can't take the square root of a negative number, we also require the part inside the square root to be non-negative. In this case, that means $x-2\geq 0$. Adding 2 to both sides of the inequality yields $x\geq 2$. Our final answer is a compound inequality combining the two simple inequalities: $x\geq 2$ and $x<18$, or $2\leq x<18$.

Note that we only get a compound inequality if the two simple inequalities are in opposite directions; otherwise, we take the one that is more restrictive.

The same technique can be used for other even roots, such as fourth roots. It is *not*, however, used for cube roots or other odd roots—negative numbers *do* have cube roots, so the condition that the quantity inside the root sign cannot be negative does not apply.

Review Video: Solving Inequalities Involving Square Roots
Visit mometrix.com/academy and enter code: 800288

Special Circumstances

Sometimes an inequality involving an absolute value or an even exponent is true for all values of x, and we don't need to do any further work to solve it. This is true if the inequality, once the absolute value or exponent term is isolated, says that term is greater than a negative number (or greater than or equal to zero). Since an absolute value or a number raised to an even exponent is *always* non-negative, this inequality is always true.

Graphical Solutions to Inequalities

Graphing Simple Inequalities

To graph a simple inequality, we first mark on the number line the value that signifies the end point of the inequality. If the inequality is strict (involves a less than or greater than), we use a hollow circle; if it is not strict (less than or equal to or greater than or equal to), we use a solid circle. We then fill in the part of the number line that satisfies the inequality: to the left of the marked point for less than (or less than or equal to), to the right for greater than (or greater than or equal to).

For example, we would graph the inequality $x<5$ by putting a hollow circle at 5 and filling in the part of the line to the left:

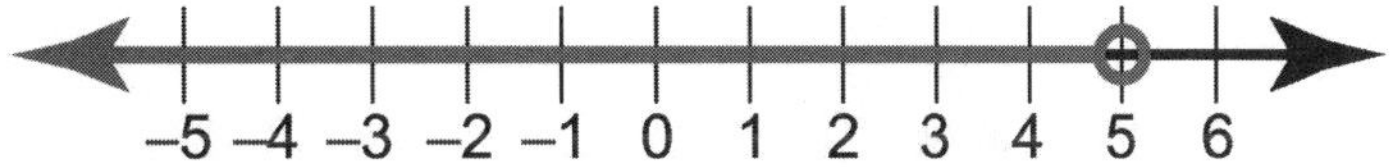

Graphing Compound Inequalities

To graph a compound inequality, we fill in both parts of the inequality for an *or* inequality, or the overlap between them for an *and* inequality. More specifically, we start by plotting the endpoints of each inequality on the number line. For an *or* inequality, we then fill in the appropriate side of the line for each inequality. Typically, the two component inequalities do not overlap, which means the shaded part is *outside* the two points. For an *and* inequality, we instead fill in the part of the line that meets both inequalities.

For the inequality "$x \leq -3$ or $x > 4$," we first put a solid circle at -3 and a hollow circle at 4. We then fill the parts of the line *outside* these circles:

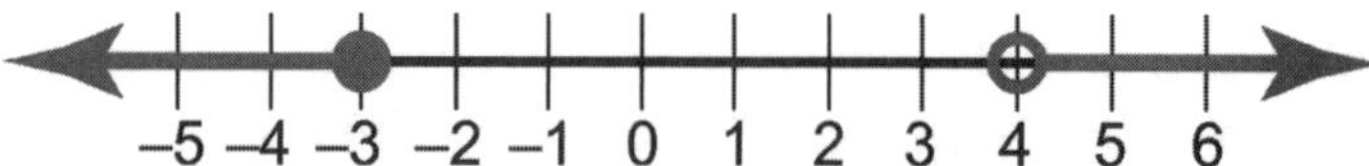

GRAPHING INEQUALITIES INCLUDING ABSOLUTE VALUES

An inequality with an absolute value can be converted to a compound inequality. To graph the inequality, first convert it to a compound inequality, and then graph that normally. If the absolute value is on the greater side of the inequality, we end up with an *or* inequality; we plot the endpoints of the inequality on the number line and fill in the part of the line *outside* those points. If the absolute value is on the smaller side of the inequality, we end up with an *and* inequality; we plot the endpoints of the inequality on the number line and fill in the part of the line *between* those points.

For example, the inequality $|x + 1| \geq 4$ can be rewritten as $x \geq 3$ or $x \leq -5$. We place solid circles at the points 3 and -5 and fill in the part of the line *outside* them:

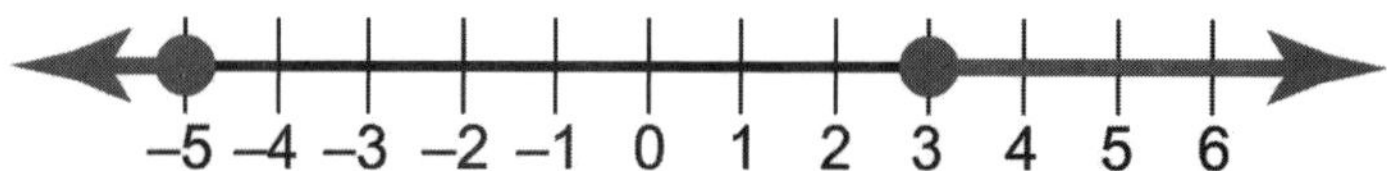

GRAPHING INEQUALITIES IN TWO VARIABLES

To graph an inequality in two variables, we first graph the border of the inequality. This means graphing the equation that we get if we replace the inequality sign with an equals sign. If the inequality is strict ($>$ or $<$), we graph the border with a dashed or dotted line; if it is not strict ($\geq$ or $\leq$), we use a solid line. We can then test any point not on the border to see if it satisfies the inequality. If it does, we shade in that side of the border; if not, we shade in the other side. As an example, consider $y > 2x + 2$. To graph this inequality, we first graph the border, $y = 2x + 2$. Since it is a strict inequality, we use a dashed line. Then, we choose a test point. This can be any point not on the border; in this case, we will choose the origin, (0,0). (This makes the calculation easy and is generally a good choice unless the border passes through the origin.) Putting this into the original inequality, we get $0 > 2(0) + 2$, i.e., $0 > 2$. This is *not* true, so we shade in the side of the border that does *not* include the point (0,0):

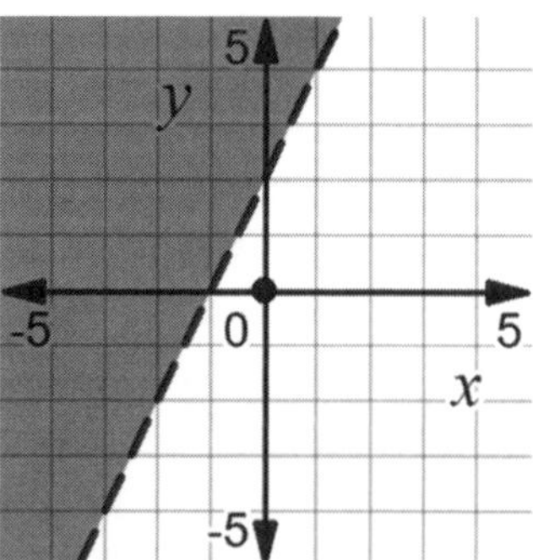

GRAPHING COMPOUND INEQUALITIES IN TWO VARIABLES

One way to graph a compound inequality in two variables is to first graph each of the component inequalities. For an *and* inequality, we then shade in only the parts where the two graphs overlap; for an *or* inequality, we shade in any region that pertains to either of the individual inequalities.

Consider the graph of "$y \geq x - 1$ and $y \leq -x$":

We first shade in the individual inequalities:

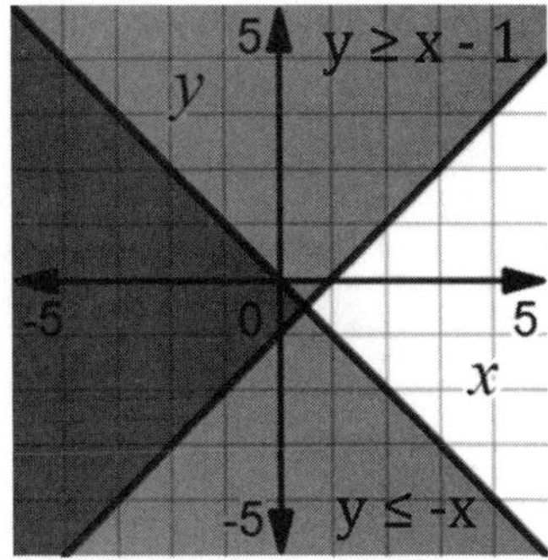

Now, since the compound inequality has an *and*, we only leave shaded the overlap—the part that pertains to *both* inequalities:

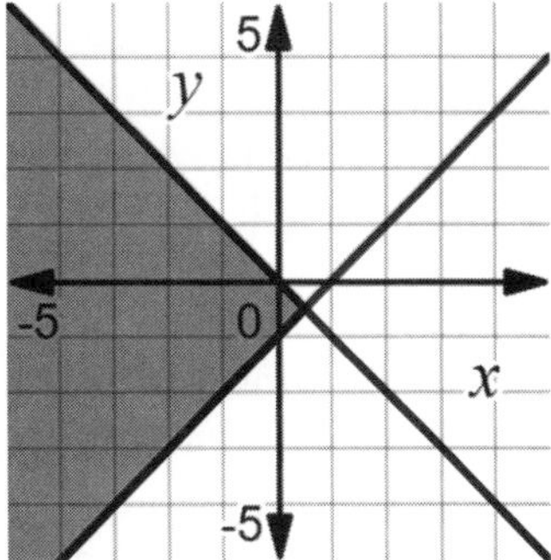

If instead the inequality had been "$y \geq x - 1$ or $y \leq -x$," our final graph would involve the *total* shaded area:

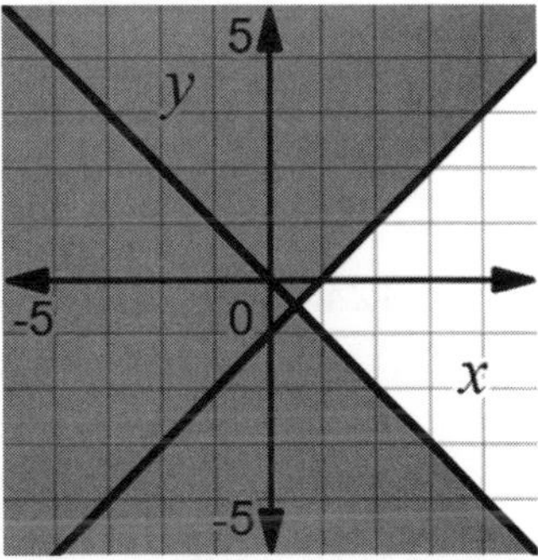

Review Video: Graphing Solutions to Inequalities
Visit mometrix.com/academy and enter code: 391281

Metric and Customary Measurements

Metric Measurement Prefixes

Giga-	One billion	1 *giga*watt is one billion watts
Mega-	One million	1 *mega*hertz is one million hertz
Kilo-	One thousand	1 *kilo*gram is one thousand grams
Deci-	One-tenth	1 *deci*meter is one-tenth of a meter
Centi-	One-hundredth	1 *centi*meter is one-hundredth of a meter
Milli-	One-thousandth	1 *milli*liter is one-thousandth of a liter
Micro-	One-millionth	1 *micro*gram is one-millionth of a gram

Review Video: Metric System Conversion - How the Metric System Works
Visit mometrix.com/academy and enter code: 163709

Measurement Conversion

When converting between units, the goal is to maintain the same meaning but change the way it is displayed. In order to go from a larger unit to a smaller unit, multiply the number of the known amount by the equivalent amount. When going from a smaller unit to a larger unit, divide the number of the known amount by the equivalent amount.

For complicated conversions, it may be helpful to set up conversion fractions. In these fractions, one fraction is the **conversion factor**. The other fraction has the unknown amount in the numerator. So, the known value is placed in the denominator. Sometimes, the second fraction has the known value from the problem in the numerator and the unknown in the denominator. Multiply the two fractions to get the converted measurement. Note that since the numerator and the denominator of the factor are equivalent, the value of the fraction is 1. That is why we can say that the result in the new units is equal to the result in the old units even though they have different numbers.

It can often be necessary to chain known conversion factors together. As an example, consider converting 512 square inches to square meters. We know that there are 2.54 centimeters in an inch and 100 centimeters in a meter, and we know we will need to square each of these factors to achieve the conversion we are looking for.

$$\frac{512\text{ in}^2}{1}\times\left(\frac{2.54\text{ cm}}{1\text{ in}}\right)^2\times\left(\frac{1\text{ m}}{100\text{ cm}}\right)^2=\frac{512\ \cancel{\text{in}^2}}{1}\times\left(\frac{6.4516\ \cancel{\text{cm}^2}}{1\ \cancel{\text{in}^2}}\right)\times\left(\frac{1\text{ m}^2}{10{,}000\ \cancel{\text{cm}^2}}\right)=0.330\text{ m}^2$$

Review Video: Measurement Conversions
Visit mometrix.com/academy and enter code: 316703

Common Units and Equivalents

Metric Equivalents

1000 μg (microgram)	1 mg
1000 mg (milligram)	1 g
1000 g (gram)	1 kg
1000 kg (kilogram)	1 metric ton
1000 mL (milliliter)	1 L
1000 μm (micrometer)	1 mm
1000 mm (millimeter)	1 m
100 cm (centimeter)	1 m
1000 m (meter)	1 km

Distance and Area Measurement

Unit	Abbreviation	US equivalent	Metric equivalent
Inch	in	1 inch	2.54 centimeters
Foot	ft	12 inches	0.305 meters
Yard	yd	3 feet	0.914 meters
Mile	mi	5280 feet	1.609 kilometers
Acre	ac	4840 square yards	0.405 hectares
Square Mile	sq. mi. or $mi.^2$	640 acres	2.590 square kilometers

Capacity Measurements

Unit	Abbreviation	US equivalent	Metric equivalent
Fluid Ounce	fl oz	8 fluid drams	29.573 milliliters
Cup	c	8 fluid ounces	0.237 liter
Pint	pt.	16 fluid ounces	0.473 liter
Quart	qt.	2 pints	0.946 liter
Gallon	gal.	4 quarts	3.785 liters
Teaspoon	t or tsp.	1 fluid dram	5 milliliters
Tablespoon	T or tbsp.	4 fluid drams	15 or 16 milliliters
Cubic Centimeter	cc or cm^3	0.271 drams	1 milliliter

Weight Measurements

Unit	Abbreviation	US equivalent	Metric equivalent
Ounce	oz	16 drams	28.35 grams
Pound	lb	16 ounces	453.6 grams
Ton	tn.	2,000 pounds	907.2 kilograms

Volume and Weight Measurement Clarifications

Always be careful when using ounces and fluid ounces. They are not equivalent.

1 pint = 16 fluid ounces	1 fluid ounce ≠ 1 ounce
1 pound = 16 ounces	1 pint ≠ 1 pound

Having one pint of something does not mean you have one pound of it. In the same way, just because something weighs one pound does not mean that its volume is one pint.

In the United States, the word "ton" by itself refers to a short ton or a net ton. Do not confuse this with a long ton (also called a gross ton) or a metric ton (also spelled *tonne*), which have different measurement equivalents.

$$1 \text{ US ton} = 2000 \text{ pounds} \quad \neq \quad 1 \text{ metric ton} = 1000 \text{ kilograms}$$

Military Time

MILITARY TIME

The **24-hour clock** is a time system used by the military and on some digital clocks. On the 24-hour clock, minutes and seconds are the same as the standard 12-hour clock. However, time is expressed in 4 figures, and the hours run from 0000 hour (12 a.m.) to 2359 hours (11:59 p.m.).

To convert from 12-hour to 24-hour time, remove the colon and:

- for a.m. times, if the time has 3 digits, add a 0 to the beginning (e.g., 8:12 a.m. becomes 0812 hours). For times between 12 a.m. and 1 a. m., replace the 12 with a pair of zeros (e.g., 12:41 a.m. becomes 0041 hours).
- for p.m. times, add 12 to the hour number (e.g., 3:40 p.m. = 1540 hours), except for times between 12 p.m. and 1 p.m., which do not require any further change.

To convert from 24-hour to 12-hour time, add a colon between the second and third digits. If the first two digits are less than 12, the time is a.m.; otherwise it is p.m. If the first two digits are zeros, the hour becomes 12 a.m. (e.g., 0020 becomes 12:20 a.m.) If only the first digit is zero, remove it (e.g., 0730 becomes 7:30 a.m.). If the first two digits are greater than 12, subtract 12 (e.g., 2325 becomes 11:25 p.m.).

Roman Numerals

ROMAN NUMERALS

Roman numerals are used today only in limited circumstances, but for the test you will still need to know what numbers they represent. Each numeral has a specific value:

Roman Numeral	Value
I	1
V	5
X	10
L	50
C	100
D	500
M	1000

When multiple numerals are placed together, their values are generally added:

$$XVI = 10 + 5 + 1 = 16$$

The exception to this rule is when a smaller number is placed in front of a larger number. In those cases, the smaller number must be subtracted from the larger number that immediately follows it:

$$IX = 10 - 1 = 9$$

$$XL = 50 - 10 = 40$$

Further complicating things, these combinations can be used as part of a larger number as well:

$$MCMXCIX = 1000 + (1000 - 100) + (100 - 10) + (10 - 1)$$

$$MCMXCIX = 1000 + 900 + 90 + 9 = 1999$$

Though it's not likely to show up on your test, a line over a Roman numeral means that its value is 1000 times its normal value:

$$\overline{V} = 5{,}000; \; \overline{X} = 10{,}000; \overline{C} = 100{,}000$$

Chapter Quiz

Ready to see how well you retained what you just read? Scan the QR code to go directly to the chapter quiz interface for this study guide. If you're using a computer, simply visit the bonus page at **mometrix.com/bonus948/hesia2** and click the Chapter Quizzes link.

Reading Comprehension

Transform passive reading into active learning! After immersing yourself in this chapter, put your comprehension to the test by taking a quiz. The insights you gained will stay with you longer this way. Scan the QR code to go directly to the chapter quiz interface for this study guide. If you're using a computer, simply visit the bonus page at **mometrix.com/bonus948/hesia2** and click the Chapter Quizzes link.

The reading comprehension portion of the exam requires the student to answer questions based on a passage that he or she has read. These questions are related to comprehension of reading and measure the student's ability to comprehend meaning, identify the main idea, find meaning of words in context, make logical inferences, etc. There are 47 reading comprehension items.

Preparation

One of the best techniques for increasing reading comprehension is to **read** as much and as often as possible. Expand your literary horizons by reading a variety of publications. Read things like fiction stories, medical journals, comic books, and newspapers. This forces your mind to encounter new words and concepts. Keep reading materials in places where you will have idle time, such as the bathroom and your car. When you are waiting in line at the bank or pumping gas, you can thumb through a news magazine or read a chapter of a book. Tuck a book or pamphlet into your purse or pocket and read while standing in line at the grocery store. If you are using the Internet to decide which movie to see, read some reviews for each movie.

Reading Comprehension

Understanding a Passage

One of the most important skills in reading comprehension is the identification of **topics** and **main ideas**. There is a subtle difference between these two features. The topic is the subject of a text (i.e., what the text is all about). The main idea, on the other hand, is the most important point being made by the author. The topic is usually expressed in a few words at the most while the main idea often needs a full sentence to be completely defined. As an example, a short passage might be written on the topic of penguins, and the main idea could be written as *Penguins are different from other birds in many ways.* In most nonfiction writing, the topic and the main idea will be **stated directly** and often appear in a sentence at the very beginning or end of the text. When being tested on an understanding of the author's topic, you may be able to skim the passage for the general idea by reading only the first sentence of each paragraph. A body paragraph's first sentence is often—but not always—the main **topic sentence** which gives you a summary of the content in the paragraph.

However, there are cases in which the reader must figure out an **unstated** topic or main idea. In these instances, you must read every sentence of the text and try to come up with an overarching idea that is supported by each of those sentences.

Note: The main idea should not be confused with the thesis statement. While the main idea gives a brief, general summary of a text, the thesis statement provides a **specific perspective** on an issue that the author supports with evidence.

Review Video: Topics and Main Ideas
Visit mometrix.com/academy and enter code: 407801

Supporting details are smaller pieces of evidence that provide backing for the main point. In order to show that a main idea is correct or valid, an author must add details that prove their point. All texts contain details, but they are only classified as supporting details when they serve to reinforce some larger point. Supporting details are most commonly found in informative and persuasive texts. In some cases, they will be clearly indicated with terms like *for example* or *for instance*, or they will be enumerated with terms like *first*, *second*, and *last*. However, you need to be prepared for texts that do not contain those indicators. As a reader, you should consider whether the author's supporting details really back up his or her main point. Details can be factual and correct, yet they may not be **relevant** to the author's point. Conversely, details can be relevant, but be ineffective because they are based on opinion or assertions that cannot be proven.

Review Video: Supporting Details
Visit mometrix.com/academy and enter code: 396297

An example of a main idea is: *Giraffes live in the Serengeti of Africa*. A supporting detail about giraffes could be: *A giraffe in this region benefits from a long neck by reaching twigs and leaves on tall trees.* The main idea gives the general idea that the text is about giraffes. The supporting detail gives a specific fact about how the giraffes eat.

Organization of the Text

The way a text is organized can help readers understand the author's intent and his or her conclusions. There are various ways to organize a text, and each one has a purpose and use. Usually, authors will organize information logically in a passage so the reader can follow and locate the information within the text. However, since not all passages are written with the same logical structure, you need to be familiar with several different types of passage structure.

Review Video: Organizational Methods to Structure Text
Visit mometrix.com/academy and enter code: 606263

Review Video: Sequence of Events in a Story
Visit mometrix.com/academy and enter code: 807512

Chronological

When using **chronological** order, the author presents information in the order that it happened. For example, biographies are typically written in chronological order. The subject's birth and childhood are presented first, followed by their adult life, and lastly the events leading up to the person's death.

Cause and Effect

One of the most common text structures is **cause and effect**. A **cause** is an act or event that makes something happen, and an **effect** is the thing that happens as a result of the cause. A cause-and-effect relationship is not always explicit, but there are some terms in English that signal causes, such as *since*, *because*, and *due to*. Furthermore, terms that signal effects include *consequently,* *therefore, this leads to*. As an example, consider the sentence *Because the sky was clear, Ron did not bring an umbrella*. The cause is the clear sky, and the effect is that Ron did not bring an umbrella. However, readers may find that sometimes the cause-and-effect relationship will not be clearly noted. For instance, the sentence *He was late and missed the meeting* does not contain any signaling words, but the sentence still contains a cause (he was late) and an effect (he missed the meeting).

Review Video: Cause and Effect
Visit mometrix.com/academy and enter code: 868099

Review Video: Rhetorical Strategy of Cause and Effect Analysis
Visit mometrix.com/academy and enter code: 725944

MULTIPLE EFFECTS

Be aware of the possibility for a single cause to have **multiple effects.** (e.g., *Single cause*: Because you left your homework on the table, your dog engulfed the assignment. *Multiple effects*: As a result, you receive a failing grade, your parents do not allow you to go out with your friends, you miss out on the new movie, and one of your classmates spoils it for you before you have another chance to watch it).

MULTIPLE CAUSES

Also, there is the possibility for a single effect to have **multiple causes.** (e.g., *Single effect*: Alan has a fever. *Multiple causes*: An unexpected cold front came through the area, and Alan forgot to take his multi-vitamin to avoid getting sick.) Additionally, an effect can in turn be the cause of another effect, in what is known as a cause-and-effect chain. (e.g., As a result of her disdain for procrastination, Lynn prepared for her exam. This led to her passing her test with high marks. Hence, her resume was accepted and her application was approved.)

CAUSE AND EFFECT IN PERSUASIVE ESSAYS

Persuasive essays, in which an author tries to make a convincing argument and change the minds of readers, usually include cause-and-effect relationships. However, these relationships should not always be taken at face value. Frequently, an author will assume a cause or take an effect for granted. To read a persuasive essay effectively, readers need to judge the cause-and-effect relationships that the author is presenting. For instance, imagine an author wrote the following: *The parking deck has been unprofitable because people would prefer to ride their bikes.* The relationship is clear: the cause is that people prefer to ride their bikes, and the effect is that the parking deck has been unprofitable. However, readers should consider whether this argument is conclusive. Perhaps there are other reasons for the failure of the parking deck: a down economy, excessive fees, etc. Too often, authors present causal relationships as if they are fact rather than opinion. Readers should be on the alert for these dubious claims.

PROBLEM-SOLUTION

Some nonfiction texts are organized to **present a problem** followed by a solution. For this type of text, the problem is often explained before the solution is offered. In some cases, as when the problem is well known, the solution may be introduced briefly at the beginning. Other passages may focus on the solution, and the problem will be referenced only occasionally. Some texts will outline multiple solutions to a problem, leaving readers to choose among them. If the author has an interest or an allegiance to one solution, he or she may fail to mention or describe accurately some of the other solutions. Readers should be careful of the author's agenda when reading a problem-solution text. Only by understanding the author's perspective and interests can one develop a proper judgment of the proposed solution.

Compare and Contrast

Many texts follow the **compare-and-contrast** model in which the similarities and differences between two ideas or things are explored. Analysis of the similarities between ideas is called **comparison**. In an ideal comparison, the author places ideas or things in an equivalent structure, i.e., the author presents the ideas in the same way. If an author wants to show the similarities between cricket and baseball, then he or she may do so by summarizing the equipment and rules for each game. Be mindful of the similarities as they appear in the passage and take note of any differences that are mentioned. Often, these small differences will only reinforce the more general similarity.

Review Video: Compare and Contrast
Visit mometrix.com/academy and enter code: 798319

Thinking critically about ideas and conclusions can seem like a daunting task. One way to ease this task is to understand the basic elements of ideas and writing techniques. Looking at the ways different ideas relate to each other can be a good way for readers to begin their analysis. For instance, sometimes authors will write about two ideas that are in opposition to each other. Or, one author will provide his or her ideas on a topic, and another author may respond in opposition. The analysis of these opposing ideas is known as **contrast**. Contrast is often marred by the author's obvious partiality to one of the ideas. A discerning reader will be put off by an author who does not engage in a fair fight. In an analysis of opposing ideas, both ideas should be presented in clear and reasonable terms. If the author does prefer a side, you need to read carefully to determine the areas where the author shows or avoids this preference. In an analysis of opposing ideas, you should proceed through the passage by marking the major differences point by point with an eye that is looking for an explanation of each side's view. For instance, in an analysis of capitalism and communism, there is an importance in outlining each side's view on labor, markets, prices, personal responsibility, etc. Additionally, as you read through the passages, you should note whether the opposing views present each side in a similar manner.

Sequence

Readers must be able to identify a text's **sequence**, or the order in which things happen. Often, when the sequence is very important to the author, the text is indicated with signal words like *first*, *then*, *next*, and *last*. However, a sequence can be merely implied and must be noted by the reader. Consider the sentence *He walked through the garden and gave water and fertilizer to the plants.* Clearly, the man did not walk through the garden before he collected water and fertilizer for the plants. So, the implied sequence is that he first collected water, then he collected fertilizer, next he walked through the garden, and last he gave water or fertilizer as necessary to the plants. Texts do not always proceed in an orderly sequence from first to last. Sometimes they begin at the end and start over at the beginning. As a reader, you can enhance your understanding of the passage by taking brief notes to clarify the sequence.

Review Video: Sequence
Visit mometrix.com/academy and enter code: 489027

Making Connections to Enhance Comprehension

Reading involves thinking. For good comprehension, readers make **text-to-self**, **text-to-text**, and **text-to-world connections**. Making connections helps readers understand text better and predict what might occur next based on what they already know, such as how characters in the story feel or what happened in another text. Text-to-self connections with the reader's life and experiences make literature more personally relevant and meaningful to readers. Readers can make connections before, during, and after reading—including whenever the text reminds them of something similar they have encountered in life or other texts. The genre, setting, characters, plot elements, literary structure and devices, and themes an author uses allow a reader to make connections to other works of literature or to people and events in their own lives. Venn diagrams and other graphic organizers help visualize connections. Readers can also make double-entry notes: key content, ideas, events, words, and quotations on one side, and the connections with these on the other.

Summarizing Literature to Support Comprehension

When reading literature, especially demanding works, **summarizing** helps readers identify important information and organize it in their minds. They can also identify themes, problems, and solutions, and can sequence the story. Readers can summarize before, during, and after they read. They should use their own words, as they do when describing a personal event or giving directions. Previewing a text's organization before reading by examining the book cover, table of contents, and illustrations also aids summarizing. Making notes of key words and ideas in a graphic organizer while reading can benefit readers in the same way. Graphic organizers are another useful method; readers skim the text to determine main ideas and then narrow the list with the aid of the organizer. Unimportant details should be omitted in summaries. Summaries can be organized using description, problem-solution, comparison-contrast, sequence, main ideas, or cause-and-effect.

Review Video: Summarizing Text
Visit mometrix.com/academy and enter code: 172903

Paraphrasing

Paraphrasing is another method that the reader can use to aid in comprehension. When paraphrasing, one puts what they have read into their own words by rephrasing what the author has written, or one "translates" all of what the author shared into their own words by including as many details as they can.

Making Predictions and Inferences

Making Predictions

When we read literature, **making predictions** about what will happen in the writing reinforces our purpose for reading and prepares us mentally. A **prediction** is a guess about what will happen next. Readers constantly make predictions based on what they have read and what they already know. We can make predictions before we begin reading and during our reading. Consider the following sentence: *Staring at the computer screen in shock, Kim blindly reached over for the brimming glass of water on the shelf to her side.* The sentence suggests that Kim is distracted, and that she is not looking at the glass that she is going to pick up. So, a reader might predict that Kim is going to knock over the glass. Of course, not every prediction will be accurate: perhaps Kim will pick the glass up cleanly. Nevertheless, the author has certainly created the expectation that the water might be spilled.

As we read on, we can test the accuracy of our predictions, revise them in light of additional reading, and confirm or refute our predictions. Predictions are always subject to revision as the reader acquires more information. A reader can make predictions by observing the title and illustrations; noting the structure, characters, and subject; drawing on existing knowledge relative to the subject; and asking "why" and "who" questions. Connecting reading to what we already know enables us to learn new information and construct meaning. For example, before third-graders read a book about Johnny Appleseed, they may start a KWL chart—a list of what they *Know*, what they *Want* to know or learn, and what they have *Learned* after reading. Activating existing background knowledge and thinking about the text before reading improves comprehension.

Review Video: Predictive Reading
Visit mometrix.com/academy and enter code: 437248

Test-taking tip: To respond to questions requiring future predictions, your answers should be based on evidence of past or present behavior and events.

Evaluating Predictions

When making predictions, readers should be able to explain how they developed their prediction. One way readers can defend their thought process is by citing textual evidence. Textual evidence to evaluate reader predictions about literature includes specific synopses of the work, paraphrases of the work or parts of it, and direct quotations from the work. These references to the text must support the prediction by indicating, clearly or unclearly, what will happen later in the story. A text may provide these indications through literary devices such as foreshadowing. Foreshadowing is anything in a text that gives the reader a hint about what is to come by emphasizing the likelihood of an event or development. Foreshadowing can occur through descriptions, exposition, and dialogue. Foreshadowing in dialogue usually occurs when a character gives a warning or expresses a strong feeling that a certain event will occur. Foreshadowing can also occur through irony. However, unlike other forms of foreshadowing, the events that seem the most likely are the opposite of what actually happens. Instances of foreshadowing and irony can be summarized, paraphrased, or quoted to defend a reader's prediction.

Review Video: Textual Evidence for Predictions
Visit mometrix.com/academy and enter code: 261070

Drawing Conclusions from Inferences

Inferences about literary text are logical conclusions that readers make based on their observations and previous knowledge. An inference is based on both what is found in a passage or a story and what is known from personal experience. For instance, a story may say that a character is frightened and can hear howling in the distance. Based on both what is in the text and personal knowledge, it is a logical conclusion that the character is frightened because he hears the sound of wolves. A good inference is supported by the information in a passage.

Implicit and Explicit Information

By inferring, readers construct meanings from text that are personally relevant. By combining their own schemas or concepts and their background information pertinent to the text with what they read, readers interpret it according to both what the author has conveyed and their own unique perspectives. Inferences are different from **explicit information**, which is clearly stated in a passage. Authors do not always explicitly spell out every meaning in what they write; many meanings are implicit. Through inference, readers can comprehend implied meanings in the text, and also derive personal significance from it, making the text meaningful and memorable to them. Inference is a natural process in everyday life. When readers infer, they can draw conclusions about what the author is saying, predict what may reasonably follow, amend these predictions as they continue to read, interpret the import of themes, and analyze the characters' feelings and motivations through their actions.

Example of Drawing Conclusions from Inferences

Read the excerpt and decide why Jana finally relaxed.

> Jana loved her job, but the work was very demanding. She had trouble relaxing. She called a friend, but she still thought about work. She ordered a pizza, but eating it did not help. Then, her kitten jumped on her lap and began to purr. Jana leaned back and began to hum a little tune. She felt better.

You can draw the conclusion that Jana relaxed because her kitten jumped on her lap. The kitten purred, and Jana leaned back and hummed a tune. Then she felt better. The excerpt does not explicitly say that this is the reason why she was able to relax. The text leaves the matter unclear, but the reader can infer or make a "best guess" that this is the reason she is relaxing. This is a logical conclusion based on the information in the passage. It is the best conclusion a reader can make based on the information he or she has read. Inferences are based on the information in a passage, but they are not directly stated in the passage.

Test-taking tip: While being tested on your ability to make correct inferences, you must look for **contextual clues**. An answer can be true, but not the best or most correct answer. The contextual clues will help you find the answer that is the **best answer** out of the given choices. Be careful in your reading to understand the context in which a phrase is stated. When asked for the implied meaning of a statement made in the passage, you should immediately locate the statement and read the **context** in which the statement was made. Also, look for an answer choice that has a similar phrase to the statement in question.

Review Video: Inference
Visit mometrix.com/academy and enter code: 379203

Review Video: How to Support a Conclusion
Visit mometrix.com/academy and enter code: 281653

Interactions with Texts

Purposes for Writing

In order to be an effective reader, one must pay attention to the author's **position** and **purpose**. Even those texts that seem objective and impartial, like textbooks, have a position and bias. Readers need to take these positions into account when considering the author's message. When an author uses emotional language or clearly favors one side of an argument, his or her position is clear. However, the author's position may be evident not only in what he or she writes, but also in what he or she doesn't write. In a normal setting, a reader would want to review some other texts on the same topic in order to develop a view of the author's position. If this was not possible, then you would want to at least acquire some background about the author. However, since you are in the middle of an exam and the only source of information is the text, you should look for language and argumentation that seems to indicate a particular stance on the subject.

Review Video: Author's Position
Visit mometrix.com/academy and enter code: 827954

Usually, identifying the author's **purpose** is easier than identifying his or her position. In most cases, the author has no interest in hiding his or her purpose. A text that is meant to entertain, for instance, should be written to please the reader. Most narratives, or stories, are written to entertain, though they may also inform or persuade. Informative texts are easy to identify, while the most difficult purpose of a text to identify is persuasion because the author has an interest in making this purpose hard to detect. When a reader discovers that the author is trying to persuade, he or she should be skeptical of the argument. For this reason, persuasive texts often try to establish an entertaining tone and hope to amuse the reader into agreement. On the other hand, an informative tone may be implemented to create an appearance of authority and objectivity.

An author's purpose is evident often in the organization of the text (e.g., section headings in bold font points to an informative text). However, you may not have such organization available to you in your exam. Instead, if the author makes his or her main idea clear from the beginning, then the likely purpose of the text is to inform. If the author begins by making a claim and provides various arguments to support that claim, then the purpose is probably to persuade. If the author tells a story or wants to gain the reader's attention more than to push a particular point or deliver information, then his or her purpose is most likely to entertain. As a reader, you must judge authors on how well they accomplish their purpose. In other words, you need to consider the type of passage (e.g., technical, persuasive, etc.) that the author has written and if the author has followed the requirements of the passage type.

Making Logical Conclusions about a Passage

A reader should always be drawing conclusions from the text. Sometimes conclusions are **implied** from written information, and other times the information is **stated directly** within the passage. One should always aim to draw conclusions from information stated within a passage, rather than to draw them from mere implications. At times an author may provide some information and then describe a counterargument. Readers should be alert for direct statements that are subsequently rejected or weakened by the author. Furthermore, you should always read through the entire passage before drawing conclusions. Many readers are trained to expect the author's conclusions at either the beginning or the end of the passage, but many texts do not adhere to this format.

Drawing conclusions from information implied within a passage requires confidence on the part of the reader. **Implications** are things that the author does not state directly, but readers can assume based on what the author does say. Consider the following passage: *I stepped outside and opened my umbrella. By the time I got to work, the cuffs of my pants were soaked.* The author never states that it is raining, but this fact is clearly implied. Conclusions based on implication must be well supported by the text. In order to draw a solid conclusion, readers should have **multiple pieces of evidence**. If readers have only one piece, they must be assured that there is no other possible explanation than their conclusion. A good reader will be able to draw many conclusions from information implied by the text, which will be a great help on the exam.

Drawing Conclusions

A common type of inference that a reader has to make is **drawing a conclusion**. The reader makes this conclusion based on the information provided within a text. Certain facts are included to help a reader come to a specific conclusion. For example, a story may open with a man trudging through the snow on a cold winter day, dragging a sled behind him. The reader can logically **infer** from the setting of the story that the man is wearing heavy winter clothes in order to stay warm. Information is implied based on the setting of a story, which is why **setting** is an important element of the text. If the same man in the example was trudging down a beach on a hot summer day, dragging a surf board behind him, the reader would assume that the man is not wearing heavy clothes. The reader makes inferences based on their own experiences and the information presented to them in the story.

Test-taking tip: When asked to identify a conclusion that may be drawn, look for critical "hedge" phrases, such as *likely*, *may*, *can*, and *will often*, among many others. When you are being tested on this knowledge, remember the question that writers insert into these hedge phrases to cover every possibility. Often an answer will be wrong simply because there is no room for exception. Extreme positive or negative answers (such as always or never) are usually not correct. When answering these questions, the reader **should not** use any outside knowledge that is not gathered directly or reasonably inferred from the passage. Correct answers can be derived straight from the passage.

EXAMPLE

Read the following sentence from *Little Women* by Louisa May Alcott and draw a conclusion based upon the information presented:

> *You know the reason Mother proposed not having any presents this Christmas was because it is going to be a hard winter for everyone; and she thinks we ought not to spend money for pleasure, when our men are suffering so in the army.*

Based on the information in the sentence, the reader can conclude, or **infer**, that the men are away at war while the women are still at home. The pronoun *our* gives a clue to the reader that the character is speaking about men she knows. In addition, the reader can assume that the character is speaking to a brother or sister, since the term "Mother" is used by the character while speaking to another person. The reader can also come to the conclusion that the characters celebrate Christmas, since it is mentioned in the **context** of the sentence. In the sentence, the mother is presented as an unselfish character who is opinionated and thinks about the wellbeing of other people.

COMPARING TWO STORIES

When presented with two different stories, there will be **similarities** and **differences** between the two. A reader needs to make a list, or other graphic organizer, of the points presented in each story. Once the reader has written down the main point and supporting points for each story, the two sets of ideas can be compared. The reader can then present each idea and show how it is the same or different in the other story. This is called **comparing and contrasting ideas**.

The reader can compare ideas by stating, for example: "In Story 1, the author believes that humankind will one day land on Mars, whereas in Story 2, the author believes that Mars is too far away for humans to ever step foot on." Note that the two viewpoints are different in each story that the reader is comparing. A reader may state that: "Both stories discussed the likelihood of humankind landing on Mars." This statement shows how the viewpoint presented in both stories is based on the same topic, rather than how each viewpoint is different. The reader will complete a comparison of two stories with a conclusion.

Review Video: How to Compare and Contrast
Visit mometrix.com/academy and enter code: 833765

OUTLINING A PASSAGE

As an aid to drawing conclusions, **outlining** the information contained in the passage should be a familiar skill to readers. An effective outline will reveal the structure of the passage and will lead to solid conclusions. An effective outline will have a title that refers to the basic subject of the text, though the title does not need to restate the main idea. In most outlines, the main idea will be the first major section. Each major idea in the passage will be established as the head of a category. For instance, the most common outline format calls for the main ideas of the passage to be indicated with Roman numerals. In an effective outline of this kind, each of the main ideas will be represented by a Roman numeral and none of the Roman numerals will designate minor details or secondary ideas. Moreover, all supporting ideas and details should be placed in the appropriate place on the outline. An outline does not need to include every detail listed in the text, but it should feature all of those that are central to the argument or message. Each of these details should be listed under the corresponding main idea.

Review Video: Outlining as an Aid to Drawing Conclusions
Visit mometrix.com/academy and enter code: 584445

Using Graphic Organizers

Ideas from a text can also be organized using **graphic organizers**. A graphic organizer is a way to simplify information and take key points from the text. A graphic organizer such as a timeline may have an event listed for a corresponding date on the timeline, while an outline may have an event listed under a key point that occurs in the text. Each reader needs to create the type of graphic organizer that works the best for him or her in terms of being able to recall information from a story. Examples include a spider-map, which takes a main idea from the story and places it in a bubble with supporting points branching off the main idea. An outline is useful for diagramming the main and supporting points of the entire story, and a Venn diagram compares and contrasts characteristics of two or more ideas.

Review Video: Graphic Organizers
Visit mometrix.com/academy and enter code: 665513

Summarizing

A helpful tool is the ability to **summarize** the information that you have read in a paragraph or passage format. This process is similar to creating an effective outline. First, a summary should accurately define the main idea of the passage, though the summary does not need to explain this main idea in exhaustive detail. The summary should continue by laying out the most important supporting details or arguments from the passage. All of the significant supporting details should be included, and none of the details included should be irrelevant or insignificant. Also, the summary should accurately report all of these details. Too often, the desire for brevity in a summary leads to the sacrifice of clarity or accuracy. Summaries are often difficult to read because they omit all of the graceful language, digressions, and asides that distinguish great writing. However, an effective summary should communicate the same overall message as the original text.

Review Video: Summarizing Text
Visit mometrix.com/academy and enter code: 172903

Evaluating a Passage

It is important to understand the logical conclusion of the ideas presented in an informational text. **Identifying a logical conclusion** can help you determine whether you agree with the writer or not. Coming to this conclusion is much like making an inference: the approach requires you to combine the information given by the text with what you already know and make a logical conclusion. If the author intended for the reader to draw a certain conclusion, then you can expect the author's argumentation and detail to be leading in that direction.

One way to approach the task of drawing conclusions is to make brief **notes** of all the points made by the author. When the notes are arranged on paper, they may clarify the logical conclusion. Another way to approach conclusions is to consider whether the reasoning of the author raises any pertinent questions. Sometimes you will be able to draw several conclusions from a passage. On occasion these will be conclusions that were never imagined by the author. Therefore, be aware that these conclusions must be **supported directly by the text**.

EVALUATION OF SUMMARIES

A summary of a literary passage is a condensation in the reader's own words of the passage's main points. Several guidelines can be used in evaluating a summary. The summary should be complete yet concise. It should be accurate, balanced, fair, neutral, and objective, excluding the reader's own opinions or reactions. It should reflect in similar proportion how much each point summarized was covered in the original passage. Summary writers should include tags of attribution, like "Macaulay argues that" to reference the original author whose ideas are represented in the summary. Summary writers should not overuse quotations; they should only quote central concepts or phrases they cannot precisely convey in words other than those of the original author. Another aspect of evaluating a summary is considering whether it can stand alone as a coherent, unified composition. In addition, evaluation of a summary should include whether its writer has cited the original source of the passage they have summarized so that readers can find it.

Arguments and Logical Errors

Author's Argument in Argumentative Writing

In argumentative writing, the argument is a belief, position, or opinion that the author wants to convince readers to believe as well. For the first step, readers should identify the **issue**. Some issues are controversial, meaning people disagree about them. Gun control, foreign policy, and the death penalty are all controversial issues. The next step is to determine the **author's position** on the issue. That position or viewpoint constitutes the author's argument. Readers should then identify the **author's assumptions**: things he or she accepts, believes, or takes for granted without needing proof. Inaccurate or illogical assumptions produce flawed arguments and can mislead readers. Readers should identify what kinds of **supporting evidence** the author offers, such as research results, personal observations or experiences, case studies, facts, examples, expert testimony and opinions, and comparisons. Readers should decide how relevant this support is to the argument.

Review Video: Argumentative Writing
Visit mometrix.com/academy and enter code: 561544

Evaluating an Author's Argument

The first three reader steps to **evaluate an author's argument** are to identify the **author's assumptions**, identify the **supporting evidence**, and decide **whether the evidence is relevant**. For example, if an author is not an expert on a particular topic, then that author's personal experience or opinion might not be relevant. The fourth step is to assess the **author's objectivity**. For example, consider whether the author introduces clear, understandable supporting evidence and facts to support the argument. The fifth step is evaluating whether the author's **argument is complete**. When authors give sufficient support for their arguments and also anticipate and respond effectively to opposing arguments or objections to their points, their arguments are complete. However, some authors omit information that could detract from their arguments. If instead they stated this information and refuted it, it would strengthen their arguments. The sixth step in evaluating an author's argumentative writing is to assess whether the **argument is valid**. Providing clear, logical reasoning makes an author's argument valid. Readers should ask themselves whether the author's points follow a sequence that makes sense, and whether each point leads to the next. The seventh step is to determine whether the author's **argument is credible**, meaning that it is convincing and believable. Arguments that are not valid are not credible, so step seven depends on step six. Readers should be mindful of their own biases as they evaluate and should not expect authors to conclusively prove their arguments, but rather to provide effective support and reason.

Evaluating an Author's Method of Appeal

To evaluate the effectiveness of an appeal, it is important to consider the author's purpose for writing. Any appeals an author uses in their argument must be relevant to the argument's goal. For example, a writer that argues for the reclassification of Pluto, but primarily uses appeals to emotion, will not have an effective argument. This writer should focus on using appeals to logic and support their argument with provable facts. While most arguments should include appeals to logic, emotion, and credibility, some arguments only call for one or two of these types of appeal. Evidence can support an appeal, but the evidence must be relevant to truly strengthen the appeal's effectiveness. If the writer arguing for Pluto's reclassification uses the reasons for Jupiter's classification as evidence, their argument would be weak. This information may seem relevant because it is related to the classification of planets. However, this classification is highly dependent on the size of the celestial object, and Jupiter is significantly bigger than Pluto. This use of evidence is illogical and does not support the appeal. Even when appropriate evidence and appeals are used, appeals and arguments lose their effectiveness when they create logical fallacies.

OPINIONS, FACTS, AND FALLACIES

Critical thinking skills are mastered through understanding various types of writing and the different purposes of authors can have for writing different passages. Every author writes for a purpose. When you understand their purpose and how they accomplish their goal, you will be able to analyze their writing and determine whether or not you agree with their conclusions.

Readers must always be aware of the difference between fact and opinion. A **fact** can be subjected to analysis and proven to be true. An **opinion**, on the other hand, is the author's personal thoughts or feelings and may not be altered by research or evidence. If the author writes that the distance from New York City to Boston is about two hundred miles, then he or she is stating a fact. If the author writes that New York City is too crowded, then he or she is giving an opinion because there is no objective standard for overpopulation. Opinions are often supported by facts. For instance, an author might use a comparison between the population density of New York City and that of other major American cities as evidence of an overcrowded population. An opinion supported by facts tends to be more convincing. On the other hand, when authors support their opinions with other opinions, readers should employ critical thinking and approach the argument with skepticism.

Review Video: Distinguishing Fact and Opinion
Visit mometrix.com/academy and enter code: 870899

RELIABLE SOURCES

When you have an argumentative passage, you need to be sure that facts are presented to the reader from **reliable sources**. An opinion is what the author thinks about a given topic. An opinion is not common knowledge or proven by expert sources, instead the information is the personal beliefs and thoughts of the author. To distinguish between fact and opinion, a reader needs to consider the type of source that is presenting information, the information that backs-up a claim, and the author's motivation to have a certain point-of-view on a given topic. For example, if a panel of scientists has conducted multiple studies on the effectiveness of taking a certain vitamin, then the results are more likely to be factual than those of a company that is selling a vitamin and simply claims that taking the vitamin can produce positive effects. The company is motivated to sell their product, and the scientists are using the scientific method to prove a theory. Remember, if you find sentences that contain phrases such as "I think...", then the statement is an opinion.

BIASES

In their attempts to persuade, writers often make mistakes in their thought processes and writing choices. These processes and choices are important to understand so you can make an informed decision about the author's credibility. Every author has a point of view, but authors demonstrate a **bias** when they ignore reasonable counterarguments or distort opposing viewpoints. A bias is evident whenever the author's claims are presented in a way that is unfair or inaccurate. Bias can be intentional or unintentional, but readers should be skeptical of the author's argument in either case. Remember that a biased author may still be correct. However, the author will be correct in spite of, not because of, his or her bias.

A **stereotype** is a bias applied specifically to a group of people or a place. Stereotyping is considered to be particularly abhorrent because it promotes negative, misleading generalizations about people. Readers should be very cautious of authors who use stereotypes in their writing. These faulty assumptions typically reveal the author's ignorance and lack of curiosity.

Review Video: Bias and Stereotype
Visit mometrix.com/academy and enter code: 644829

Vocabulary and Word Relationships

Synonyms and Antonyms

When you understand how words relate to each other, you will discover more in a passage. This is explained by understanding **synonyms** (e.g., words that mean the same thing) and **antonyms** (e.g., words that mean the opposite of one another). As an example, *dry* and *arid* are synonyms, and *dry* and *wet* are antonyms.

There are many pairs of words in English that can be considered synonyms, despite having slightly different definitions. For instance, the words *friendly* and *collegial* can both be used to describe a warm interpersonal relationship, and one would be correct to call them synonyms. However, *collegial* (kin to *colleague*) is often used in reference to professional or academic relationships, and *friendly* has no such connotation.

If the difference between the two words is too great, then they should not be called synonyms. *Hot* and *warm* are not synonyms because their meanings are too distinct. A good way to determine whether two words are synonyms is to substitute one word for the other word and verify that the meaning of the sentence has not changed. Substituting *warm* for *hot* in a sentence would convey a different meaning. Although warm and hot may seem close in meaning, warm generally means that the temperature is moderate, and hot generally means that the temperature is excessively high.

Antonyms are words with opposite meanings. *Light* and *dark*, *up* and *down*, *right* and *left*, *good* and *bad*: these are all sets of antonyms. Be careful to distinguish between antonyms and pairs of words that are simply different. *Black* and *gray*, for instance, are not antonyms because gray is not the opposite of black. *Black* and *white*, on the other hand, are antonyms.

Not every word has an antonym. For instance, many nouns do not. What would be the antonym of *chair*? During your exam, the questions related to antonyms are more likely to concern adjectives. You will recall that adjectives are words that describe a noun. Some common adjectives include *purple*, *fast*, *skinny*, and *sweet*. From those four adjectives, *purple* is the item that lacks a group of obvious antonyms.

Review Video: What Are Synonyms and Antonyms?
Visit mometrix.com/academy and enter code: 105612

Affixes

Affixes in the English language are morphemes that are added to words to create related but different words. Derivational affixes form new words based on and related to the original words. For example, the affix *-ness* added to the end of the adjective *happy* forms the noun *happiness*. Inflectional affixes form different grammatical versions of words. For example, the plural affix *-s* changes the singular noun *book* to the plural noun *books*, and the past tense affix *-ed* changes the present tense verb *look* to the past tense *looked*. Prefixes are affixes placed in front of words. For example, *heat* means to make hot; *preheat* means to heat in advance. Suffixes are affixes placed at the ends of words. The *happiness* example above contains the suffix *-ness*. Circumfixes add parts both before and after words, such as how *light* becomes *enlighten* with the prefix *en-* and the suffix *-en.* Interfixes create compound words via central affixes: *speed* and *meter* become *speedometer* via the interfix *-o-*.

> **Review Video: Affixes**
> Visit mometrix.com/academy and enter code: 782422

Word Roots, Prefixes, and Suffixes to Help Determine Meanings of Words

Many English words were formed from combining multiple sources. For example, the Latin *habēre* means "to have," and the prefixes *in-* and *im-* mean a lack or prevention of something, as in *insufficient* and *imperfect.* Latin combined *in-* with *habēre* to form *inhibēre,* whose past participle was *inhibitus.* This is the origin of the English word *inhibit,* meaning to prevent from having. Hence by knowing the meanings of both the prefix and the root, one can decipher the word meaning. In Greek, the root *enkephalo-* refers to the brain. Many medical terms are based on this root, such as encephalitis and hydrocephalus. Understanding the prefix and suffix meanings (*-itis* means inflammation; *hydro-* means water) allows a person to deduce that encephalitis refers to brain inflammation and hydrocephalus refers to water (or other fluid) in the brain.

> **Review Video: Determining Word Meanings**
> Visit mometrix.com/academy and enter code: 894894

Prefixes

While knowing prefix meanings helps ESL and beginning readers learn new words, other readers take for granted the meanings of known words. However, prefix knowledge will also benefit them for determining meanings or definitions of unfamiliar words. For example, native English speakers and readers familiar with recipes know what *preheat* means. Knowing that *pre-* means in advance can also inform them that *presume* means to assume in advance, that *prejudice* means advance judgment, and that this understanding can be applied to many other words beginning with *pre-*. Knowing that the prefix *dis-* indicates opposition informs the meanings of words like *disbar, disagree, disestablish,* and many more. Knowing *dys-* means bad, impaired, abnormal, or difficult informs *dyslogistic, dysfunctional, dysphagia,* and *dysplasia.*

Suffixes

In English, certain suffixes generally indicate both that a word is a noun, and that the noun represents a state of being or quality. For example, *-ness* is commonly used to change an adjective into its noun form, as with *happy* and *happiness, nice* and *niceness,* and so on. The suffix *-tion* is commonly used to transform a verb into its noun form, as with *converse* and *conversation or move* and *motion.* Thus, if readers are unfamiliar with the second form of a word, knowing the meaning of the transforming suffix can help them determine meaning.

Prefixes for Numbers

Prefix	Definition	Examples
bi-	two	bisect, biennial
mono-	one, single	monogamy, monologue
poly-	many	polymorphous, polygamous
semi-	half, partly	semicircle, semicolon
uni-	one	uniform, unity

PREFIXES FOR TIME, DIRECTION, AND SPACE

Prefix	Definition	Examples
a-	in, on, of, up, to	abed, afoot
ab-	from, away, off	abdicate, abjure
ad-	to, toward	advance, adventure
ante-	before, previous	antecedent, antedate
anti-	against, opposing	antipathy, antidote
cata-	down, away, thoroughly	catastrophe, cataclysm
circum-	around	circumspect, circumference
com-	with, together, very	commotion, complicate
contra-	against, opposing	contradict, contravene
de-	from	depart
dia-	through, across, apart	diameter, diagnose
dis-	away, off, down, not	dissent, disappear
epi-	upon	epilogue
ex-	out	extract, excerpt
hypo-	under, beneath	hypodermic, hypothesis
inter-	among, between	intercede, interrupt
intra-	within	intramural, intrastate
ob-	against, opposing	objection
per-	through	perceive, permit
peri-	around	periscope, perimeter
post-	after, following	postpone, postscript
pre-	before, previous	prevent, preclude
pro-	forward, in place of	propel, pronoun
retro-	back, backward	retrospect, retrograde
sub-	under, beneath	subjugate, substitute
super-	above, extra	supersede, supernumerary
trans-	across, beyond, over	transact, transport
ultra-	beyond, excessively	ultramodern, ultrasonic

NEGATIVE PREFIXES

Prefix	Definition	Examples
a-	without, lacking	atheist, agnostic
in-	not, opposing	incapable, ineligible
non-	not	nonentity, nonsense
un-	not, reverse of	unhappy, unlock

Extra Prefixes

Prefix	Definition	Examples
for-	away, off, from	forget, forswear
fore-	previous	foretell, forefathers
homo-	same, equal	homogenized, homonym
hyper-	excessive, over	hypercritical, hypertension
in-	in, into	intrude, invade
mal-	bad, poorly, not	malfunction, malpractice
mis-	bad, poorly, not	misspell, misfire
neo-	new	Neolithic, neoconservative
omni-	all, everywhere	omniscient, omnivore
ortho-	right, straight	orthogonal, orthodox
over-	above	overbearing, oversight
pan-	all, entire	panorama, pandemonium
para-	beside, beyond	parallel, paradox
re-	backward, again	revoke, recur
sym-	with, together	sympathy, symphony

Below is a list of common suffixes and their meanings:

Adjective Suffixes

Suffix	Definition	Examples
-able (-ible)	capable of being	toler*able*, ed*ible*
-esque	in the style of, like	picturesque, grotesque
-ful	filled with, marked by	thankful, zestful
-ific	make, cause	terrific, beatific
-ish	suggesting, like	churlish, childish
-less	lacking, without	hopeless, countless
-ous	marked by, given to	religious, riotous

Noun Suffixes

Suffix	Definition	Examples
-acy	state, condition	accuracy, privacy
-ance	act, condition, fact	acceptance, vigilance
-ard	one that does excessively	drunkard, sluggard
-ation	action, state, result	occupation, starvation
-dom	state, rank, condition	serfdom, wisdom
-er (-or)	office, action	teach*er*, elevat*or*, hon*or*
-ess	feminine	waitress, duchess
-hood	state, condition	manhood, statehood
-ion	action, result, state	union, fusion
-ism	act, manner, doctrine	barbarism, socialism
-ist	worker, follower	monopolist, socialist
-ity (-ty)	state, quality, condition	acid*ity*, civil*ity*, twen*ty*
-ment	result, action	Refreshment
-ness	quality, state	greatness, tallness
-ship	position	internship, statesmanship
-sion (-tion)	state, result	revi*sion*, expedi*tion*
-th	act, state, quality	warmth, width
-tude	quality, state, result	magnitude, fortitude

Verb Suffixes

Suffix	Definition	Examples
-ate	having, showing	separate, desolate
-en	cause to be, become	deepen, strengthen
-fy	make, cause to have	glorify, fortify
-ize	cause to be, treat with	sterilize, mechanize

Denotative vs. Connotative Meaning

The **denotative** meaning of a word is the literal meaning. The **connotative** meaning goes beyond the denotative meaning to include the emotional reaction that a word may invoke. The connotative meaning often takes the denotative meaning a step further due to associations the reader makes with the denotative meaning. Readers can differentiate between the denotative and connotative meanings by first recognizing how authors use each meaning. Most non-fiction, for example, is fact-based and authors do not use flowery, figurative language. The reader can assume that the writer is using the denotative meaning of words. In fiction, the author may use the connotative meaning. Readers can determine whether the author is using the denotative or connotative meaning of a word by implementing context clues.

Review Video: Connotation and Denotation
Visit mometrix.com/academy and enter code: 310092

Nuances of Word Meaning Relative to Connotation, Denotation, Diction, and Usage

A word's denotation is simply its objective dictionary definition. However, its connotation refers to the subjective associations, often emotional, that specific words evoke in listeners and readers. Two or more words can have the same dictionary meaning, but very different connotations. Writers use diction (word choice) to convey various nuances of thought and emotion by selecting synonyms for other words that best communicate the associations they want to trigger for readers. For example, a car engine is naturally greasy; in this sense, "greasy" is a neutral term. But when a person's smile, appearance, or clothing is described as "greasy," it has a negative connotation. Some words have even gained additional or different meanings over time. For example, *awful* used to be used to describe things that evoked a sense of awe. When *awful* is separated into its root word, awe, and suffix, -ful, it can be understood to mean "full of awe." However, the word is now commonly used to describe things that evoke repulsion, terror, or another intense, negative reaction.

Review Video: Word Usage in Sentences
Visit mometrix.com/academy and enter code: 197863

Context Clues

Readers of all levels will encounter words that they have either never seen or have encountered only on a limited basis. The best way to define a word in **context** is to look for nearby words that can assist in revealing the meaning of the word. For instance, unfamiliar nouns are often accompanied by examples that provide a definition. Consider the following sentence: *Dave arrived at the party in hilarious garb: a leopard-print shirt, buckskin trousers, and bright green sneakers.* If a reader was unfamiliar with the meaning of garb, he or she could read the examples (i.e., a leopard-print shirt, buckskin trousers, and high heels) and quickly determine that the word means *clothing*. Examples will not always be this obvious. Consider this sentence: *Parsley, lemon, and flowers were just a few of the items he used as garnishes.* Here, the word *garnishes* is exemplified by parsley, lemon, and flowers. Readers who have eaten in a variety of restaurants will probably be able to identify a garnish as something used to decorate a plate.

Review Video: Reading Comprehension: Using Context Clues
Visit mometrix.com/academy and enter code: 613660

Using Contrast in Context Clues

In addition to looking at the context of a passage, readers can use contrast to define an unfamiliar word in context. In many sentences, the author will not describe the unfamiliar word directly; instead, he or she will describe the opposite of the unfamiliar word. Thus, you are provided with some information that will bring you closer to defining the word. Consider the following example: *Despite his intelligence, Hector's low brow and bad posture made him look obtuse.* The author writes that Hector's appearance does not convey intelligence. Therefore, *obtuse* must mean unintelligent. Here is another example: *Despite the horrible weather, we were beatific about our trip to Alaska.* The word *despite* indicates that the speaker's feelings were at odds with the weather. Since the weather is described as *horrible*, then *beatific* must mean something positive.

Substitution to Find Meaning

In some cases, there will be very few contextual clues to help a reader define the meaning of an unfamiliar word. When this happens, one strategy that readers may employ is **substitution**. A good reader will brainstorm some possible synonyms for the given word, and he or she will substitute these words into the sentence. If the sentence and the surrounding passage continue to make sense, then the substitution has revealed at least some information about the unfamiliar word. Consider the sentence: *Frank's admonition rang in her ears as she climbed the mountain.* A reader unfamiliar with *admonition* might come up with some substitutions like *vow, promise, advice, complaint,* or *compliment.* All of these words make general sense of the sentence, though their meanings are diverse. However, this process has suggested that an admonition is some sort of message. The substitution strategy is rarely able to pinpoint a precise definition, but this process can be effective as a last resort.

Occasionally, you will be able to define an unfamiliar word by looking at the descriptive words in the context. Consider the following sentence: *Fred dragged the recalcitrant boy kicking and screaming up the stairs.* The words *dragged*, *kicking*, and *screaming* all suggest that the boy does not want to go up the stairs. The reader may assume that *recalcitrant* means something like unwilling or protesting. In this example, an unfamiliar adjective was identified.

Additionally, using description to define an unfamiliar noun is a common practice compared to unfamiliar adjectives, as in this sentence: *Don's wrinkled frown and constantly shaking fist identified him as a curmudgeon of the first order.* Don is described as having a *wrinkled frown and constantly shaking fist*, suggesting that a *curmudgeon* must be a grumpy person. Contrasts do not always provide detailed information about the unfamiliar word, but they at least give the reader some clues.

Words with Multiple Meanings

When a word has more than one meaning, readers can have difficulty determining how the word is being used in a given sentence. For instance, the verb *cleave*, can mean either *join* or *separate*. When readers come upon this word, they will have to select the definition that makes the most sense. Consider the following sentence: *Hermione's knife cleaved the bread cleanly.* Since a knife cannot join bread together, the word must indicate separation. A slightly more difficult example would be the sentence: *The birds cleaved to one another as they flew from the oak tree.* Immediately, the presence of the words *to one another* should suggest that in this sentence *cleave* is being used to mean *join*. Discovering the intent of a word with multiple meanings requires the same tricks as defining an unknown word: look for contextual clues and evaluate the substituted words.

Context Clues to Help Determine Meanings of Words

If readers simply bypass unknown words, they can reach unclear conclusions about what they read. However, looking for the definition of every unfamiliar word in the dictionary can slow their reading progress. Moreover, the dictionary may list multiple definitions for a word, so readers must search the word's context for meaning. Hence context is important to new vocabulary regardless of reader methods. Four types of context clues are examples, definitions, descriptive words, and opposites. Authors may use a certain word, and then follow it with several different examples of what it describes. Sometimes authors actually supply a definition of a word they use, which is especially true in informational and technical texts. Authors may use descriptive words that elaborate upon a vocabulary word they just used. Authors may also use opposites with negation that help define meaning.

Examples and Definitions

An author may use a word and then give examples that illustrate its meaning. Consider this text: "Teachers who do not know how to use sign language can help students who are deaf or hard of hearing understand certain instructions by using gestures instead, like pointing their fingers to indicate which direction to look or go; holding up a hand, palm outward, to indicate stopping; holding the hands flat, palms up, curling a finger toward oneself in a beckoning motion to indicate 'come here'; or curling all fingers toward oneself repeatedly to indicate 'come on', 'more', or 'continue.'" The author of this text has used the word "gestures" and then followed it with examples, so a reader unfamiliar with the word could deduce from the examples that "gestures" means "hand motions." Readers can find examples by looking for signal words "for example," "for instance," "like," "such as," and "e.g."

While readers sometimes have to look for definitions of unfamiliar words in a dictionary or do some work to determine a word's meaning from its surrounding context, at other times an author may make it easier for readers by defining certain words. For example, an author may write, "The company did not have sufficient capital, that is, available money, to continue operations." The author defined "capital" as "available money," and heralded the definition with the phrase "that is." Another way that authors supply word definitions is with appositives. Rather than being introduced by a signal phrase like "that is," "namely," or "meaning," an appositive comes after the vocabulary word it defines and is enclosed within two commas. For example, an author may write, "The Indians introduced the Pilgrims to pemmican, cakes they made of lean meat dried and mixed with fat, which proved greatly beneficial to keep settlers from starving while trapping." In this example, the appositive phrase following "pemmican" and preceding "which" defines the word "pemmican."

Descriptions

When readers encounter a word they do not recognize in a text, the author may expand on that word to illustrate it better. While the author may do this to make the prose more picturesque and vivid, the reader can also take advantage of this description to provide context clues to the meaning of the unfamiliar word. For example, an author may write, "The man sitting next to me on the airplane was obese. His shirt stretched across his vast expanse of flesh, strained almost to bursting." The descriptive second sentence elaborates on and helps to define the previous sentence's word "obese" to mean extremely fat. A reader unfamiliar with the word "repugnant" can decipher its meaning through an author's accompanying description: "The way the child grimaced and shuddered as he swallowed the medicine showed that its taste was particularly repugnant."

Opposites

Text authors sometimes introduce a contrasting or opposing idea before or after a concept they present. They may do this to emphasize or heighten the idea they present by contrasting it with something that is the reverse. However, readers can also use these context clues to understand familiar words. For example, an author may write, "Our conversation was not cheery. We sat and talked very solemnly about his experience and a number of similar events." The reader who is not familiar with the word "solemnly" can deduce by the author's preceding use of "not cheery" that "solemn" means the opposite of cheery or happy, so it must mean serious or sad. Or if someone writes, "Don't condemn his entire project because you couldn't find anything good to say about it," readers unfamiliar with "condemn" can understand from the sentence structure that it means the opposite of saying anything good, so it must mean reject, dismiss, or disapprove. "Entire" adds another context clue, meaning total or complete rejection.

Syntax to Determine Part of Speech and Meanings of Words

Syntax refers to sentence structure and word order. Suppose that a reader encounters an unfamiliar word when reading a text. To illustrate, consider an invented word like "splunch." If this word is used in a sentence like "Please splunch that ball to me," the reader can assume from syntactic context that "splunch" is a verb. We would not use a noun, adjective, adverb, or preposition with the object "that ball," and the prepositional phrase "to me" further indicates "splunch" represents an action. However, in the sentence, "Please hand that splunch to me," the reader can assume that "splunch" is a noun. Demonstrative adjectives like "that" modify nouns. Also, we hand someone some*thing*—a thing being a noun; we do not hand someone a verb, adjective, or adverb. Some sentences contain further clues. For example, from the sentence, "The princess wore the glittering splunch on her head," the reader can deduce that it is a crown, tiara, or something similar from the syntactic context, without knowing the word.

Syntax to Indicate Different Meanings of Similar Sentences

The syntax, or structure, of a sentence affords grammatical cues that aid readers in comprehending the meanings of words, phrases, and sentences in the texts that they read. Seemingly minor differences in how the words or phrases in a sentence are ordered can make major differences in meaning. For example, two sentences can use exactly the same words but have different meanings based on the word order:

- "The man with a broken arm sat in a chair."
- "The man sat in a chair with a broken arm."

While both sentences indicate that a man sat in a chair, differing syntax indicates whether the man's or chair's arm was broken.

Determining Meaning of Phrases and Paragraphs

Like unknown words, the meanings of phrases, paragraphs, and entire works can also be difficult to discern. Each of these can be better understood with added context. However, for larger groups of words, more context is needed. Unclear phrases are similar to unclear words, and the same methods can be used to understand their meaning. However, it is also important to consider how the individual words in the phrase work together. Paragraphs are a bit more complicated. Just as words must be compared to other words in a sentence, paragraphs must be compared to other paragraphs in a composition or a section.

Determining Meaning in Various Types of Compositions

To understand the meaning of an entire composition, the type of composition must be considered. **Expository writing** is generally organized so that each paragraph focuses on explaining one idea, or part of an idea, and its relevance. **Persuasive writing** uses paragraphs for different purposes to organize the parts of the argument. **Unclear paragraphs** must be read in the context of the paragraphs around them for their meaning to be fully understood. The meaning of full texts can also be unclear at times. The purpose of composition is also important for understanding the meaning of a text. To quickly understand the broad meaning of a text, look to the introductory and concluding paragraphs. Fictional texts are different. Some fictional works have implicit meanings, but some do not. The target audience must be considered for understanding texts that do have an implicit meaning, as most children's fiction will clearly state any lessons or morals. For other fiction, the application of literary theories and criticism may be helpful for understanding the text.

Additional Resources for Determining Word Meaning and Usage

While these strategies are useful for determining the meaning of unknown words and phrases, sometimes additional resources are needed to properly use the terms in different contexts. Some words have multiple definitions, and some words are inappropriate in particular contexts or modes of writing. The following tools are helpful for understanding all meanings and proper uses for words and phrases.

- **Dictionaries** provide the meaning of a multitude of words in a language. Many dictionaries include additional information about each word, such as its etymology, its synonyms, or variations of the word.
- **Glossaries** are similar to dictionaries, as they provide the meanings of a variety of terms. However, while dictionaries typically feature an extensive list of words and comprise an entire publication, glossaries are often included at the end of a text and only include terms and definitions that are relevant to the text they follow.

- **Spell Checkers** are used to detect spelling errors in typed text. Some spell checkers may also detect the misuse of plural or singular nouns, verb tenses, or capitalization. While spell checkers are a helpful tool, they are not always reliable or attuned to the author's intent, so it is important to review the spell checker's suggestions before accepting them.
- **Style Manuals** are guidelines on the preferred punctuation, format, and grammar usage according to different fields or organizations. For example, the Associated Press Stylebook is a style guide often used for media writing. The guidelines within a style guide are not always applicable across different contexts and usages, as the guidelines often cover grammatical or formatting situations that are not objectively correct or incorrect.

Chapter Quiz

Ready to see how well you retained what you just read? Scan the QR code to go directly to the chapter quiz interface for this study guide. If you're using a computer, simply visit the bonus page at **mometrix.com/bonus948/hesia2** and click the Chapter Quizzes link.

Vocabulary and General Knowledge

Transform passive reading into active learning! After immersing yourself in this chapter, put your comprehension to the test by taking a quiz. The insights you gained will stay with you longer this way. Scan the QR code to go directly to the chapter quiz interface for this study guide. If you're using a computer, simply visit the bonus page at **mometrix.com/bonus948/hesia2** and click the Chapter Quizzes link.

The Vocabulary and General Knowledge exam has 50 items, and contains basic vocabulary that is often used in health care fields.

Increasing Verbal Ability

Nursing, like many professions, requires the ability to **communicate effectively**. Students should prepare for standardized testing and their nursing careers by utilizing some basic techniques for increasing vocabulary. Writing down new words is a good way to increase vocabulary. While reading, watching TV, or talking to others, make a note of any unfamiliar words you encounter. Look up the definition of those words and then attempt to use them in conversation. This will help the word become part of your general store of knowledge. Reading new and different material will also increase vocabulary. For example, if you normally read only for leisure or entertainment, try thumbing through a professional journal of archaeology or mathematics. This will introduce new words that you would not encounter in everyday life. Playing games like Scrabble and solving crossword puzzles can also help build verbal ability.

Etymology

Etymology is the study of words. It specifically focuses on the **origins** of words: how they have developed over time and between languages. Language is made up of words from different cultures and areas of the world. Some words we use today mean something completely different from what they meant hundreds of years ago. Words are constantly being redefined, changed, and created. New words appear as technology increases. Some words are formed by combining root words with prefixes and suffixes. Students who must improve verbal ability for standardized testing can do so by studying common prefixes and suffixes. By understanding the prefix pre, a student increases their chances of understanding words like predate. The prefix pre means "before", so it can be reasoned that predate means to date something in advance, such as predating a check.

Glossary of Important Terms

A

Abrupt: describes a sudden change that occurs without warning

Abstain: the deliberate effort to refrain from an action, such as drinking alcohol or eating junk food

Access: the freedom to use something as one chooses; the permission or ability to enter or approach a specific entity or area

Accountable: responsible for actions or explanations

Acute: experiencing something to a sharp or intense degree

Adhere: the process of binding one thing to another using glue, tape, or another agent; refers to the action of maintaining loyalty or support

Adverse: in a contrary fashion; can cause harm; may also refer to something that is in opposition to one's interests

Affect: a clear influence on one's emotions

Ambivalent: being uncertain; having conflicting thoughts or feelings about something

Ambulate: to walk or move around without assistance

Annual: the duration of a single year; an occurrence that takes place once each year

Apply: to put something to use; having a relevant or valid connection to something else

Assent: to agree to or endorse something

Audible: capable of being heard

B

Bacteria: microscopic, free-living, single-celled organisms with a simple structure and no distinct nucleus

Bilateral: having two sides; may refer to something that affects both side of the human body

C

Cardiac: concerning the heart

Cast: the process by which something is given shape through the pouring of a liquid substance into a mold; may also refer to the throwing of an object

Cavity: a pocket or hollow space; often referring to an empty space or hole in the human body (e.g., the chest cavity, or a cavity in a tooth caused by decay)

Cease: to bring about a gradual end; refers to something that dies out or becomes extinct

Chronic: persisting for a long period of time or happening over and over again

Chronology: events arranged in the order of their occurrence in time

Compensatory: an equivalent; the action of making a payment that serves as a counterbalance for another action

Complications: a factor that presents a degree of difficulty; may also refer to a secondary disease or condition

Comply: to carry out the wishes of another person; to perform in the manner prescribed by law

Concave: a surface that is rounded inward like a bowl; surface that is arched or curved

Concise: straightforward and to the point; absent of all excessive detail

Congenital: having a certain trait or disease from birth

Consistency: the agreement of each of the parts that constitute a whole

Constrict: to make something narrow by squeezing or compressing

Contingent: something that may happen; may also refer to something that is dependent upon or conditioned by something else

Contour: the line that represents the shape of a curvy figure

Contract: an agreement between two parties that binds each to perform certain actions

Contraindication: the presence of a symptom or condition that will make a specific treatment unadvisable

Convulsive: causing or consisting of sudden involuntary movement

Cursory: brief or hasty; not in-depth or thorough

D

Defecate: to have feces removed from the bowels

Deficit: a lack in an amount or quality of something, such as money or rainfall

Depress: to press down; the lessening of activity or strength; an action in which something moves to a lower position

Depth: a quality of being complete and thorough

Deteriorating: to make inferior in quality; to diminish in function or condition

Device: something that is devised or thought up; may be a piece of equipment designed for a specific task

Diagnosis: determining the dysfunction/disease

Diameter: the length of a line that passes through the body of an object

Diffuse: spread out over a wide area

Dilate: to enlarge, extend, or widen; to become wide like the pupil of the eye

Dilute: to make a substance thinner or less potent; diminish in flavor or intensity

Discrete: a separate entity; unique and separate from other things

Distal: located away from the central point or distant from the place of attachment

Distended: something that has been enlarged by the force of internal pressure

Dysfunction: a hindered function a body system or organ

E

Elevate: to lift or make something higher; to lift in rank or title

Empathy: being able to understand and take part in another person's feelings

Endogenous: the growth from a deep tissue; refers to conditions that arise from factors that are internal to an organism

Equilibrium: a balanced state

Etiology: the origin, cause, or reason by which something exists

Exacerbate: to cause something to become more intense in nature; especially an increase in violence or severity

Excess: surpassing usual limitations; unnecessary indulgence

Exogenous: the growth from superficial or shallow tissue; refers to conditions caused by factors that are external to an organism

Expand: to open or unfold; refers to an increase in number, size, or scope; may refer to the expression of an idea in greater depth

Exposure: being subject to a condition or influence; making a secret fact known publicly

Extension: an elongation or addition to a preexisting entity

External: being outside the human body; existing outside the confines of a specific space or institution

F

Fatal: something that may cause death; relating to fate or proceeding in a manner that follows a fixed sequence of events

Fatigue: the state of tiredness brought on by labor, exertion, or stress; the tendency of a specified material to break under stress

Febrile: related to fever, or displaying flushed or feverish symptoms

Flaccid: the state of not being firm; lacking vigor, force, or youthful firmness

Flexion: bending or the state of being bent, particularly in reference to joints or limbs

Flushed: blushing or an area of the body that becomes reddened

G

Gaping: something that is wide open and exposed

Gastrointestinal: concerning the stomach and intestines

Gender: the behavioral, cultural, or psychological traits that are associated with a specific sex

H

Hematologic: concerning blood

Hydration: the process of taking in water; the introduction or replenishing of fluids

Hygiene: the science of health: inducing practices; the condition or practice of activities that can maintain physical health

I

Impaired: a condition in which one cannot perform or function properly; often refers to a person who is under the influence of drugs or alcohol

Impending: hanging overhead threateningly; bound to occur in the near future

Impervious: resistant, unaffected, watertight; not allowing entrance or passage of fluid

Imply: to suggest or insinuate something without directly stating it

Incidence: the arrival of something at a surface; something that occurs or affects something else

Infection: an area of body tissue that been invaded with pathogenic organisms

Infer: to make a judgment or come to a conclusion based on evidence and reasoning

Inflamed: to incite an intensely emotional state; also refers to something that has been set on fire

Ingest: to take into one's mouth for digestion

Initiate: to cause something to begin or to set events in motion; as initiation, can also refer to the process through which a person is allowed entry into a club or organization

Insidious: something or someone who is enticing but dangerous; slow: developing dangerousness

Intact: something that remains whole or untouched by destructive forces; having no relevant part removed or altered

Internal: things inside of the body or the mind; something that exists within the limits and confines of something else

Intubate: to insert a tube, often to circumvent an obstructed airway

Invasive: tending to spread or infringe upon something; may also refer to something that will enter the human body

K

Kinetic: resulting from or relating to objects in motion; the forces and energy associated with that motion

L

Labile: unstable; constantly undergoing a chemical or physical change or breakdown

Laceration: wound with irregular borders, knife like in appearance

Latent: not presently active but with the potential to become active

Lateral: referring to or affecting the side or sides of a body

Lethargic: sluggish, indifferent, or apathetic

M

Manifestation: the act of becoming outwardly visible; can refer to the occult phenomenon of a supernatural materialization

Musculoskeletal: concerning the connections of the muscle and the skeleton

N

Neurologic: concerning the nervous system

Neurovascular: concerning the blood vessels and the nerves

Nutrient: something that provides nourishment

O

Occluded: closed or blocked off

Ominous: exhibiting an omen; refers to something evil or disastrous that appears likely to occur

Ongoing: in the process of occurring; continuously advancing or moving ahead

Oral: spoken by the mouth; of or relating to the mouth

Otic: relating to, or located in the region of the ear

Overt: something that is openly displayed or obvious

P

Parameter: a limit or boundary; in math, it is an arbitrary value that is used to describe a statistical population

Paroxysmal: characterized by a sudden fit or attack of symptoms; may be a sudden emotion or uncontrollable action

Patent: a clear and easily accessible passage

Pathogenic: disease causing

Pathology: the study of diseases

Posterior: related to the rear/back position

Potent: able to copulate as a male; refers to something that is chemically or medically effective

Potential: having the possibility of becoming a reality

Precaution: the act of taking care in advance; refers to measures taken in advance in order to prevent harm

Precipitous: very steep or difficult to climb or overcome

Predispose: to dispose in advance of or to make susceptible to

Preexisting: the state of existing before or previous to something else

Primary: first in order; a rank of importance

Priority: the state of being before; coming first in order of date or position; a preferential rating

Prognosis: the possibility of recovery after the diagnosis of an illness or disease

R

Rationale: an explanation regarding the principles, opinions, beliefs, or practices held by a specific party

Recur: something that is revisited for consideration; a thought or idea that enters one's mind for a second time

Renal: concerning the kidneys

Residual: a small part remaining after most is removed

Respiration: the act of breathing in and out of air

Restrict: to confine something or someone within specific limitations or boundaries

Retain: to keep in one's possession; to maintain an item or person in security

S

Site: the physical location of a structure; the physical space reserved for a building; the place or scene of an occurrence

Status: the position or rank held in relation to others; a person or object's condition with respect to circumstances

Strict: inflexible; maintained in such a manner that cannot be changed or altered

Subcutaneous: occurring, living, being situated, or applied under the skin

Sublingual: beneath the tongue

Supplement: an item that completes something else

Suppress: to restrain by authority or force; to omit something from memory; to keep from public knowledge

Symmetric: exhibiting symmetry; capable of being divided by a longitudinal plane into equal sections

Symptom: the evidence of a disease or illness; the presence of a symptom is indicative of something else

Syndrome: a group of symptoms that happen close together and suggest an illness or irregular condition

T

Therapeutic: concerning the treatment of an illness or irregular condition

Toxic: poisonous, damaging, and harmful to organisms; exhibiting symptoms of infection or toxicosis

Transdermal: passing through skin

Transmission: passing something from one place to another

Trauma: an injury done by an outside object

Triage: a system that helps to determine which patients need the most care by evaluating their condition and chances of responding positively to treatment

U

Ubiquitous: common, widespread, or present everywhere

Untoward: difficult to manage; marked by trouble or unpleasantness

Urinate: to expel urine

V

Vascular: concerning the blood vessels

Verbal: relating to or consisting of words; involving words rather than meaning or substance

Virulent: highly infective; producing extremely harmful or damaging results

Virus: a microscopic pathogen that replicates in living cells and can cause disease

Vital: necessary or essential to the existence of life

Void: not occupied or empty; of no legal force or effect

Volume: printed pages bound in a book form; space occupied by a three-dimensional form; degree of loudness

Chapter Quiz

Ready to see how well you retained what you just read? Scan the QR code to go directly to the chapter quiz interface for this study guide. If you're using a computer, simply visit the bonus page at **mometrix.com/bonus948/hesia2** and click the Chapter Quizzes link.

Grammar

Transform passive reading into active learning! After immersing yourself in this chapter, put your comprehension to the test by taking a quiz. The insights you gained will stay with you longer this way. Scan the QR code to go directly to the chapter quiz interface for this study guide. If you're using a computer, simply visit the bonus page at **mometrix.com/bonus948/hesia2** and click the Chapter Quizzes link.

The grammar section of the exam has 50 items and focuses on basic grammar.

Foundations of Grammar

The Eight Parts of Speech

Nouns

When you talk about a person, place, thing, or idea, you are talking about a **noun**. The two main types of nouns are **common** and **proper** nouns. Also, nouns can be abstract (i.e., general) or concrete (i.e., specific).

Common Nouns

Common nouns are generic names for people, places, and things. Common nouns are not usually capitalized.

Examples of common nouns:

> *People*: boy, girl, worker, manager
>
> *Places*: school, bank, library, home
>
> *Things*: dog, cat, truck, car

Review Video: What is a Noun?
Visit mometrix.com/academy and enter code: 344028

Proper Nouns

Proper nouns name specific people, places, or things. All proper nouns are capitalized.

Examples of proper nouns:

> *People*: Abraham Lincoln, George Washington, Martin Luther King, Jr.
>
> *Places*: Los Angeles, California; New York; Asia
>
> *Things*: Statue of Liberty, Earth, Lincoln Memorial

Note: When referring to the planet that we live on, capitalize *Earth*. When referring to the dirt, rocks, or land, lowercase *earth*.

General and Specific Nouns

General nouns are the names of conditions or ideas. **Specific nouns** name people, places, and things that are understood by using your senses.

General nouns:

Condition: beauty, strength

Idea: truth, peace

Specific nouns:

People: baby, friend, father

Places: town, park, city hall

Things: rainbow, cough, apple, silk, gasoline

Collective Nouns

Collective nouns are the names for a group of people, places, or things that may act as a whole. The following are examples of collective nouns: *class, company, dozen, group, herd, team,* and *public*. Collective nouns usually require an article, which denotes the noun as being a single unit. For instance, a choir is a group of singers. Even though there are many singers in a choir, the word choir is grammatically treated as a single unit. If we refer to the members of the group, and not the group itself, it is no longer a collective noun.

Incorrect: The *choir are* going to compete nationally this year.

Correct: The *choir is* going to compete nationally this year.

Incorrect: The *members* of the choir *is* competing nationally this year.

Correct: The *members* of the choir *are* competing nationally this year.

Pronouns

Pronouns are words that are used to stand in for nouns. A pronoun may be classified as personal, intensive, relative, interrogative, demonstrative, indefinite, and reciprocal.

Personal: *Nominative* is the case for nouns and pronouns that are the subject of a sentence. *Objective* is the case for nouns and pronouns that are an object in a sentence. *Possessive* is the case for nouns and pronouns that show possession or ownership.

Singular

	Nominative	Objective	Possessive
First Person	I	me	my, mine
Second Person	you	you	your, yours
Third Person	he, she, it	him, her, it	his, her, hers, its

Plural

	Nominative	Objective	Possessive
First Person	we	us	our, ours
Second Person	you	you	your, yours
Third Person	they	them	their, theirs

Intensive: I myself, you yourself, he himself, she herself, the (thing) itself, we ourselves, you yourselves, they themselves

Relative: which, who, whom, whose

Interrogative: what, which, who, whom, whose

Demonstrative: this, that, these, those

Indefinite: all, any, each, everyone, either/neither, one, some, several

Reciprocal: each other, one another

Review Video: Nouns and Pronouns
Visit mometrix.com/academy and enter code: 312073

VERBS

If you want to write a sentence, then you need a verb. Without a verb, you have no sentence. The verb of a sentence indicates action or being. In other words, the verb shows something's action or state of being or the action that has been done to something.

TRANSITIVE AND INTRANSITIVE VERBS

A **transitive verb** is a verb whose action (e.g., drive, run, jump) indicates a receiver (e.g., car, dog, kangaroo). **Intransitive verbs** do not indicate a receiver of an action. In other words, the action of the verb does not point to a subject or object.

Transitive: He plays the piano. | The piano was played by him.

Intransitive: He plays. | John plays well.

A dictionary will tell you whether a verb is transitive or intransitive. Some verbs can be transitive and intransitive.

ACTION VERBS AND LINKING VERBS

Action verbs show what the subject is doing. In other words, an action verb shows action. Unlike most types of words, a single action verb, in the right context, can be an entire sentence. **Linking verbs** link the subject of a sentence to a noun or pronoun, or they link a subject with an adjective. You always need a verb if you want a complete sentence. However, linking verbs on their own cannot be a complete sentence.

Common linking verbs include *appear, be, become, feel, grow, look, seem, smell, sound,* and *taste.* However, any verb that shows a condition and connects to a noun, pronoun, or adjective that describes the subject of a sentence is a linking verb.

Action: He sings. | Run! | Go! | I talk with him every day. | She reads.

Linking:

Incorrect: I am.

Correct: I am John. | The roses smell lovely. | I feel tired.

Note: Some verbs are followed by words that look like prepositions, but they are a part of the verb and a part of the verb's meaning. These are known as phrasal verbs, and examples include *call off, look up*, and *drop off.*

Review Video: Action Verbs and Linking Verbs
Visit mometrix.com/academy and enter code: 743142

Voice

Transitive verbs come in active or passive **voice**. If something does an action or is acted upon, then you will know whether a verb is active or passive. When the subject of the sentence is doing the action, the verb is in **active voice**. When the subject is acted upon, the verb is in **passive voice**.

Active: Jon drew the picture. (The subject *Jon* is doing the action of *drawing a picture.*)

Passive: The picture is drawn by Jon. (The subject *picture* is receiving the action from Jon.)

Verb Tenses

A verb **tense** shows the different form of a verb to point to the time of an action. The present and past tense are indicated by the verb's form. An action in the present, *I talk,* can change form for the past: *I talked*. However, for the other tenses, an auxiliary (i.e., helping) verb is needed to show the change in form. These helping verbs include *am, are, is* | *have, has, had* | *was, were, will* (or *shall*).

Present: I talk	Present perfect: I have talked
Past: I talked	Past perfect: I had talked
Future: I will talk	Future perfect: I will have talked

Present: The action happens at the current time.

Example: He *walks* to the store every morning.

To show that something is happening right now, use the progressive present tense: I *am walking.*

Past: The action happened in the past.

Example: He *walked* to the store an hour ago.

Future: The action is going to happen later.

Example: I *will walk* to the store tomorrow.

Present perfect: The action started in the past and continues into the present or took place previously at an unspecified time.

Example: I *have walked* to the store three times today.

Past perfect: The second action happened in the past. The first action came before the second.

Example: Before I walked to the store (Action 2), I *had walked* to the library (Action 1).

Future perfect: An action that uses the past and the future. In other words, the action is complete before a future moment.

> Example: When she comes for the supplies (future moment), I *will have walked* to the store (action completed before the future moment).

Review Video: Present Perfect, Past Perfect, and Future Perfect Verb Tenses
Visit mometrix.com/academy and enter code: 269472

CONJUGATING VERBS

When you need to change the form of a verb, you are **conjugating** a verb. The key forms of a verb are singular, present tense (dream); singular, past tense (dreamed); and the past participle (have dreamed). Note: the past participle needs a helping verb to make a verb tense. For example, I *have dreamed* of this day. The following tables demonstrate some of the different ways to conjugate a verb:

Singular

Tense	First Person	Second Person	Third Person
Present	I dream	You dream	He, she, it dreams
Past	I dreamed	You dreamed	He, she, it dreamed
Past Participle	I have dreamed	You have dreamed	He, she, it has dreamed

Plural

Tense	First Person	Second Person	Third Person
Present	We dream	You dream	They dream
Past	We dreamed	You dreamed	They dreamed
Past Participle	We have dreamed	You have dreamed	They have dreamed

MOOD

There are three **moods** in English: the indicative, the imperative, and the subjunctive.

The **indicative mood** is used for facts, opinions, and questions.

> Fact: You can do this.
>
> Opinion: I think that you can do this.
>
> Question: Do you know that you can do this?

The **imperative** is used for orders or requests.

> Order: You are going to do this!
>
> Request: Will you do this for me?

The **subjunctive mood** is for wishes and statements that go against fact.

Wish: I wish that I were famous.

Statement against fact: If I were you, I would do this. (This goes against fact because I am not you. You have the chance to do this, and I do not have the chance.)

ADJECTIVES

An **adjective** is a word that is used to modify a noun or pronoun. An adjective answers a question: *Which one? What kind?* or *How many?* Usually, adjectives come before the words that they modify, but they may also come after a linking verb.

Which one? The *third* suit is my favorite.

What kind? This suit is *navy blue*.

How many? I am going to buy *four* pairs of socks to match the suit.

> **Review Video: Descriptive Text**
> Visit mometrix.com/academy and enter code: 174903

ARTICLES

Articles are adjectives that are used to distinguish nouns as definite or indefinite. **Definite** nouns are preceded by the article *the* and indicate a specific person, place, thing, or idea. **Indefinite** nouns are preceded by *a* or *an* and do not indicate a specific person, place, thing, or idea. *A*, *an*, and *the* are the only articles. Note: *An* comes before words that start with a vowel sound. For example, "Are you going to get an **u**mbrella?"

Definite: I lost *the* bottle that belongs to me.

Indefinite: Does anyone have *a* bottle to share?

> **Review Video: Function of Articles in a Sentence**
> Visit mometrix.com/academy and enter code: 449383

COMPARISON WITH ADJECTIVES

Some adjectives are relative and other adjectives are absolute. Adjectives that are **relative** can show the comparison between things. **Absolute** adjectives can also show comparison, but they do so in a different way. Let's say that you are reading two books. You think that one book is perfect, and the other book is not exactly perfect. It is not possible for one book to be more perfect than the other. Either you think that the book is perfect, or you think that the book is imperfect. In this case, perfect and imperfect are absolute adjectives.

Relative adjectives will show the different **degrees** of something or someone to something else or someone else. The three degrees of adjectives include positive, comparative, and superlative.

The **positive** degree is the normal form of an adjective.

Example: This work is *difficult*. | She is *smart*.

The **comparative** degree compares one person or thing to another person or thing.

Example: This work is *more difficult* than your work. | She is *smarter* than me.

The **superlative** degree compares more than two people or things.

Example: This is the *most difficult* work of my life. | She is the *smartest* lady in school.

Review Video: What is an Adjective?
Visit mometrix.com/academy and enter code: 470154

ADVERBS

An **adverb** is a word that is used to **modify** a verb, adjective, or another adverb. Usually, adverbs answer one of these questions: *When? Where? How?* and *Why?* The negatives *not* and *never* are considered adverbs. Adverbs that modify adjectives or other adverbs **strengthen** or **weaken** the words that they modify.

Examples:

He walks *quickly* through the crowd.

The water flows *smoothly* on the rocks.

Note: Adverbs are usually indicated by the morpheme *-ly*, which has been added to the root word. For instance, *quick* can be made into an adverb by adding *-ly* to construct *quickly*. Some words that end in *-ly* do not follow this rule and can behave as other parts of speech. Examples of adjectives ending in *-ly* include: *early, friendly, holy, lonely, silly*, and *ugly*. To know if a word that ends in *-ly* is an adjective or adverb, check your dictionary. Also, while many adverbs end in *-ly*, you need to remember that not all adverbs end in *-ly*.

Examples:

He is *never* angry.

You are *too* irresponsible to travel alone.

Review Video: What is an Adverb?
Visit mometrix.com/academy and enter code: 713951

Review Video: Adverbs that Modify Adjectives
Visit mometrix.com/academy and enter code: 122570

COMPARISON WITH ADVERBS

The rules for comparing adverbs are the same as the rules for adjectives.

The **positive** degree is the standard form of an adverb.

Example: He arrives *soon.* | She speaks *softly* to her friends.

The **comparative** degree compares one person or thing to another person or thing.

Example: He arrives *sooner* than Sarah. | She speaks *more softly* than him.

The **superlative** degree compares more than two people or things.

Example: He arrives *soonest* of the group. | She speaks the *most softly* of any of her friends.

Prepositions

A **preposition** is a word placed before a noun or pronoun that shows the relationship between an object and another word in the sentence.

Common prepositions:

about	before	during	on	under
after	beneath	for	over	until
against	between	from	past	up
among	beyond	in	through	with
around	by	of	to	within
at	down	off	toward	without

Examples:

The napkin is *in* the drawer.

The Earth rotates *around* the Sun.

The needle is *beneath* the haystack.

Can you find "me" *among* the words?

Review Video: Prepositions
Visit mometrix.com/academy and enter code: 946763

Conjunctions

Conjunctions join words, phrases, or clauses and they show the connection between the joined pieces. **Coordinating conjunctions** connect equal parts of sentences. **Correlative conjunctions** show the connection between pairs. **Subordinating conjunctions** join subordinate (i.e., dependent) clauses with independent clauses.

Coordinating Conjunctions

The **coordinating conjunctions** include: *and, but, yet, or, nor, for,* and *so*

Examples:

The rock was small, *but* it was heavy.

She drove in the night, *and* he drove in the day.

Correlative Conjunctions

The **correlative conjunctions** are: *either...or* | *neither...nor* | *not only...but also*

Examples:

Either you are coming *or* you are staying.

He *not only* ran three miles *but also* swam 200 yards.

Review Video: Coordinating and Correlative Conjunctions
Visit mometrix.com/academy and enter code: 390329

Review Video: Adverb Equal Comparisons
Visit mometrix.com/academy and enter code: 231291

Subordinating Conjunctions

Common **subordinating conjunctions** include:

after	since	whenever
although	so that	where
because	unless	wherever
before	until	whether
in order that	when	while

Examples:

I am hungry *because* I did not eat breakfast.

He went home *when* everyone left.

Review Video: Subordinating Conjunctions
Visit mometrix.com/academy and enter code: 958913

Interjections

Interjections are words of exclamation (i.e., audible expression of great feeling) that are used alone or as a part of a sentence. Often, they are used at the beginning of a sentence for an introduction. Sometimes, they can be used in the middle of a sentence to show a change in thought or attitude.

Common Interjections: Hey! | Oh, | Ouch! | Please! | Wow!

Agreement and Sentence Structure

Subjects and Predicates

Subjects

The **subject** of a sentence names who or what the sentence is about. The subject may be directly stated in a sentence, or the subject may be the implied *you*. The **complete subject** includes the simple subject and all of its modifiers. To find the complete subject, ask *Who* or *What* and insert the verb to complete the question. The answer, including any modifiers (adjectives, prepositional phrases, etc.), is the complete subject. To find the **simple subject**, remove all of the modifiers in the complete subject. Being able to locate the subject of a sentence helps with many problems, such as those involving sentence fragments and subject-verb agreement.

Examples:

The small, red car (simple subject: car) is the one that he wants for Christmas. (complete subject: The small, red car)

The young artist (simple subject: artist) is coming over for dinner. (complete subject: The young artist)

Review Video: Subjects in English
Visit mometrix.com/academy and enter code: 444771

In **imperative** sentences, the verb's subject is understood (e.g., [You] Run to the store), but is not actually present in the sentence. Normally, the subject comes before the verb. However, the subject comes after the verb in sentences that begin with *There are* or *There was*.

Direct:

John knows the way to the park.	Who knows the way to the park?	John
The cookies need ten more minutes.	What needs ten minutes?	The cookies
By five o'clock, Bill will need to leave.	Who needs to leave?	Bill
There are five letters on the table for him.	What is on the table?	Five letters
There were coffee and doughnuts in the house.	What was in the house?	Coffee and doughnuts

Implied:

Go to the post office for me.	Who is going to the post office?	You
Come and sit with me, please?	Who needs to come and sit?	You

PREDICATES

In a sentence, you always have a predicate and a subject. The subject tells what the sentence is about, and the **predicate** explains or describes the subject.

Think about the sentence *He sings*. In this sentence, we have a subject (He) and a predicate (sings). This is all that is needed for a sentence to be complete. Most sentences contain more information, but if this is all the information that you are given, then you have a complete sentence.

Now, let's look at another sentence: *John and Jane sing on Tuesday nights at the dance hall.*

subject — John and Jane; predicate — sing on Tuesday nights at the dance hall.

John and Jane sing on Tuesday nights at the dance hall.

SUBJECT-VERB AGREEMENT

Verbs **agree** with their subjects in number. In other words, singular subjects need singular verbs. Plural subjects need plural verbs. **Singular** is for **one** person, place, or thing. **Plural** is for **more than one** person, place, or thing. Subjects and verbs must also share the same point of view, as in first, second, or third person. The present tense ending *-s* is used on a verb if its subject is third person singular; otherwise, the verb's ending is not modified.

Review Video: Subject-Verb Agreement
Visit mometrix.com/academy and enter code: 479190

NUMBER AGREEMENT EXAMPLES:

Single Subject and Verb: Dan (singular subject) calls (singular verb) home.

Dan is one person. So, the singular verb *calls* is needed.

Plural Subject and Verb: Dan and Bob (plural subject) call (plural verb) home.

More than one person needs the plural verb *call.*

PERSON AGREEMENT EXAMPLES:

First Person: I *am* walking.

Second Person: You *are* walking.

Third Person: He *is* walking.

COMPLICATIONS WITH SUBJECT-VERB AGREEMENT

WORDS BETWEEN SUBJECT AND VERB

Words that come between the simple subject and the verb have no bearing on subject-verb agreement.

Examples:

The joy (singular subject) of my life returns (singular verb) home tonight.

The phrase *of my life* does not influence the verb *returns.*

The question (singular subject) that still remains unanswered is (singular verb) "Who are you?"

Don't let the phrase "*that still remains...*" trouble you. The subject *question* goes with *is.*

Compound Subjects

A compound subject is formed when two or more nouns joined by *and*, *or*, or *nor* jointly act as the subject of the sentence.

Joined by And

When a compound subject is joined by *and*, it is treated as a plural subject and requires a plural verb.

Examples:

plural subject: You and Jon; plural verb: are

You and Jon are invited to come to my house.

plural subject: pencil and paper; plural verb: belong

The pencil and paper belong to me.

Joined by Or/Nor

For a compound subject joined by *or* or *nor*, the verb must agree in number with the part of the subject that is closest to the verb (italicized in the examples below).

Examples:

subject: Today or tomorrow; verb: is

Today or tomorrow is the day.

subject: Stan or Phil; verb: wants

Stan or Phil wants to read the book.

subject: the pen nor the book; verb: is

Neither the pen nor the book is on the desk.

subject: blanket or pillows; verb: arrive

Either the blanket or pillows arrive this afternoon.

Indefinite Pronouns as Subject

An indefinite pronoun is a pronoun that does not refer to a specific noun. Different indefinite pronouns may only function as a singular noun, only function as a plural noun, or change depending on how they are used.

Always Singular

Pronouns such as *each*, *either*, *everybody*, *anybody*, *somebody*, and *nobody* are always singular.

Examples:

singular subject: Each; singular verb: has

Each of the runners has a different bib number.

singular verb: Is; singular subject: either

Is either of you ready for the game?

Note: The words *each* and *either* can also be used as adjectives (e.g., *each* person is unique). When one of these adjectives modifies the subject of a sentence, it is always a singular subject.

singular subject / singular verb
Everybody grows a day older every day.

singular subject / singular verb
Anybody is welcome to bring a tent.

Always Plural

Pronouns such as *both*, *several*, and *many* are always plural.

Examples:

plural subject / plural verb
Both of the siblings were too tired to argue.

plural subject / plural verb
Many have tried, but none have succeeded.

Depend on Context

Pronouns such as *some*, *any*, *all*, *none*, *more*, and *most* can be either singular or plural depending on what they are representing in the context of the sentence.

Examples:

singular subject / singular verb
All of my dog's food was still there in his bowl.

plural subject / plural verb
By the end of the night, all of my guests were already excited about coming to my next party.

Other Cases Involving Plural or Irregular Form

Some nouns are **singular in meaning but plural in form**: news, mathematics, physics, and economics.

The *news is* coming on now.

Mathematics is my favorite class.

Some nouns are plural in form and meaning, and have **no singular equivalent**: scissors and pants.

Do these *pants come* with a shirt?

The *scissors are* for my project.

Mathematical operations are **irregular** in their construction, but are normally considered to be **singular in meaning**.

> *One plus one is* two.
>
> *Three times three is* nine.

Note: Look to your **dictionary** for help when you aren't sure whether a noun with a plural form has a singular or plural meaning.

COMPLEMENTS

A complement is a noun, pronoun, or adjective that is used to give more information about the subject or verb in the sentence.

DIRECT OBJECTS

A direct object is a noun or pronoun that takes or receives the **action** of a verb. (Remember: a complete sentence does not need a direct object, so not all sentences will have them. A sentence needs only a subject and a verb.) When you are looking for a direct object, find the verb and ask *who* or *what.*

Examples:

> I took *the blanket.*
>
> Jane read *books.*

INDIRECT OBJECTS

An indirect object is a word or group of words that show how an action had an **influence** on someone or something. If there is an indirect object in a sentence, then you always have a direct object in the sentence. When you are looking for the indirect object, find the verb and ask *to/for whom or what.*

Examples:

> We taught the old dog (indirect object) a new trick (direct object).
>
> I gave them (indirect object) a math lesson (direct object).

Review Video: Direct and Indirect Objects
Visit mometrix.com/academy and enter code: 817385

PREDICATE NOMINATIVES AND PREDICATE ADJECTIVES

As we looked at previously, verbs may be classified as either action verbs or linking verbs. A linking verb is so named because it links the subject to words in the predicate that describe or define the subject. These words are called predicate nominatives (if nouns or pronouns) or predicate adjectives (if adjectives).

Examples:

My father (subject) is a lawyer (predicate nominative).

Your mother (subject) is patient (predicate adjective).

Pronoun Usage

The **antecedent** is the noun that has been replaced by a pronoun. A pronoun and its antecedent **agree** when they have the same number (singular or plural) and gender (male, female, or neutral).

Examples:

Singular agreement: John (antecedent) came into town, and he (pronoun) played for us.

Plural agreement: John and Rick (antecedent) came into town, and they (pronoun) played for us.

To determine which is the correct pronoun to use in a compound subject or object, try each pronoun **alone** in place of the compound in the sentence. Your knowledge of pronouns will tell you which one is correct.

Example:

Bob and (I, me) will be going.

Test: (1) *I will be going* or (2) *Me will be going*. The second choice cannot be correct because *me* cannot be used as the subject of a sentence. Instead, *me* is used as an object.

Answer: Bob and I will be going.

When a pronoun is used with a noun immediately following (as in "we boys"), try the sentence **without the added noun**.

Example:

(We/Us) boys played football last year.

Test: (1) *We played football last ye*ar or (2) *Us played football last year*. Again, the second choice cannot be correct because *us* cannot be used as a subject of a sentence. Instead, *us* is used as an object.

Answer: We boys played football last year.

Review Video: Pronoun Usage
Visit mometrix.com/academy and enter code: 666500

Review Video: What is Pronoun-Antecedent Agreement?
Visit mometrix.com/academy and enter code: 919704

A pronoun should point clearly to the **antecedent**. Here is how a pronoun reference can be unhelpful if it is puzzling or not directly stated.

> antecedent — pronoun
>
> **Unhelpful**: Ron and Jim went to the store, and he bought soda.
>
> Who bought soda? Ron or Jim?
>
> antecedent — pronoun
>
> **Helpful**: Jim went to the store, and he bought soda.
>
> The sentence is clear. Jim bought the soda.

Some pronouns change their form by their placement in a sentence. A pronoun that is a **subject** in a sentence comes in the **subjective case**. Pronouns that serve as **objects** appear in the **objective case**. Finally, the pronouns that are used as **possessives** appear in the **possessive case**.

Examples:

> **Subjective case**: *He* is coming to the show.
>
> The pronoun *He* is the subject of the sentence.
>
> **Objective case**: Josh drove *him* to the airport.
>
> The pronoun *him* is the object of the sentence.
>
> **Possessive case**: The flowers are *mine*.
>
> The pronoun *mine* shows ownership of the flowers.

The word *who* is a subjective-case pronoun that can be used as a **subject**. The word *whom* is an objective-case pronoun that can be used as an **object**. The words *who* and *whom* are common in subordinate clauses or in questions.

Examples:

> subject — verb
>
> He knows who wants to come.
>
> object — verb
>
> He knows the man whom we want at the party.

CLAUSES

A clause is a group of words that contains both a subject and a predicate (verb). There are two types of clauses: independent and dependent. An **independent clause** contains a complete thought, while a **dependent (or subordinate) clause** does not. A dependent clause includes a subject and a verb, and may also contain objects or complements, but it cannot stand as a complete thought without being joined to an independent clause. Dependent clauses function within sentences as adjectives, adverbs, or nouns.

Example:

independent clause: I am running | dependent clause: because I want to stay in shape.

I am running because I want to stay in shape.

The clause *I am running* is an independent clause: it has a subject and a verb, and it gives a complete thought. The clause *because I want to stay in shape* is a dependent clause: it has a subject and a verb, but it does not express a complete thought. It adds detail to the independent clause to which it is attached.

Review Video: What is a Clause?
Visit mometrix.com/academy and enter code: 940170

Review Video: Independent and Dependent Clauses
Visit mometrix.com/academy and enter code: 556903

Types of Dependent Clauses

Adjective Clauses

An **adjective clause** is a dependent clause that modifies a noun or a pronoun. Adjective clauses begin with a relative pronoun (*who, whose, whom, which,* and *that*) or a relative adverb (*where, when,* and *why*).

Also, adjective clauses come after the noun that the clause needs to explain or rename. This is done to have a clear connection to the independent clause.

Examples:

independent clause: I learned the reason | adjective clause: why I won the award.

I learned the reason why I won the award.

independent clause: This is the place | adjective clause: where I started my first job.

This is the place where I started my first job.

An adjective clause can be an essential or nonessential clause. An essential clause is very important to the sentence. **Essential clauses** explain or define a person or thing. **Nonessential clauses** give more information about a person or thing but are not necessary to define them. Nonessential clauses are set off with commas while essential clauses are not.

Examples:

essential clause: who works hard at first

A person who works hard at first can often rest later in life.

nonessential clause: who walked on the moon

Neil Armstrong, who walked on the moon, is my hero.

Review Video: Adjective Clauses and Phrases
Visit mometrix.com/academy and enter code: 520888

ADVERB CLAUSES

An **adverb clause** is a dependent clause that modifies a verb, adjective, or adverb. In sentences with multiple dependent clauses, adverb clauses are usually placed immediately before or after the independent clause. An adverb clause is introduced with words such as *after, although, as, before, because, if, since, so, unless, when, where*, and *while.*

Examples:

> When you walked outside (adverb clause), I called the manager.

> I will go with you unless you want to stay (adverb clause).

NOUN CLAUSES

A **noun clause** is a dependent clause that can be used as a subject, object, or complement. Noun clauses begin with words such as *how, that, what, whether, which, who,* and *why*. These words can also come with an adjective clause. Unless the noun clause is being used as the subject of the sentence, it should come after the verb of the independent clause.

Examples:

> The real mystery is how you avoided serious injury (noun clause).

> What you learn from each other (noun clause) depends on your honesty with others.

SUBORDINATION

When two related ideas are not of equal importance, the ideal way to combine them is to make the more important idea an independent clause and the less important idea a dependent or subordinate clause. This is called **subordination**.

Example:

> **Separate ideas**: The team had a perfect regular season. The team lost the championship.

> **Subordinated**: Despite having a perfect regular season, *the team lost the championship*.

PHRASES

A phrase is a group of words that functions as a single part of speech, usually a noun, adjective, or adverb. A **phrase** is not a complete thought, but it adds detail or explanation to a sentence, or renames something within the sentence.

PREPOSITIONAL PHRASES

One of the most common types of phrases is the prepositional phrase. A **prepositional phrase** begins with a preposition and ends with a noun or pronoun that is the object of the preposition. Normally, the prepositional phrase functions as an **adjective** or an **adverb** within the sentence.

Examples:

The picnic is on the blanket. (prepositional phrase: on the blanket)

I am sick with a fever today. (prepositional phrase: with a fever)

Among the many flowers, John found a four-leaf clover. (prepositional phrase: Among the many flowers)

VERBAL PHRASES

A **verbal** is a word or phrase that is formed from a verb but does not function as a verb. Depending on its particular form, it may be used as a noun, adjective, or adverb. A verbal does **not** replace a verb in a sentence.

Examples:

Correct: Walk a mile daily. (verb: Walk)

This is a complete sentence with the implied subject *you*.

Incorrect: To walk a mile. (verbal: To walk)

This is not a sentence since there is no functional verb.

There are three types of verbal: **participles**, **gerunds**, and **infinitives**. Each type of verbal has a corresponding **phrase** that consists of the verbal itself along with any complements or modifiers.

PARTICIPLES

A **participle** is a type of verbal that always functions as an adjective. The present participle always ends with *-ing*. Past participles end with *-d, -ed, -n,* or *-t*.

Examples: dance (verb) | dancing (present participle) | danced (past participle)

Participial phrases most often come right before or right after the noun or pronoun that they modify.

Examples:

participial phrase

Shipwrecked on an island, the boys started to fish for food.

participial phrase

Having been seated for five hours, we got out of the car to stretch our legs.

participial phrase

Praised for their work, the group accepted the first-place trophy.

GERUNDS

A **gerund** is a type of verbal that always functions as a **noun**. Like present participles, gerunds always end with *-ing*, but they can be easily distinguished from one another by the part of speech they represent (participles always function as adjectives). Since a gerund or gerund phrase always functions as a noun, it can be used as the subject of a sentence, the predicate nominative, or the object of a verb or preposition.

Examples:

gerund

We want to be known for teaching the poor.

object of preposition

gerund

Coaching this team is the best job of my life.

subject

gerund

We like practicing our songs in the basement.

object of verb

INFINITIVES

An **infinitive** is a type of verbal that can function as a noun, an adjective, or an adverb. An infinitive is made of the word *to* and the basic form of the verb. As with all other types of verbal phrases, an infinitive phrase includes the verbal itself and all of its complements or modifiers.

Examples:

infinitive
To join the team is my goal in life.
noun

infinitive
The animals have enough food to eat for the night.
adjective

infinitive
People lift weights to exercise their muscles.
adverb

Review Video: Verbals
Visit mometrix.com/academy and enter code: 915480

Appositive Phrases

An **appositive** is a word or phrase that is used to explain or rename nouns or pronouns. Noun phrases, gerund phrases, and infinitive phrases can all be used as appositives.

Examples:

appositive
Terriers, hunters at heart, have been dressed up to look like lap dogs.

The noun phrase *hunters at heart* renames the noun *terriers*.

appositive
His plan, to save and invest his money, was proven as a safe approach.

The infinitive phrase explains what the plan is.

Appositive phrases can be **essential** or **nonessential**. An appositive phrase is essential if the person, place, or thing being described or renamed is too general for its meaning to be understood without the appositive.

Examples:

essential
Two of America's Founding Fathers, George Washington and Thomas Jefferson, served as presidents.

nonessential
George Washington and Thomas Jefferson, two Founding Fathers, served as presidents.

Absolute Phrases

An absolute phrase is a phrase that consists of **a noun followed by a participle**. An absolute phrase provides **context** to what is being described in the sentence, but it does not modify or explain any particular word; it is essentially independent.

Examples:

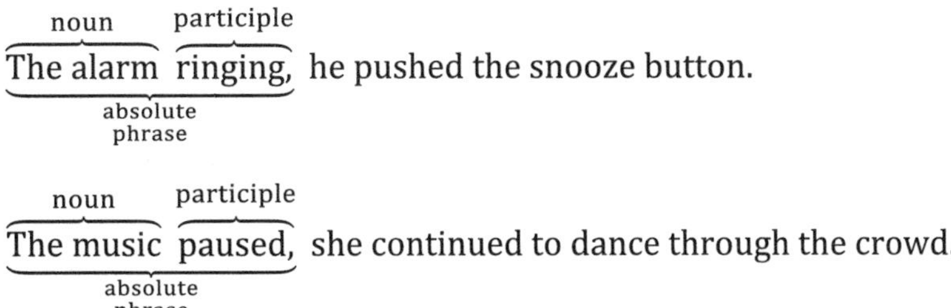

Parallelism

When multiple items or ideas are presented in a sentence in series, such as in a list, the items or ideas must be stated in grammatically equivalent ways. In other words, if one idea is stated in gerund form, the second cannot be stated in infinitive form. For example, to write, *I enjoy reading and to study* would be incorrect. An infinitive and a gerund are not equivalent. Instead, you should write *I enjoy reading and studying*. In lists of more than two, all items must be parallel.

Example:

> **Incorrect**: He stopped at the office, grocery store, and the pharmacy before heading home.
>
> The first and third items in the list of places include the article *the*, so the second item needs it as well.
>
> **Correct**: He stopped at the office, *the* grocery store, and the pharmacy before heading home.

Example:

> **Incorrect**: While vacationing in Europe, she went biking, skiing, and climbed mountains.
>
> The first and second items in the list are gerunds, so the third item must be as well.
>
> **Correct**: While vacationing in Europe, she went biking, skiing, and *mountain climbing.*

Review Video: Parallel Sentence Construction
Visit mometrix.com/academy and enter code: 831988

Sentence Purpose

There are four types of sentences: declarative, imperative, interrogative, and exclamatory.

A **declarative** sentence states a fact and ends with a period.

> *The football game starts at seven o'clock.*

An **imperative** sentence tells someone to do something and generally ends with a period. An urgent command might end with an exclamation point instead.

> *Don't forget to buy your ticket.*

An **interrogative** sentence asks a question and ends with a question mark.

> *Are you going to the game on Friday?*

An **exclamatory** sentence shows strong emotion and ends with an exclamation point.

I can't believe we won the game!

Sentence Structure

Sentences are classified by structure based on the type and number of clauses present. The four classifications of sentence structure are the following:

Simple: A simple sentence has one independent clause with no dependent clauses. A simple sentence may have **compound elements** (i.e., compound subject or verb).

Examples:

single subject | single verb

Judy watered the lawn.

compound subject | single verb

Judy and Alan watered the lawn.

single subject | compound verb | compound verb

Judy watered the lawn and pulled weeds.

compound subject | compound verb | compound verb

Judy and Alan watered the lawn and pulled weeds.

Compound: A compound sentence has two or more independent clauses with no dependent clauses. Usually, the independent clauses are joined with a comma and a coordinating conjunction or with a semicolon.

Examples:

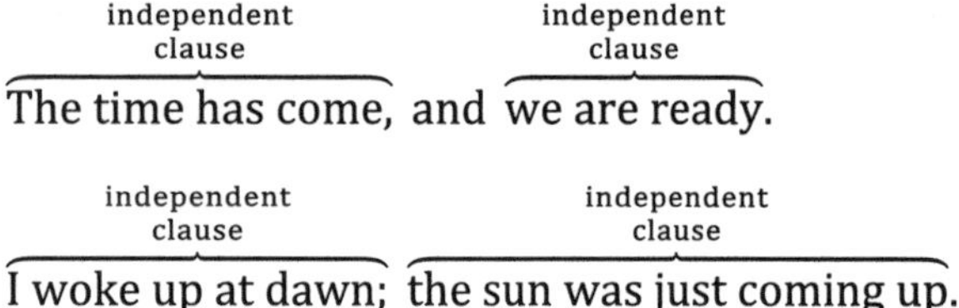

Complex: A complex sentence has one independent clause and at least one dependent clause.

Examples:

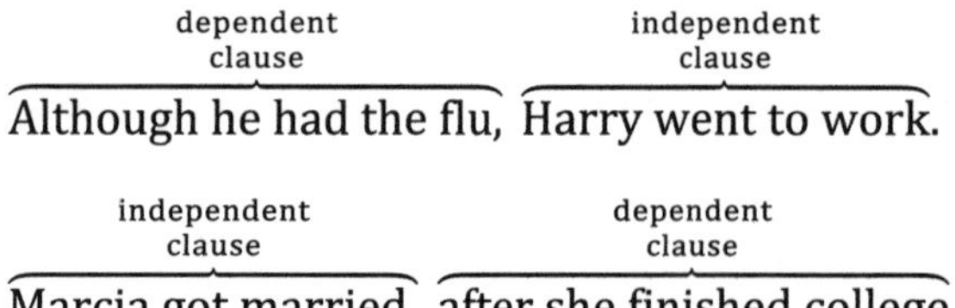

Compound-Complex: A compound-complex sentence has at least two independent clauses and at least one dependent clause.

Examples:

John is my friend (independent clause) who went to India, (dependent clause) and he brought back souvenirs. (independent clause)

You may not realize this, (independent clause) but we heard the music (independent clause) that you played last night. (dependent clause)

Review Video: Sentence Structure
Visit mometrix.com/academy and enter code: 700478

Sentence variety is important to consider when writing an essay or speech. A variety of sentence lengths and types creates rhythm, makes a passage more engaging, and gives writers an opportunity to demonstrate their writing style. Writing that uses the same length or type of sentence without variation can be boring or difficult to read. To evaluate a passage for effective sentence variety, it is helpful to note whether the passage contains diverse sentence structures and lengths. It is also important to pay attention to the way each sentence starts and avoid beginning with the same words or phrases.

Sentence Fragments

Recall that a group of words must contain at least one **independent clause** in order to be considered a sentence. If it doesn't contain even one independent clause, it is called a **sentence fragment**.

The appropriate process for **repairing** a sentence fragment depends on what type of fragment it is. If the fragment is a dependent clause, it can sometimes be as simple as removing a subordinating word (e.g., when, because, if) from the beginning of the fragment. Alternatively, a dependent clause can be incorporated into a closely related neighboring sentence. If the fragment is missing some required part, like a subject or a verb, the fix might be as simple as adding the missing part.

Examples:

Fragment: Because he wanted to sail the Mediterranean.

Removed subordinating word: He wanted to sail the Mediterranean.

Combined with another sentence: Because he wanted to sail the Mediterranean, he booked a Greek island cruise.

Run-on Sentences

Run-on sentences consist of multiple independent clauses that have not been joined together properly. Run-on sentences can be corrected in several different ways:

Join clauses properly: This can be done with a comma and coordinating conjunction, with a semicolon, or with a colon or dash if the second clause is explaining something in the first.

Example:

Incorrect: I went on the trip, we visited lots of castles.

Corrected: I went on the trip, and we visited lots of castles.

Split into separate sentences: This correction is most effective when the independent clauses are very long or when they are not closely related.

Example:

Incorrect: The drive to New York takes ten hours, my uncle lives in Boston.

Corrected: The drive to New York takes ten hours. My uncle lives in Boston.

Make one clause dependent: This is the easiest way to make the sentence correct and more interesting at the same time. It's often as simple as adding a subordinating word between the two clauses or before the first clause.

Example:

Incorrect: I finally made it to the store and I bought some eggs.

Corrected: When I finally made it to the store, I bought some eggs.

Reduce to one clause with a compound verb: If both clauses have the same subject, remove the subject from the second clause, and you now have just one clause with a compound verb.

Example:

Incorrect: The drive to New York takes ten hours, it makes me very tired.

Corrected: The drive to New York takes ten hours and makes me very tired.

Note: While these are the simplest ways to correct a run-on sentence, often the best way is to completely reorganize the thoughts in the sentence and rewrite it.

Review Video: Fragments and Run-on Sentences
Visit mometrix.com/academy and enter code: 541989

Dangling and Misplaced Modifiers

Dangling Modifiers

A dangling modifier is a dependent clause or verbal phrase that does not have a clear logical connection to a word in the sentence.

Example:

dangling modifier

Incorrect: Reading each magazine article, the stories caught my attention.

The word *stories* cannot be modified by *Reading each magazine article*. People can read, but stories cannot read. Therefore, the subject of the sentence must be a person.

dependent clause

Corrected: Reading each magazine article, I was entertained by the stories.

Example:

dangling modifier

Incorrect: Ever since childhood, my grandparents have visited me for Christmas.

The speaker in this sentence can't have been visited by her grandparents when *they* were children, since she wouldn't have been born yet. Either the modifier should be clarified or the sentence should be rearranged to specify whose childhood is being referenced.

dependent clause

Clarified: Ever since I was a child, my grandparents have visited for Christmas.

dependent clause

Rearranged: I have enjoyed my grandparents visiting for Christmas, ever since childhood.

Misplaced Modifiers

Because modifiers are grammatically versatile, they can be put in many different places within the structure of a sentence. The danger of this versatility is that a modifier can accidentally be placed where it is modifying the wrong word or where it is not clear which word it is modifying.

Example:

modifier

Incorrect: She read the book to a crowd that was filled with beautiful pictures.

The book was filled with beautiful pictures, not the crowd.

modifier

Corrected: She read the book that was filled with beautiful pictures to a crowd.

Example:

modifier
Ambiguous: Derek saw a bus nearly hit a man on his way to work.

Was Derek on his way to work or was the other man?

modifier
Derek: On his way to work, Derek saw a bus nearly hit a man.

modifier
The other man: Derek saw a bus nearly hit a man who was on his way to work.

Split Infinitives

A split infinitive occurs when a modifying word comes between the word *to* and the verb that pairs with *to*.

Example: To *clearly* explain vs. *To explain* clearly | To *softly* sing vs. *To sing* softly

Though considered improper by some, split infinitives may provide better clarity and simplicity in some cases than the alternatives. As such, avoiding them should not be considered a universal rule.

Double Negatives

Standard English allows **two negatives** only when a **positive** meaning is intended. For example, *The team was not displeased with their performance.* Double negatives to emphasize negation are not used in standard English.

Negative modifiers (e.g., never, no, and not) should not be paired with other negative modifiers or negative words (e.g., none, nobody, nothing, or neither). The modifiers *hardly, barely*, and *scarcely* are also considered negatives in standard English, so they should not be used with other negatives.

Punctuation

End Punctuation

Periods

Use a period to end all sentences except direct questions and exclamations. Periods are also used for abbreviations.

Examples: 3 p.m. | 2 a.m. | Mr. Jones | Mrs. Stevens | Dr. Smith | Bill, Jr. | Pennsylvania Ave.

Note: An abbreviation is a shortened form of a word or phrase.

Question Marks

Question marks should be used following a **direct question**. A polite request can be followed by a period instead of a question mark.

Direct Question: What is for lunch today? | How are you? | Why is that the answer?

Polite Requests: Can you please send me the item tomorrow. | Will you please walk with me on the track.

Review Video: Question Marks
Visit mometrix.com/academy and enter code: 118471

Exclamation Marks

Exclamation marks are used after a word group or sentence that shows much feeling or has special importance. Exclamation marks should not be overused. They are saved for proper **exclamatory interjections**.

Example: We're going to the finals! | You have a beautiful car! | "That's crazy!" she yelled.

Review Video: Exclamation Points
Visit mometrix.com/academy and enter code: 199367

Commas

The comma is a punctuation mark that can help you understand connections in a sentence. Not every sentence needs a comma. However, if a sentence needs a comma, you need to put it in the right place. A comma in the wrong place (or an absent comma) will make a sentence's meaning unclear. These are some of the rules for commas:

Use Case	Example
Before a **coordinating conjunction** joining independent clauses	Bob caught three fish, and I caught two fish.
After an **introductory phrase**	After the final out, we went to a restaurant to celebrate.
After an **adverbial clause**	Studying the stars, I was awed by the beauty of the sky.
Between **items in a series**	I will bring the turkey, the pie, and the coffee.
For **interjections**	Wow, you know how to play this game.
After ***yes*** **and** ***no*** **responses**	No, I cannot come tomorrow.
Separate **nonessential modifiers**	John Frank, who coaches the team, was promoted today.
Separate **nonessential appositives**	Thomas Edison, an American inventor, was born in Ohio.
Separate **nouns of direct address**	You, John, are my only hope in this moment.
Separate **interrogative tags**	This is the last time, correct?
Separate **contrasts**	You are my friend, not my enemy.
Writing **dates**	July 4, 1776, is an important date to remember.
Writing **addresses**	He is meeting me at 456 Delaware Avenue, Washington, D.C., tomorrow morning.
Writing **geographical names**	Paris, France, is my favorite city.
Writing **titles**	John Smith, PhD, will be visiting your class today.
Separate **expressions like** ***he said***	"You can start," she said, "with an apology."

Also, you can use a comma **between coordinate adjectives** not joined with *and*. However, not all adjectives are coordinate (i.e., equal or parallel).

Incorrect: The kind, brown dog followed me home.

Correct: The kind, loyal dog followed me home.

There are two simple ways to know if your adjectives are coordinate. One, you can join the adjectives with *and*: *The kind and loyal dog*. Two, you can change the order of the adjectives: *The loyal, kind dog*.

Review Video: When to Use a Comma
Visit mometrix.com/academy and enter code: 786797

SEMICOLONS

The semicolon is used to connect major sentence pieces of equal value. Some rules for semicolons include:

Use Case	Example
Between closely connected independent clauses **not connected with a coordinating conjunction**	You are right; we should go with your plan.
Between independent clauses **linked with a transitional word**	I think that we can agree on this; however, I am not sure about my friends.
Between items in a **series that has internal punctuation**	I have visited New York, New York; Augusta, Maine; and Baltimore, Maryland.

Review Video: How to Use Semicolons
Visit mometrix.com/academy and enter code: 370605

COLONS

The colon is used to call attention to the words that follow it. A colon must come after a **complete independent clause**. The rules for colons are as follows:

Use Case	Example
After an independent clause to **make a list**	I want to learn many languages: Spanish, German, and Italian.
For **explanations**	There is one thing that stands out on your resume: responsibility.
To give a **quote**	He started with an idea: "We are able to do more than we imagine."
After the **greeting in a formal letter**	To Whom It May Concern:
Show **hours and minutes**	It is 3:14 p.m.
Separate a **title and subtitle**	The essay is titled "America: A Short Introduction to a Modern Country."

Review Video: Colons
Visit mometrix.com/academy and enter code: 868673

Parentheses

Parentheses are used for additional information. Also, they can be used to put labels for letters or numbers in a series. Parentheses should be not be used very often. If they are overused, parentheses can be a distraction instead of a help.

Examples:

Extra Information: The rattlesnake (see Image 2) is a dangerous snake of North and South America.

Series: Include in the email (1) your name, (2) your address, and (3) your question for the author.

Review Video: Parentheses
Visit mometrix.com/academy and enter code: 947743

Quotation Marks

Use quotation marks to close off **direct quotations** of a person's spoken or written words. Do not use quotation marks around indirect quotations. An indirect quotation gives someone's message without using the person's exact words. Use **single quotation marks** to close off a quotation inside a quotation.

Direct Quote: Nancy said, "I am waiting for Henry to arrive."

Indirect Quote: Henry said that he is going to be late to the meeting.

Quote inside a Quote: The teacher asked, "Has everyone read 'The Gift of the Magi'?"

Quotation marks should be used around the titles of **short works**: newspaper and magazine articles, poems, short stories, songs, television episodes, radio programs, and subdivisions of books or websites.

Examples:

"Rip Van Winkle" (short story by Washington Irving)

"O Captain! My Captain!" (poem by Walt Whitman)

Although it is not standard usage, quotation marks are sometimes used to highlight **irony** or the use of words to mean something other than their dictionary definition. This type of usage should be employed sparingly, if at all.

Examples:

The boss warned Frank that he was walking on "thin ice."	Frank is not walking on real ice. Instead, he is being warned to avoid mistakes.
The teacher thanked the young man for his "honesty."	The quotation marks around *honesty* show that the teacher does not believe the young man's explanation.

Review Video: Quotation Marks
Visit mometrix.com/academy and enter code: 884918

Periods and commas are put **inside** quotation marks. Colons and semicolons are put **outside** the quotation marks. Question marks and exclamation points are placed inside quotation marks when they are part of a quote. When the question or exclamation mark goes with the whole sentence, the mark is left outside of the quotation marks.

Examples:

Period and comma	We read "The Gift of the Magi," "The Skylight Room," and "The Cactus."
Semicolon	They watched "The Nutcracker"; then, they went home.
Exclamation mark that is a part of a quote	The crowd cheered, "Victory!"
Question mark that goes with the whole sentence	Is your favorite short story "The Tell-Tale Heart"?

Apostrophes

An apostrophe is used to show **possession** or the **deletion of letters in contractions**. An apostrophe is not needed with the possessive pronouns *his, hers, its, ours, theirs, whose*, and *yours*.

Singular Nouns: David's car | a book's theme | my brother's board game

Plural Nouns that end with -*s*: the scissors' handle | boys' basketball

Plural Nouns that end without -*s*: Men's department | the people's adventure

Review Video: When to Use an Apostrophe
Visit mometrix.com/academy and enter code: 213068

Review Video: Punctuation Errors in Possessive Pronouns
Visit mometrix.com/academy and enter code: 221438

Hyphens

Hyphens are used to **separate compound words**. Use hyphens in the following cases:

Use Case	Example
Compound numbers from 21 to 99 when written out in words	This team needs twenty-five points to win the game.
Written-out fractions that are used as adjectives	The recipe says that we need a three-fourths cup of butter.
Compound adjectives that come before a noun	The well-fed dog took a nap.
Unusual compound words that would be hard to read or easily confused with other words	This is the best anti-itch cream on the market.

Note: This is not a complete set of the rules for hyphens. A dictionary is the best tool for knowing if a compound word needs a hyphen.

Review Video: Hyphens
Visit mometrix.com/academy and enter code: 981632

Dashes

Dashes are used to show a **break** or a **change in thought** in a sentence or to act as parentheses in a sentence. When typing, use two hyphens to make a dash. Do not put a space before or after the dash. The following are the functions of dashes:

Use Case	Example
Set off parenthetical statements or an **appositive with internal punctuation**	The three trees—oak, pine, and magnolia—are coming on a truck tomorrow.
Show a **break or change in tone or thought**	The first question—how silly of me—does not have a correct answer.

Ellipsis Marks

The ellipsis mark has **three** periods (…) to show when **words have been removed** from a quotation. If a **full sentence or more** is removed from a quoted passage, you need to use **four** periods to show the removed text and the end punctuation mark. The ellipsis mark should not be used at the beginning of a quotation. The ellipsis mark should also not be used at the end of a quotation unless some words have been deleted from the end of the final sentence.

Example:

> "Then he picked up the groceries…paid for them…later he went home."

Brackets

There are two main reasons to use brackets:

Use Case	Example
Placing **parentheses inside of parentheses**	The hero of this story, Paul Revere (a silversmith and industrialist [see Ch. 4]), rode through towns of Massachusetts to warn of advancing British troops.
Adding **clarification or detail to a quotation** that is not part of the quotation	The father explained, "My children are planning to attend my alma mater [State University]."

Review Video: Brackets
Visit mometrix.com/academy and enter code: 727546

Common Mistakes

Word Confusion

Which, That, and Who

The words *which*, *that*, and *who* can act as **relative pronouns** to help clarify or describe a noun.

Which is used for things only.

Example: Andrew's car, *which is old and rusty,* broke down last week.

That is used for people or things. *That* is usually informal when used to describe people.

Example: Is this the only book *that Louis L'Amour wrote?*

Example: Is Louis L'Amour the author *that wrote Western novels?*

Who is used for people or for animals that have an identity or personality.

Example: Mozart was the composer *who wrote those operas.*

Example: John's dog, *who is called Max,* is large and fierce.

Homophones

Homophones are words that sound alike (or similar) but have different **spellings** and **definitions**. A homophone is a type of **homonym**, which is a pair or group of words that are pronounced or spelled the same, but do not mean the same thing.

To, Too, and Two

To can be an adverb or a preposition for showing direction, purpose, and relationship. See your dictionary for the many other ways to use *to* in a sentence.

Examples: I went to the store. | I want to go with you.

Too is an adverb that means *also, as well, very,* or *in excess.*

Examples: I can walk a mile too. | You have eaten too much.

Two is a number.

Example: You have two minutes left.

There, Their, and They're

There can be an adjective, adverb, or pronoun. Often, *there* is used to show a place or to start a sentence.

Examples: I went there yesterday. | There is something in his pocket.

Their is a pronoun that is used to show ownership.

Examples: He is their father. | This is their fourth apology this week.

They're is a contraction of *they are.*

Example: Did you know that they're in town?

Knew and New

Knew is the past tense of *know*.

Example: I knew the answer.

New is an adjective that means something is current, has not been used, or is modern.

Example: This is my new phone.

Then and Than

Then is an adverb that indicates sequence or order:

Example: I'm going to run to the library and then come home.

Than is special-purpose word used only for comparisons:

Example: Susie likes chips more than candy.

Its and It's

Its is a pronoun that shows ownership.

Example: The guitar is in its case.

It's is a contraction of *it is.*

Example: It's an honor and a privilege to meet you.

Note: The *h* in honor is silent, so *honor* starts with the vowel sound *o*, which must have the article *an*.

Your and You're

Your is a pronoun that shows ownership.

Example: This is your moment to shine.

You're is a contraction of *you are.*

Example: Yes, you're correct.

Saw and Seen

Saw is the past-tense form of *see.*

Example: I saw a turtle on my walk this morning.

Seen is the past participle of *see.*

Example: I have seen this movie before.

Affect and Effect

There are two main reasons that *affect* and *effect* are so often confused: 1) both words can be used as either a noun or a verb, and 2) unlike most homophones, their usage and meanings are closely related to each other. Here is a quick rundown of the four usage options:

Affect (n): feeling, emotion, or mood that is displayed

Example: The patient had a flat *affect*. (i.e., his face showed little or no emotion)

Affect (v): to alter, to change, to influence

Example: The sunshine *affects* the plant's growth.

Effect (n): a result, a consequence

Example: What *effect* will this weather have on our schedule?

Effect (v): to bring about, to cause to be

Example: These new rules will *effect* order in the office.

The noun form of *affect* is rarely used outside of technical medical descriptions, so if a noun form is needed on the test, you can safely select *effect*. The verb form of *effect* is not as rare as the noun form of *affect*, but it's still not all that likely to show up on your test. If you need a verb and you can't decide which to use based on the definitions, choosing *affect* is your best bet.

Homographs

Homographs are words that share the same spelling, but have different meanings and sometimes different pronunciations. To figure out which meaning is being used, you should be looking for context clues. The context clues give hints to the meaning of the word. For example, the word *spot* has many meanings. It can mean "a place" or "a stain or blot." In the sentence "After my lunch, I saw a spot on my shirt," the word *spot* means "a stain or blot." The context clues of "After my lunch" and "on my shirt" guide you to this decision. A homograph is another type of homonym.

Bank

(noun): an establishment where money is held for savings or lending

(verb): to collect or pile up

Content

(noun): the topics that will be addressed within a book

(adjective): pleased or satisfied

(verb): to make someone pleased or satisfied

Fine

(noun): an amount of money that acts a penalty for an offense

(adjective): very small or thin

(adverb): in an acceptable way

(verb): to make someone pay money as a punishment

Incense

(noun): a material that is burned in religious settings and makes a pleasant aroma

(verb): to frustrate or anger

LEAD

(noun): the first or highest position

(noun): a heavy metallic element

(verb): to direct a person or group of followers

(adjective): containing lead

OBJECT

(noun): a lifeless item that can be held and observed

(verb): to disagree

PRODUCE

(noun): fruits and vegetables

(verb): to make or create something

REFUSE

(noun): garbage or debris that has been thrown away

(verb): to not allow

SUBJECT

(noun): an area of study

(verb): to force or subdue

TEAR

(noun): a fluid secreted by the eyes

(verb): to separate or pull apart

Chapter Quiz

Ready to see how well you retained what you just read? Scan the QR code to go directly to the chapter quiz interface for this study guide. If you're using a computer, simply visit the bonus page at **mometrix.com/bonus948/hesia2** and click the Chapter Quizzes link.

Biology

Transform passive reading into active learning! After immersing yourself in this chapter, put your comprehension to the test by taking a quiz. The insights you gained will stay with you longer this way. Scan the QR code to go directly to the chapter quiz interface for this study guide. If you're using a computer, simply visit the bonus page at **mometrix.com/bonus948/hesia2** and click the Chapter Quizzes link.

The Biology section of the HESI A^2 exam consists of 25 questions. This section may or may not be included on your specific test, depending on the requirements where you are applying. **Some of the concepts that will appear on the Biology section of the exam are covered in greater depth in the Anatomy and Physiology chapter**, so we recommend reading both even if you only have to take the Biology section.

Macromolecules

Macromolecules are large and complex, and play an important role in cell structure and function. The four basic organic macromolecules produced by anabolic reactions are **carbohydrates** (polysaccharides), **nucleic acids**, **proteins**, and **lipids**. The four basic building blocks involved in catabolic reactions are **monosaccharides** (glucose), **amino acids**, **fatty acids** (glycerol), and **nucleotides**.

An **anabolic reaction** is one that builds larger and more complex molecules (macromolecules) from smaller ones. **Catabolic reactions** are the opposite. Larger molecules are broken down into smaller, simpler molecules. Catabolic reactions *release energy*, while anabolic ones *require energy*.

Endothermic reactions are chemical reactions that *absorb* heat and **exothermic reactions** are chemical reactions that *release* heat.

Review Video: Macromolecules
Visit mometrix.com/academy and enter code: 220156

Carbohydrate

Carbohydrates are the primary source of energy and are responsible for providing energy as they can be easily converted to **glucose**. It is the oxidation of carbohydrates that provides the cells with most of their energy. Glucose can be further broken down by respiration or fermentation by **glycolysis**. They are involved in the metabolic energy cycles of photosynthesis and respiration.

Structurally, carbohydrates usually take the form of some variation of CH_2O as they are made of carbon, hydrogen, and oxygen. Carbohydrates (**polysaccharides**) are broken down into sugars or glucose.

The simple sugars can be grouped into monosaccharides (glucose, fructose, and galactose) and disaccharides. These are both types of carbohydrates. Monosaccharides have one monomer of sugar and disaccharides have two. Monosaccharides (CH_2O) have one carbon for every water molecule.

A **monomer** is a small molecule. It is a single compound that forms chemical bonds with other monomers to make a polymer. A **polymer** is a compound of large molecules formed by repeating monomers. Carbohydrates, proteins, and nucleic acids are groups of macromolecules that are polymers.

LIPIDS

Lipids are molecules that are soluble in nonpolar solvents, but are hydrophobic, meaning they do not bond well with water or mix well with water solutions. Lipids have numerous **C–H bonds.** In this way, they are similar to **hydrocarbons** (substances consisting only of carbon and hydrogen). The major roles of lipids include *energy storage and structural functions*. Examples of lipids include fats, phospholipids, steroids, and waxes. **Fats** (which are triglycerides) are made of long chains of fatty acids (three fatty acids bound to a glycerol). **Fatty acids** are chains with reduced carbon at one end and a carboxylic acid group at the other. An example is soap, which contains the sodium salts of free fatty acids. **Phospholipids** are lipids that have a phosphate group rather than a fatty acid. **Glycerides** are another type of lipid. Examples of glycerides are fat and oil. Glycerides are formed from fatty acids and glycerol (a type of alcohol).

PROTEINS

Proteins are macromolecules formed from amino acids. They are **polypeptides**, which consist of many (10 to 100) peptides linked together. The peptide connections are the result of condensation reactions. A **condensation reaction** results in a loss of water when two molecules are joined together. A **hydrolysis reaction** is the opposite of a condensation reaction. During hydrolysis, water is added. –H is added to one of the smaller molecules and OH is added to another molecule being formed. A **peptide** is a compound of two or more amino acids. **Amino acids** are formed by the partial hydrolysis of protein, which forms an **amide bond**. This partial hydrolysis involves an amine group and a carboxylic acid. In the carbon chain of amino acids, there is a **carboxylic acid group** (–COOH), an **amine group** ($-NH_2$), a **central carbon atom** between them with an attached hydrogen, and an attached **"R" group** (side chain), which is different for different amino acids. It is the "R" group that determines the properties of the protein.

ENZYMES

Enzymes are proteins with strong **catalytic** power. They greatly accelerate the speed at which specific reactions approach equilibrium. Although enzymes do not start chemical reactions that would not eventually occur by themselves, they do make these reactions happen *faster and more often*. This acceleration can be substantial, sometimes making reactions happen a million times faster. Each type of enzyme deals with **reactants**, also called **substrates**. Each enzyme is highly selective, only interacting with substrates that are a match for it at an active site on the enzyme. This is the "key in the lock" analogy: a certain enzyme only fits with certain substrates. Even with a matching substrate, sometimes an enzyme must reshape itself to fit well with the substrate, forming a strong bond that aids in catalyzing a reaction before it returns to its original shape. An unusual quality of enzymes is that they are not permanently consumed in the reactions they speed up. They can be used again and again, providing a constant source of energy accelerants for cells. This allows for a tremendous increase in the number and rate of reactions in cells.

NUCLEIC ACIDS

Nucleic acids are macromolecules that are composed of **nucleotides**. **Hydrolysis** is a reaction in which water is broken down into **hydrogen cations** (H or H^+) and **hydroxide anions** (OH or OH^-). This is part of the process by which nucleic acids are broken down by enzymes to produce shorter strings of RNA and DNA (oligonucleotides). **Oligonucleotides** are broken down into smaller sugar nitrogenous units called **nucleosides**. These can be digested by cells since the sugar is divided from the nitrogenous base. This, in turn, leads to the formation of the five types of nitrogenous bases, sugars, and the preliminary substances involved in the synthesis of new RNA and DNA. DNA and RNA have a helix shape.

Macromolecular nucleic acid polymers, such as RNA and DNA, are formed from nucleotides, which are monomeric units joined by **phosphodiester bonds**. Cells require energy in the form of ATP to synthesize proteins from amino acids and replicate DNA. **Nitrogen fixation** is used to synthesize nucleotides for DNA and amino acids for proteins. Nitrogen fixation uses the enzyme nitrogenase in the reduction of dinitrogen gas (N_2) to ammonia (NH_3).

Nucleic acids store information and energy and are also important catalysts. It is the **RNA** that catalyzes the transfer of **DNA genetic information** into protein coded information. ATP is an RNA nucleotide. **Nucleotides** are used to form the nucleic acids. Nucleotides are made of a five-carbon sugar, such as ribose or deoxyribose, a nitrogenous base, and one or more phosphates. Nucleotides consisting of more than one phosphate can also store energy in their bonds.

DNA

Chromosomes consist of **genes**, which are single units of genetic information. Genes are made up of deoxyribonucleic acid (DNA). DNA is a nucleic acid located in the cell nucleus. There is also DNA in the **mitochondria**. DNA replicates to pass on genetic information. The DNA in almost all cells is the same. It is also involved in the biosynthesis of proteins.

Review Video: Chromosomes
Visit mometrix.com/academy and enter code: 132083

The model or structure of DNA is described as a **double helix**. A helix is a curve, and a double helix is two congruent curves connected by horizontal members. The model can be likened to a spiral staircase. It is right-handed. The British scientist Rosalind Elsie Franklin is credited with taking the x-ray diffraction image in 1952 that was used by Francis Crick and James Watson to formulate the double-helix model of DNA and speculate about its important role in carrying and transferring genetic information.

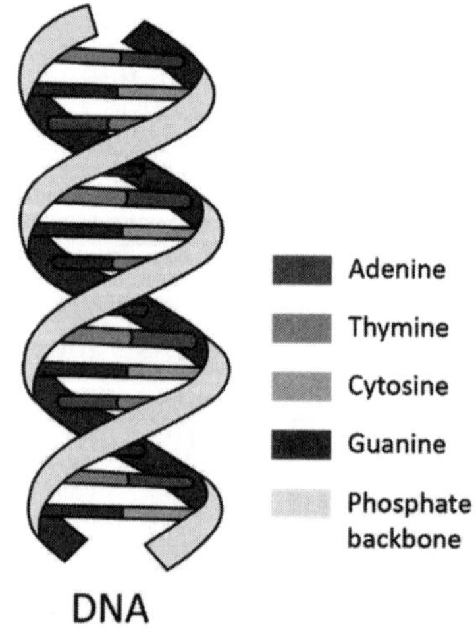

DNA

Review Video: DNA
Visit mometrix.com/academy and enter code: 639552

DNA Structure

DNA has a double helix shape, resembles a twisted ladder, and is compact. It consists of **nucleotides**. Nucleotides consist of a **five-carbon sugar** (pentose), a **phosphate group**, and a **nitrogenous base**. Two bases pair up to form the rungs of the ladder. The "side rails" or backbone consists of the covalently bonded sugar and phosphate. The bases are attached to each other with hydrogen bonds, which are easily dismantled so replication can occur. Each base is attached to a phosphate and to a sugar. There are four types of nitrogenous bases: **adenine** (A), **guanine** (G), **cytosine** (C), and **thymine** (T). There are about 3 billion bases in human DNA. The bases are mostly the same in everybody, but their order is different. It is the order of these bases that creates diversity in people. *Adenine (A) pairs with thymine (T)*, and *cytosine (C) pairs with guanine (G)*.

Purines and Pyrimidines

The five bases in DNA and RNA can be categorized as either pyrimidine or purine according to their structure. The **pyrimidine bases** include *cytosine, thymine, and uracil*. They are six-sided and have a single ring shape. The **purine bases** are *adenine and guanine*, which consist of two attached rings. One ring has five sides and the other has six. When combined with a sugar, any of the five bases become **nucleosides**. Nucleosides formed from purine bases end in "osine" and those formed from pyrimidine bases end in "idine." **Adenosine** and **thymidine** are examples of nucleosides. Bases are the most basic components, followed by nucleosides, nucleotides, and then DNA or RNA.

Codons

Codons are groups of three nucleotides on the messenger RNA, and can be visualized as three rungs of a ladder. A **codon** has the code for a single amino acid. There are 64 codons but 20 amino acids. More than one combination, or triplet, can be used to synthesize the necessary amino acids. For example, AAA (adenine-adenine-adenine) or AAG (adenine-adenine-guanine) can serve as codons for lysine. These groups of three occur in strings, and might be thought of as frames. For example, AAAUCUUCGU, if read in groups of three from the beginning, would be AAA, UCU, UCG, which are codons for lysine, serine, and serine, respectively. If the same sequence was read in groups of three starting from the second position, the groups would be AAU (asparagine), CUU (proline), and so on. The resulting amino acids would be completely different. For this reason, there are **start and stop codons** that indicate the beginning and ending of a sequence (or frame). **AUG** (methionine) is the start codon. **UAA**, **UGA**, and **UAG**, also known as ocher, opal, and amber, respectively, are stop codons.

Review Video: Codons
Visit mometrix.com/academy and enter code: 978172

DNA Replication

Pairs of chromosomes are composed of DNA, which is tightly wound to conserve space. When replication starts, it unwinds. The steps in **DNA replication** are controlled by enzymes. The enzyme **helicase** instigates the deforming of hydrogen bonds between the bases to split the two strands. The splitting starts at the A-T bases (adenine and thymine) as there are only two hydrogen bonds. The cytosine-guanine base pair has three bonds. The term "**origin of replication**" is used to refer to where the splitting starts. The portion of the DNA that is unwound to be replicated is called the

replication fork. Each strand of DNA is transcribed by an mRNA. It copies the DNA onto itself, base by base, in a complementary manner. The exception is that uracil replaces thymine.

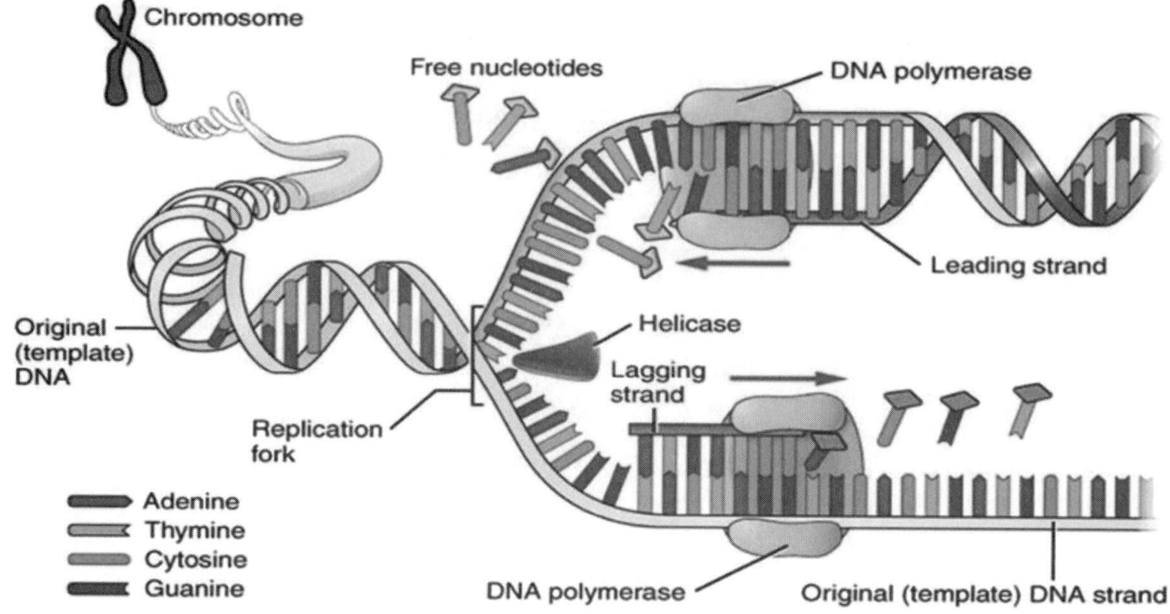

RNA

Types of RNA

RNA acts as a *helper* to DNA and carries out a number of other functions. Types of RNA include ribosomal RNA (rRNA), transfer RNA (tRNA), and messenger RNA (mRNA). Viruses can use RNA to carry their genetic material to DNA. **Ribosomal RNA** is not believed to have changed much over time. For this reason, it can be used to study relationships in organisms. **Messenger RNA** carries a copy of a strand of DNA and transports it from the nucleus to the cytoplasm. **Transcription** is the process in which RNA polymerase copies DNA into RNA. DNA unwinds itself and serves as a template while RNA is being assembled. The DNA molecules are copied to RNA. **Translation** is the process whereby ribosomes use transcribed RNA to put together the needed protein. **Transfer RNA** is a molecule that helps in the translation process, and is found in the cytoplasm.

Differences between RNA and DNA

RNA and DNA differ in terms of structure and function. RNA has a different sugar than DNA. It has **ribose** rather than **deoxyribose** sugar. The RNA nitrogenous bases are adenine (A), guanine (G), cytosine (C), and uracil (U). **Uracil** is found only in RNA and **thymine** in found only in DNA. RNA consists of a single strand and DNA has two strands. If straightened out, DNA has two side rails. RNA only has one "backbone," or strand of sugar and phosphate group components. RNA uses the fully hydroxylated sugar **pentose**, which includes an extra oxygen compared to deoxyribose, which is the sugar used by DNA. RNA supports the functions carried out by DNA. It aids in gene expression, replication, and transportation.

Review Video: DNA vs. RNA
Visit mometrix.com/academy and enter code: 184871

Mendel's Laws

Mendel's laws are the law of segregation (the first law), the law of independent assortment (the second law), and the law of dominance (the third law). The **law of segregation** states that there are two **alleles** and that half of the total number of alleles are contributed by each parent organism. The **law of independent assortment** states that traits are passed on randomly and are not influenced by other traits. The exception to this is linked traits. A **Punnett square** can illustrate how alleles combine from the contributing genes to form various **phenotypes**. One set of a parent's genes are put in columns, while the genes from the other parent are placed in rows. The allele combinations are shown in each cell. The **law of dominance** states that when two different alleles are present in a pair, the **dominant** one is expressed. A Punnett square can be used to predict the outcome of crosses.

Gene, Genotype, Phenotype, and Allele

A gene is a portion of DNA that identifies how traits are expressed and passed on in an organism. A gene is part of the **genetic code**. Collectively, all genes form the **genotype** of an individual. The genotype includes genes that may not be expressed, such as **recessive genes**. The **phenotype** is the physical, visual manifestation of genes. It is determined by the basic genetic information and how genes have been affected by their environment.

An **allele** is a variation of a gene. Also known as a trait, it determines the manifestation of a gene. This manifestation results in a specific physical appearance of some facet of an organism, such as eye color or height. For example, the genetic information for eye color is a gene. The gene variations responsible for blue, green, brown, or black eyes are called alleles. **Locus** (pl. loci) refers to the location of a gene or alleles.

Review Video: Genotype vs Phenotype
Visit mometrix.com/academy and enter code: 922853

Dominant and Recessive

Gene traits are represented in pairs with an upper-case letter for the dominant trait (A) and a lower-case letter for the recessive trait (a). Genes occur in pairs (AA, Aa, or aa). There is one gene on each chromosome half supplied by each parent organism. Since half the genetic material is from each parent, the offspring's traits are represented as a combination of these. A dominant trait only requires one gene of a gene pair for it to be expressed in a phenotype, whereas a recessive trait requires both genes in order to be manifested. For example, if the mother's genotype is Dd and the father's is dd, the possible combinations are Dd and dd. The dominant trait will be manifested if the genotype is DD or Dd. The recessive trait will be manifested if the genotype is dd. Both DD and dd are homozygous pairs. Dd is heterozygous.

Monohybrid and Hybrid Crosses

Genetic crosses are the possible combinations of alleles, and can be represented using Punnett squares. A **monohybrid cross** refers to a cross involving only one trait. Typically, the ratio is 3:1 (DD, Dd, Dd, dd), which is the ratio of dominant gene manifestation to recessive gene manifestation. This ratio occurs when both parents have a pair of dominant and recessive genes. If one parent has a pair of dominant genes (DD) and the other has a pair of recessive (dd) genes, the recessive trait cannot be expressed in the next generation because the resulting crosses all have the Dd genotype.

A **dihybrid cross** refers to one involving more than one trait, which means more combinations are possible. The ratio of genotypes for a dihybrid cross is 9:3:3:1 when the traits are not linked. The ratio for incomplete dominance is 1:2:1, which corresponds to dominant, mixed, and recessive phenotypes.

MONOHYBRID CROSS EXAMPLE

A monohybrid cross is a genetic cross for a single trait that has two alleles. A monohybrid cross can be used to show which allele is **dominant** for a single trait. The first monohybrid cross typically occurs between two **homozygous** parents. Each parent is homozygous for a separate allele for a particular trait. For example, in pea plants, green pods (G) are dominant over yellow pods (g). In a genetic cross of two pea plants that are homozygous for pod color, the F_1 generation will be 100% heterozygous green pods.

	g	**g**
G	Gg	Gg
G	Gg	Gg

If the plants with the heterozygous green pods are crossed, the F_2 generation should be 50% heterozygous green, 25% homozygous green, and 25% homozygous yellow.

	G	**g**
G	GG	Gg
g	Gg	gg

DIHYBRID CROSS EXAMPLE

A dihybrid cross is a genetic cross for **two traits** that each have two alleles. For example, in pea plants, green pods (G) are dominant over yellow pods (g), and yellow seeds (Y) are dominant over green seeds (y). In a genetic cross of two pea plants that are homozygous for pod color and seed color, the F_1 generation will be 100% heterozygous green pods and yellow seeds (GgYy). If these F_1 plants are crossed, the resulting F_2 generation is shown below. There are nine genotypes for green-pod, yellow-seed plants: one GGYY, two GGYy, two GgYY, and four GgYy. There are three genotypes for green-pod, green-seed plants: one GGyy and two Ggyy. There are three genotypes for yellow-pod, yellow-seed plants: one ggYY and two ggYy. There is only one genotype for yellow-pod, green-seed plants: ggyy. This cross has a 9:3:3:1 ratio.

	GY	**Gy**	**gY**	**gy**
GY	GGYY	GGYy	GgYY	GgYy
Gy	GGYy	GGyy	GgYy	Ggyy
gY	GgYY	GgYy	ggYY	ggYy
gy	GgYy	Ggyy	ggYy	ggyy

Non-Mendelian Concepts

CO-DOMINANCE

Co-dominance refers to the expression of *both alleles* so that both traits are shown. Cows, for example, can have hair colors of red, white, or red and white (not pink). In the latter color, both traits are fully expressed. The ABO human blood typing system is also co-dominant.

INCOMPLETE DOMINANCE

Incomplete dominance is when both the **dominant** and **recessive** genes are expressed, resulting in a phenotype that is a mixture of the two. The fact that snapdragons can be red, white, or pink is a good example. The dominant red gene (RR) results in a red flower because of large amounts of red pigment. White (rr) occurs because both genes call for no pigment. Pink (Rr) occurs because one gene is for red and one is for no pigment. The colors blend to produce pink flowers. A cross of pink flowers (Rr) can result in red (RR), white (rr), or pink (Rr) flowers.

Review Video: Mendelian and Non-Mendelian Genetics
Visit mometrix.com/academy and enter code: 113159

POLYGENIC INHERITANCE

Polygenic inheritance goes beyond the simplistic Mendelian concept that one gene influences one trait. It refers to traits that are influenced by *more than one gene*, and takes into account environmental influences on development.

MULTIPLE ALLELES

Each gene is made up of only two alleles, but in some cases, there are more than two possibilities for what those two alleles might be. For example, in blood typing, there are three alleles (A, B, O), but each person has only two of them. A gene with more than two possible alleles is known as a multiple allele. A gene that can result in two or more possible forms or expressions is known as a polymorphic gene.

Chapter Quiz

Ready to see how well you retained what you just read? Scan the QR code to go directly to the chapter quiz interface for this study guide. If you're using a computer, simply visit the bonus page at **mometrix.com/bonus948/hesia2** and click the Chapter Quizzes link.

Chemistry

Transform passive reading into active learning! After immersing yourself in this chapter, put your comprehension to the test by taking a quiz. The insights you gained will stay with you longer this way. Scan the QR code to go directly to the chapter quiz interface for this study guide. If you're using a computer, simply visit the bonus page at **mometrix.com/bonus948/hesia2** and click the Chapter Quizzes link.

The Chemistry section of the HESI A^2 exam consists of 25 questions. This section may or may not be included on your specific test, depending on the requirements where you are applying.

Metric System and Scientific Reasoning

Metric System

The metric system is generally accepted as the preferred method for taking measurements. Having a universal standard allows individuals to interpret measurements more easily, regardless of where they are located.

The basic units of measurement are: the **meter**, which measures length; the **liter**, which measures volume; and the **gram**, which measures mass. The metric system starts with a **base unit** and increases or decreases in units of 10. The prefix and the base unit combined are used to indicate an amount.

For example, deka is 10 times the base unit. A dekameter is 10 meters; a dekaliter is 10 liters; and a dekagram is 10 grams. The prefix hecto refers to 100 times the base amount; kilo is 1,000 times the base amount. The prefixes that indicate a fraction of the base unit are deci, which is 1/10 of the base unit; centi, which is 1/100 of the base unit; and milli, which is 1/1000 of the base unit.

SI Units of Measurement

SI uses the **second** (s) to measure time. Fractions of seconds are usually measured in metric terms using prefixes such as millisecond (1/1,000 of a second) or nanosecond (1/1,000,000,000 of a second). Increments of time larger than a second are measured in minutes and hours, which are multiples of 60 and 24. An example of this is a swimmer's time in the 800-meter freestyle being described as 7:32.67, meaning 7 minutes, 32 seconds, and 67 one-hundredths of a second. One second is equal to 1/60 of a minute, 1/3,600 of an hour, and 1/86,400 of a day.

Other SI base units are the **ampere** (A) (used to measure electric current), the **kelvin** (K) (used to measure thermodynamic temperature), the **candela** (cd) (used to measure luminous intensity), and the **mole** (mol) (used to measure the amount of a substance at a molecular level). **Meter** (m) is used to measure length and **kilogram** (kg) is used to measure mass.

METRIC PREFIXES FOR MULTIPLES AND SUBDIVISIONS

The prefixes for multiples are as follows:

Deka	(da)	**10^1** (deka is the American spelling, but deca is also used)
Hecto	(h)	10^2
Kilo	(k)	10^3
Mega	(M)	10^6
Giga	(G)	10^9
Tera	(T)	10^{12}

The prefixes for subdivisions are as follows:

Deci	(d)	**10^{-1}**
Centi	(c)	10^{-2}
Milli	(m)	10^{-3}
Micro	(μ)	10^{-6}
Nano	(n)	10^{-9}
Pico	(p)	10^{-12}

The rule of thumb is that prefixes greater than 10^3 are capitalized when abbreviating. Abbreviations do not need a period after them. A decimeter (dm) is a tenth of a meter, a deciliter (dL) is a tenth of a liter, and a decigram (dg) is a tenth of a gram. Pluralization is understood. For example, when referring to 5 mL of water, no "s" needs to be added to the abbreviation.

REVIEW A SCIENTIFIC EXPLANATION WITH LOGIC AND EVIDENCE

DATA COLLECTION

A valid experiment must be measurable. **Data tables** should be formed, and meticulous, detailed data should be collected for every trial. First, the researcher must determine exactly what data are needed and why those data are needed. The researcher should know in advance what will be done with those data at the end of the experimental research. The data should be *repeatable, reproducible, and accurate.* The researcher should be sure that the procedure for data collection will be reliable and consistent. The researcher should validate the measurement system by performing **practice tests** and making sure that all of the equipment is correctly **calibrated** and periodically retesting the procedure and equipment to ensure that all data being collected are still valid.

SCIENTIFIC PROCESS SKILLS

Perhaps the most important skill in science is that of **observation**. Scientists must be able to take accurate data from their experimental setup or from nature without allowing bias to alter the results. Another important skill is **hypothesizing**. Scientists must be able to combine their knowledge of theory and of other experimental results to logically determine what should occur in their own tests.

The **data-analysis process** requires the twin skills of ordering and categorizing. Gathered data must be arranged in such a way that it is readable and readily shows the key results. A skill that may be integrated with the previous two is comparing. Scientists should be able to **compare** their own results with other published results. They must also be able to **infer**, or draw logical conclusions, from their results. They must be able to **apply** their knowledge of theory and results to create logical experimental designs and determine cases of special behavior.

Lastly, scientists must be able to **communicate** their results and their conclusions. The greatest scientific progress is made when scientists are able to review and test one another's work and offer advice or suggestions.

Scientific Statements

Hypotheses are educated guesses about what is likely to occur, and are made to provide a starting point from which to begin design of the experiment. They may be based on results of previously observed experiments or knowledge of theory, and follow logically forth from these.

Assumptions are statements that are taken to be fact without proof for the purpose of performing a given experiment. They may be entirely true, or they may be true only for a given set of conditions under which the experiment will be conducted. Assumptions are necessary to simplify experiments; indeed, many experiments would be impossible without them.

Scientific models are mathematical statements that describe a physical behavior. Models are only as good as our knowledge of the actual system. Often models will be discarded when new discoveries are made that show the model to be inaccurate. While a model can never perfectly represent an actual system, it is useful for simplifying a system to allow for better understanding of its behavior.

Scientific laws are statements of natural behavior that have stood the test of time and have been found to produce accurate and repeatable results in all testing. A **theory** is a statement of behavior that consolidates all current observations. Theories are similar to laws in that they describe natural behavior, but are more recently developed and are more susceptible to being proved wrong. Theories may eventually become laws if they stand up to scrutiny and testing.

Events and Objects

Events

A **cause** is an act or event that makes something happen, and an **effect** is the thing that happens as a result of the cause. A cause-and-effect relationship is not always explicit, but there are some terms in English that signal causes, such as *since*, *because*, and *due to*. Terms that signal effects include *consequently, therefore, this lead(s) to*.

Remember the chance for a single cause to have many effects. (e.g., *Single cause*: Because you left your homework on the table, your dog eats the homework. *Many effects*: (1) As a result, you fail your homework. (2) Your parents do not let you see your friends. (3) You miss out on the new movie. (4) You miss holding the hand of an important person.)

Also, there is a chance of a single effect to have many causes. (e.g., *Single effect*: Alan has a fever. *Many causes*: (1) An unexpected cold front came through the area, and (2) Alan forgot to take his multi-vitamin.)

Now, an effect can become the cause of another effect. This is known as a cause and effect chain. (e.g., As a result of her hatred for not doing work, Lynn got ready for her exam. This led to her passing her test with high marks. Hence, her resume was accepted, and her application was accepted.)

Scale

From the largest objects in outer space to the smallest pieces of the human body, there are objects that can come in many different sizes and shapes. Many of those objects need to be measured in different ways. So, it is important to know which **unit of measurement** is needed to record the length or width and the weight of an object.

An example is taking the measurements of a patient. When measuring the total height of a patient or finding the length of an extremity, the accepted measure is given in meters. However, when one is asked for the diameter of a vein, the accepted measure is given in millimeters. Another example would be measuring the weight of a patient which would be given in kilograms, while the measurement of a human heart would be given in grams. The same idea for scale holds true with time as well. When measuring the lifespan of a patient, the accepted measure is given in days, months, or years. However, when measuring the number of breaths that a patient takes, the accepted measure is given in terms of minutes (e.g., breaths per minute).

Scientific Inquiry

Scientific Method

The scientific method of inquiry is a general method by which ideas are tested and either confirmed or refuted by experimentation. The first step in the scientific method is **formulating the problem** that is to be addressed. It is essential to define clearly the limits of what is to be observed, since that allows for a more focused analysis.

Once the problem has been defined, it is necessary to form a **hypothesis**. This educated guess should be a possible solution to the problem that was formulated in the first step.

The next step is to test that hypothesis by **experimentation**. This often requires the scientist to design a complete experiment. The key to making the best possible use of an experiment is observation. Observations may be **quantitative**, that is, when a numeric measurement is taken, or they may be **qualitative**, that is, when something is evaluated based on feeling or preference. This measurement data will then be examined to find trends or patterns that are present.

From these trends, the scientist will draw **conclusions** or make **generalizations** about the results, intended to predict future results. If these conclusions support the original hypothesis, the experiment is complete and the scientist will publish his conclusions to allow others to test them by repeating the experiment. If they do not support the hypothesis, the results should then be used to develop a new hypothesis, which can then be verified by a new or redesigned experiment.

Experimental Design

Designing relevant experiments that allow for meaningful results is not a simple task. Every stage of the experiment must be carefully planned to ensure that the right data can be safely and accurately taken.

Ideally, an experiment should be **controlled** so that all of the conditions except the ones being manipulated are held **constant**. This helps to ensure that the results are not skewed by unintended consequences of shifting conditions. A good example of this is a placebo group in a drug trial. All other conditions are the same, but that group is not given the medication.

In addition to proper control, it is important that the experiment be designed with **data collection** in mind. For instance, if the quantity to be measured is temperature, there must be a temperature device such as a thermocouple integrated into the experimental setup. While the data are being collected, they should periodically be checked for obvious errors. If there are data points that are orders of magnitude from the expected value, then it might be a good idea to make sure that no experimental errors are being made, either in data collection or condition control.

Once all the data have been gathered, they must be **analyzed**. The way in which this should be done depends on the type of data and the type of trends observed. It may be useful to fit curves to the data to determine if the trends follow a common mathematical form. It may also be necessary to perform a statistical analysis of the results to determine what effects are significant. Data should be clearly presented.

CONTROLS

A valid experiment must be carefully **controlled**. All variables except the one being tested must be carefully maintained. This means that all conditions must be kept exactly the same except for the independent variable.

Additionally, a set of data is usually needed for a **control group**. The control group represents the "normal" state or condition of the variable being manipulated. Controls can be negative or positive. **Positive controls** are the variables that the researcher expects to have an effect on the outcome of the experiment. A positive control group can be used to verify that an experiment is set up properly. **Negative control groups** are typically thought of as placebos. A negative control group should verify that a variable has no effect on the outcome of the experiment.

The better an experiment is controlled, the more valid the conclusions from that experiment will be. A researcher is more likely to draw a valid conclusion if all variables other than the one being manipulated are being controlled.

VARIABLES

Every experiment has several **variables**; however, only one variable should be purposely changed and tested. This variable is the **manipulated** or **independent variable**. As this variable is manipulated or changed, another variable, called the **responding** or **dependent variable**, is observed and recorded.

All other variables in the experiment must be carefully controlled and are usually referred to as **constants**. For example, when testing the effect of temperature on solubility of a solute, the independent variable is the temperature, and the dependent variable is the solubility. All other factors in the experiment such as pressure, amount of stirring, type of solvent, type of solute, and particle size of the solute are the constants.

Review Video: Identifying Independent and Dependent Variables
Visit mometrix.com/academy and enter code: 627181

Atomic Structure

Pieces of an Atom

All matter consists of atoms. Atoms consist of a **nucleus** and **electrons**. The nucleus consists of **protons** and **neutrons**. The properties of these are measurable; they have mass and an electrical charge. The nucleus is **positively charged** due to the presence of protons. Electrons are **negatively charged** and orbit the nucleus. The nucleus has considerably more mass than the surrounding electrons. Atoms can bond together to make **molecules**. Atoms that have an equal number of protons and electrons are electrically **neutral**. If the number of protons and electrons in an atom is not equal, the atom has a positive or negative charge and is an **ion**.

Review Video: Structure of Atoms
Visit mometrix.com/academy and enter code: 905932

Models of Atoms

Atoms are extremely small. A hydrogen atom is about 5×10^{-8} mm in diameter. According to some estimates, five trillion hydrogen atoms could fit on the head of a pin. **Atomic radius** refers to the average distance between the nucleus and the outermost electron. Models of atoms that include the proton, nucleus, and electrons typically show the electrons very close to the nucleus and revolving around it, similar to how the Earth orbits the sun. However, another model relates the Earth as the nucleus and its atmosphere as electrons, which is the basis of the term "**electron cloud**." Another description is that electrons swarm around the nucleus. It should be noted that these atomic models are not to scale. A more accurate representation would be a nucleus with a diameter of about 2 cm in a stadium. The electrons would be in the bleachers. This model is similar to the not-to-scale solar system model. In reference to the periodic table, atomic radius increases as energy levels are added and decreases as more protons are added (because they pull the electrons closer to the nucleus). Essentially, atomic radius increases toward the left and toward the bottom of the periodic table (i.e., Francium (Fr) has the largest atomic radius while Helium (He) has the smallest).

Atomic Number

The atomic number of an element refers to the **number of protons** in the nucleus of an atom. It is a unique identifier. It can be represented as Z. Atoms with a neutral charge have an atomic number that is equal to the **number of electrons**.

Atomic Mass

Atomic mass is also known as the **mass number**. The atomic mass is the *total number of protons and neutrons* in the nucleus of an atom. It is referred to as "A." The atomic mass (A) is equal to the number of protons (Z) plus the number of neutrons (N). This can be represented by the equation $A = Z + N$. The mass of electrons in an atom is basically insignificant because it is so small. Atomic weight may sometimes be referred to as "**relative atomic mass**," but should not be confused with atomic mass. Atomic weight is the ratio of the average mass per atom of a sample (which can include various isotopes of an element) to 1/12 of the mass of an atom of carbon-12.

Isotopes

Isotopes are atoms of the same element that vary in their number of neutrons. Isotopes of the same element have the same number of protons and thus the same atomic number. They are denoted by the element symbol, preceded in superscript and subscript by the mass number and atomic number, respectively. For instance, the notations for protium, deuterium, and tritium are, respectively: ${}^{1}_{1}H$, ${}^{2}_{1}H$, and ${}^{3}_{1}H$.

Isotopes that have not been observed to decay are **stable**, or non-radioactive, isotopes. It is not known whether some stable isotopes may have such long decay times that observing decay is not possible. Currently, 80 elements have one or more stable isotopes. There are 256 known stable isotopes in total. Carbon, for example, has three isotopes. Two (carbon-12 and carbon-13) are stable and one (carbon-14) is radioactive. **Radioactive isotopes** have unstable nuclei and can undergo spontaneous nuclear reactions, which results in particles or radiation being emitted. It cannot be predicted when a specific nucleus will decay, but large groups of identical nuclei decay at predictable rates. Knowledge about rates of decay can be used to *estimate the age of materials* that contain radioactive isotopes.

Bonding

Electrons

Electrons are subatomic particles that orbit the nucleus at various levels commonly referred to as **layers, shells**, or **clouds**. The orbiting electron or electrons account for only a fraction of the atom's mass. They are much smaller than the nucleus, are negatively charged, and exhibit wave-like characteristics. Electrons are part of the **lepton** family of elementary particles. Electrons can occupy orbits that are varying distances away from the nucleus, and tend to occupy the lowest energy level they can. If an atom has all its electrons in the lowest available positions, it has a **stable** electron arrangement. The outermost electron shell of an atom in its uncombined state is known as the **valence shell**. The electrons there are called **valence electrons**, and it is their number that determines **bonding behavior**. Atoms tend to react in a manner that will allow them to fill or empty their valence shells.

Chemical Bonds and Electron Shells

Chemical bonds involve a negative-positive attraction between an electron or electrons and the nucleus of an atom or nuclei of more than one atom. The attraction keeps the atom cohesive, but also enables the formation of bonds among other atoms and molecules. Each of the four **energy levels** (or shells) of an atom has a maximum number of electrons they can contain. Each level must be completely filled before electrons can be added to the **valence level**. The farther away from the nucleus an electron is, the more energy it has. The first shell, or K-shell, can hold a maximum of 2 electrons; the second, the L-shell, can hold 8; the third, the M-shell, can hold 18; the fourth, the N-shell, can hold 32. The shells can also have **subshells**. Chemical bonds form and break between atoms when atoms gain, lose, or share an electron in the outer valence shell. **Polar bond** refers to a covalent type of bond with a separation of charge. One end is negative and the other is positive. The hydrogen-oxygen bond in water is one example of a polar bond.

Ions

Most atoms are **neutral** since the positive charge of the protons in the nucleus is balanced by the negative charge of the surrounding electrons. Electrons are transferred between atoms when they come into contact with each other. This creates a molecule or atom in which the number of electrons does not equal the number of protons, which gives it a positive or negative charge. A **negative ion** is created when an atom gains electrons, while a **positive ion** is created when an atom loses electrons. An **ionic bond** is formed between ions with opposite charges. The resulting compound is neutral. **Ionization** refers to the process by which neutral particles are ionized into charged particles. Gases and plasmas can be partially or fully ionized through ionization.

Chemical Bonds between Atoms

Atoms of the same element may bond together to form **molecules** or **crystalline solids**. When two or more different types of atoms bind together chemically, a **compound** is made. The physical properties of compounds reflect the nature of the interactions among their molecules. These interactions are determined by the structure of the molecule, including the atoms they consist of and the distances and angles between them.

A union between the electron structures of atoms is called **chemical bonding**. An atom may gain, surrender, or share its electrons with another atom it bonds with. Listed below are three types of chemical bonding.

- **Ionic bonding** – When an atom gains or loses electrons it becomes negatively or positively charged, turning it into an ion. An ionic bond is a relationship between two *oppositely charged ions.*
- **Covalent bonding** – Atoms that share electrons have what is called a covalent bond. Electrons shared equally have a *non-polar bond*, while electrons shared unequally have a *polar bond.*
- **Hydrogen bonding** – The atom of a molecule interacts with a hydrogen atom in the same area. Hydrogen bonds can also form between two different parts of the same molecule, as in the structure of DNA and other large molecules.

A **cation** or positive ion is formed when an atom loses one or more electrons. An **anion** or negative ion is formed when an atom gains one or more electrons.

Ionic Bonding

The transfer of electrons from one atom to another is called **ionic bonding**. Atoms that lose or gain electrons are referred to as **ions**. The gain or loss of electrons will result in an ion having a positive or negative charge. Here is an example:

> Take an atom of sodium (Na) and an atom of chlorine (Cl). The sodium atom has a total of 11 electrons (including one electron in its outer shell). The chlorine has 17 electrons (including 7 electrons in its outer shell). From this, the atomic number, or number of protons, of sodium can be calculated as 11 because the number of protons equals the number of electrons in an atom. When sodium chloride (NaCl) is formed, one electron from sodium transfers to chlorine. Ions have charges. They are written with a plus (+) or minus (–) symbol. Ions in a compound are attracted to each other because they have *opposite charges*.

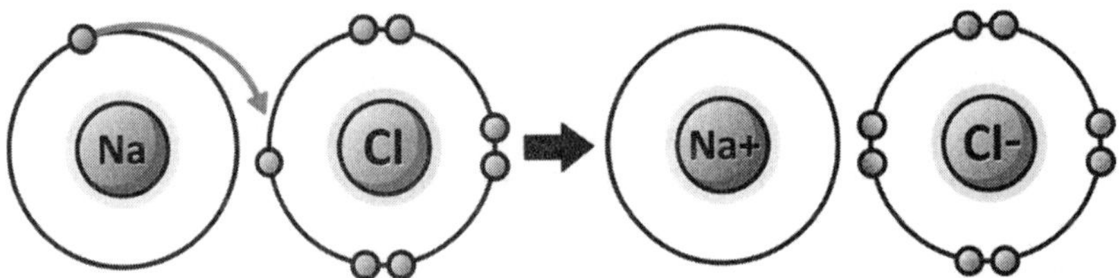

Covalent Bonding

Covalent bonding is characterized by the sharing of one or more pairs of electrons between two atoms or between an atom and another **covalent bond**. This produces an attraction to repulsion stability that holds these molecules together.

Atoms have the tendency to share electrons with each other so that all outer electron shells are filled. The resultant bonds are always stronger than the **intermolecular hydrogen bond** and are similar in strength to ionic bonds.

Review Video: Covalent Bonds
Visit mometrix.com/academy and enter code: 482899

Covalent bonding occurs most frequently between atoms with similar **electronegativities**. **Nonmetals** are more likely to form covalent bonds than metals since it is more difficult for nonmetals to liberate an electron. **Electron sharing** takes place when one species encounters another species with similar electronegativity. Covalent bonding of metals is important in both *process chemistry* and *industrial catalysis.*

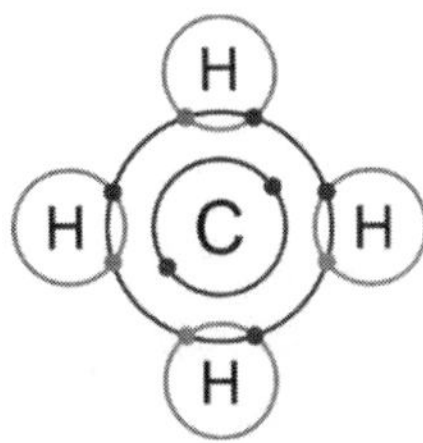

ELECTRONEGATIVITY

Electronegativity is a measure of how capable an atom is of attracting a pair of bonding electrons. It refers to the fact that one atom exerts slightly more force in a bond than another, creating a **dipole**. If the electronegative difference between two atoms is small, the atoms will form a **polar covalent bond**. If the difference is large, the atoms will form an **ionic bond**. When there is no electronegativity, a **pure nonpolar covalent bond** is formed.

Review Video: Electronegativity
Visit mometrix.com/academy and enter code: 823348

COMPOUNDS

An **element** is the most basic type of matter. It has unique properties and cannot be broken down into other elements. The smallest unit of an element is the **atom**. A chemical combination of two or more types of elements is called a **compound**.

Compounds often have properties that are very different from those of their constituent elements. The smallest independent unit of an element or compound is known as a **molecule**. Most elements are found somewhere in nature in single-atom form, but a few elements only exist naturally in pairs. These are called **diatomic elements**, of which some of the most common are hydrogen, nitrogen, and oxygen.

Elements and compounds are represented by **chemical symbols**, one or two letters, most often the first in the element name. More than one atom of the same element in a compound is represented with a subscript number designating how many atoms of that element are present. Water, for instance, contains two hydrogens and one oxygen. Thus, the chemical formula is H_2O. Methane contains one carbon and four hydrogens, so its formula is CH_4.

The Periodic Table

Period ↓ / Group →	1	2	3	4	5	6	7	8	9	10	11	12	13	14	15	16	17	18
1	1 H																	2 He
2	3 Li	4 Be											5 B	6 C	7 N	8 O	9 F	10 Ne
3	11 Na	12 Mg											13 Al	14 Si	15 P	16 S	17 Cl	18 Ar
4	19 K	20 Ca	21 Sc	22 Ti	23 V	24 Cr	25 Mn	26 Fe	27 Co	28 Ni	29 Cu	30 Zn	31 Ga	32 Ge	33 As	34 Se	35 Br	36 Kr
5	37 Rb	38 Sr	39 Y	40 Zr	41 Nb	42 Mo	43 Tc	44 Ru	45 Rh	46 Pd	47 Ag	48 Cd	49 In	50 Sn	51 Sb	52 Te	53 I	54 Xe
6	55 Cs	56 Ba	*	72 Hf	73 Ta	74 W	75 Re	76 Os	77 Ir	78 Pt	79 Au	80 Hg	81 Tl	82 Pb	83 Bi	84 Po	85 At	86 Rn
7	87 Fr	88 Ra	**	104 Rf	105 Db	106 Sg	107 Bh	108 Hs	109 Mt	110 Ds	111 Rg	112 Cn	113 Nh	114 Fl	115 Mc	116 Lv	117 Ts	118 Og

*	57 La	58 Ce	59 Pr	60 Nd	61 Pm	62 Sm	63 Eu	64 Gd	65 Tb	66 Dy	67 Ho	68 Er	69 Tm	70 Yb	71 Lu
**	89 Ac	90 Th	91 Pa	92 U	93 Np	94 Pu	95 Am	96 Cm	97 Bk	98 Cf	99 Es	100 Fm	101 Md	102 No	103 Lr

The **periodic table** is a tabular arrangement of the elements and is organized according to **periodic law**. The properties of the elements depend on their **atomic structure** and vary with **atomic number**. It shows periodic trends of physical and chemical properties and identifies families of elements with similar properties. In the periodic table, the elements are arranged by atomic number in horizontal rows called **periods** and vertical columns called **groups** or **families**. They are further categorized as metals, metalloids, or nonmetals. The majority of known elements are metals; there are seventeen nonmetals and eight metalloids. **Metals** are situated at the left end of the periodic table, **nonmetals** to the right and **metalloids** between the two.

A typical periodic table shows the elements' symbols and atomic number, the number of protons in the atomic nucleus. Some more detailed tables also list **atomic mass**, **electronegativity**, and other data. The position of an element in the table reveals its group, its block, and whether it is a representative, transition, or inner transition element. Its position also shows the element as a metal, nonmetal, or metalloid.

For the representative elements, the last digit of the **group number** reveals the number of outer-level electrons. Roman numerals for the A groups also reveal the number of outer level electrons within the group. The position of the element in the table reveals its **electronic configuration** and how it differs in atomic size from neighbors in its period or group. In this example, Boron has an atomic number of 5 and an atomic weight of 10.811. It is found in group 13, in which all atoms of the group have 3 valence electrons; the group's Roman numeral representation is IIIA.

Review Video: Periodic Table
Visit mometrix.com/academy and enter code: 154828

Important Features and Structure

The most important feature of the table is its arrangement according to **periodicity**, or the predictable trends observable in atoms. The arrangement enables classification, organization, and prediction of important elemental properties.

The table is organized in horizontal rows called **Periods**, and vertical columns called **Groups** or **Families**. Groups of elements share predictable characteristics, the most important of which is that their outer energy levels have the same configuration of electrons. For example, the highest group is group 18, the noble gases. Each element in this group has a full complement of electrons in its outer level, making the reactivity low. Elements in periods also share some common properties, but most classifications rely more heavily on groups.

Chemical Reactivity

Reactivity refers to the tendency of a substance to engage in **chemical reactions**. If that tendency is high, the substance is said to be highly reactive, or to have **high reactivity**. Because the basis of a chemical reaction is the transfer of electrons, reactivity depends upon the presence of uncommitted electrons which are available for transfer. **Periodicity** allows us to predict an element's reactivity based on its position on the periodic table. High numbered groups on the right side of the table have a fuller complement of electrons in their outer levels, making them less likely to react. Noble gases, on the far right of the table, each have eight electrons in the outer level, with the exception of He, which has two. Because atoms tend to lose or gain electrons to reach an ideal of eight in the outer level, these elements have very low reactivity.

Groups and Periods in Terms of Reactivity

Reading left to right within a period, each element contains one more electron than the one preceding it. (Note that H and He are in the same period, though nothing is between them and they are in different groups.) As electrons are added, their attraction to the nucleus increases, meaning that as we read to the right in a period, each atom's electrons are more densely compacted, more strongly bound to the nucleus, and less likely to be pulled away in reactions. As we read down a group, each successive atom's outer electrons are less tightly bound to the nucleus, thus increasing their reactivity, because the principal energy levels are increasingly full as we move downward within the group. **Principal energy levels** shield the outer energy levels from nuclear attraction, allowing the valence electrons to react. For this reason, noble gases farther down the group can react under certain circumstances.

Metals, Nonmetals, and Metalloids in the Periodic Table

The metals are located on the left side and center of the periodic table, and the nonmetals are located on the right side of the periodic table. The metalloids or semimetals form a zigzag line between the metals and nonmetals. Metals include the **alkali metals** such as lithium, sodium, and potassium and the **alkaline earth metals** such as beryllium, magnesium, and calcium. Metals also include the **transition metals** such as iron, copper, and nickel and the **inner transition metals** such as thorium, uranium, and plutonium. **Nonmetals** include the **chalcogens** such as oxygen and sulfur, the **halogens** such as fluorine and chlorine, and the **noble gases** such as helium and argon. Carbon, nitrogen, and phosphorus are also nonmetals. **Metalloids** or **semimetals** include boron, silicon, germanium, antimony, and polonium.

Properties of Substances

Intensive and Extensive Properties

Physical properties are categorized as either intensive or extensive. **Intensive properties** *do not* depend on the amount of matter or quantity of the sample. This means that intensive properties will not change if the sample size is increased or decreased. Intensive properties include color, hardness, melting point, boiling point, density, ductility, malleability, specific heat, temperature, concentration, and magnetization.

Extensive properties *do* depend on the amount of matter or quantity of the sample. Therefore, extensive properties do change if the sample size is increased or decreased. If the sample size is increased, the property increases. If the sample size is decreased, the property decreases. Extensive properties include volume, mass, weight, energy, entropy, number of moles, and electrical charge.

Physical Properties of Matter

Physical properties are any property of matter that can be **observed** or **measured**. These include properties such as color, elasticity, mass, volume, and temperature. **Mass** is a measure of the amount of substance in an object. **Weight** is a measure of the gravitational pull of Earth on an object. **Volume** is a measure of the amount of space occupied. There are many formulas to determine volume. For example, the volume of a cube is the length of one side cubed (a^3) and the volume of a rectangular prism is length times width times height ($l \times w \times h$). The volume of an irregular shape can be determined by how much water it displaces. **Density** is a measure of the amount of mass per unit volume. The formula to find density is mass divided by volume ($D = m/V$). It is expressed in terms of mass per cubic unit (e.g., grams per cubic centimeter $\frac{g}{cm^3}$). **Specific gravity** is a measure of the ratio of a substance's density compared to the density of water.

Density

The density of an object is equal to its *mass divided by its volume* ($d = m/v$). It is important to note the difference between an *object's density* and a *material's density*. Water has a density of one gram per cubic centimeter, while steel has a density approximately eight times that. Despite having a much higher material density, an object made of steel may still float. A hollow steel sphere, for instance, will float easily because the density of the object includes the air contained within the sphere.

Specific Heat Capacity

Specific heat capacity, also known as **specific heat**, is the *heat capacity per unit mass*. Each element and compound has its own specific heat. For example, it takes different amounts of heat energy to raise the temperature of the same amounts of magnesium and lead by one degree. The equation for relating heat energy to specific heat capacity is $Q = mc\Delta T$, where m represents the mass of the object, and c represents its specific heat capacity.

Review Video: Specific Heat Capacity
Visit mometrix.com/academy and enter code: 736791

Conduction

Heat always flows from a region of higher temperature to a region of lower temperature. If two regions are at the same temperature, there is a **thermal equilibrium** between them and there will be **no net heat transfer** between them. **Conduction** is a form of heat transfer that requires contact.

Since heat is a measure of kinetic energy, most commonly vibration, at the atomic level, it may be transferred from one location to another or one object to another by contact.

Chemical Properties of Matter

If a chemical change must be carried out in order to observe and measure a property, then the property is a **chemical property**. For example, when hydrogen gas is burned in oxygen, it forms water. This is a chemical property of hydrogen because after burning, a different chemical substance – water – is all that remains. The hydrogen cannot be recovered from the water by means of a physical change such as freezing or boiling.

> **Review Video: Physical and Chemical Properties of Matter**
> Visit mometrix.com/academy and enter code: 717349

Properties of Water

The important properties of water (H_2O) are high polarity, hydrogen bonding, cohesiveness, adhesiveness, high specific heat, high latent heat, and high heat of vaporization. Water is vital to life as we know it. The reason is that water is one of the main parts of many living things.

Water is a liquid at room temperature. The high specific heat of water means that it does not easily break its hydrogen bonds. Also, it resists heat and motion. This is why it has a high boiling point and high vaporization point.

Most substances are denser in their solid forms. However, water is different because its solid-state floats in its liquid state. Water is cohesive. This means that it is drawn to itself. It is also adhesive. This means that it draws in other molecules. If water will attach to another substance, the substance is said to be hydrophilic. Because of its cohesive and adhesive properties, water makes a good solvent. Substances with polar ions and molecules easily dissolve in water.

> **Review Video: Properties of Water**
> Visit mometrix.com/academy and enter code: 279526

Hydrogen Bonds

Hydrogen bonds are weaker than covalent and ionic bonds, and refer to the type of attraction in an **electronegative atom** such as oxygen, fluorine, or nitrogen. Hydrogen bonds can form within a single molecule or between molecules. A water molecule is **polar**, meaning it is partially positively charged on one end (the hydrogen end) and partially negatively charged on the other (the oxygen end). This is because the hydrogen atoms are arranged around the oxygen atom in a close tetrahedron. Hydrogen is **oxidized** (its number of electrons is reduced) when it bonds with oxygen to form water. Hydrogen bonds tend not only to be weak but also short-lived. They also tend to be numerous. Hydrogen bonds give water many of its important properties, including its high specific heat and high heat of vaporization, its solvent qualities, its adhesiveness and cohesiveness, its hydrophobic qualities, and its ability to float in its solid form. Hydrogen bonds are also an important component of *proteins, nucleic acids, and DNA*.

Passive Transport Mechanisms: Diffusion and Osmosis

Transport mechanisms allow for the movement of substances through membranes. **Passive transport mechanisms** include simple and facilitated diffusion and osmosis. They do not require energy from the cell. **Diffusion** occurs when particles are transported from areas of higher concentration to areas of lower concentration. When equilibrium is reached, diffusion stops. Examples are gas exchange (carbon dioxide and oxygen) during photosynthesis and the transport of oxygen from air to blood and from blood to tissue. **Facilitated diffusion** occurs when specific molecules are transported by a specific carrier protein. **Carrier proteins** vary in terms of size, shape, and charge. Glucose and amino acids are examples of substances transported by carrier proteins.

Review Video: Passive Transport: Diffusion and Osmosis
Visit mometrix.com/academy and enter code: 642038

Osmosis is the diffusion of water through a semi-permeable membrane from an area of lower solute concentration to one of higher solute concentration. Examples of osmosis include the absorption of water by plant roots and the alimentary canal. Plants lose and gain water through osmosis. A plant cell that swells because of water retention is said to be **turgid**.

States of Matter

Matter refers to substances that *have mass and occupy space* (or volume). The traditional definition of matter describes it as having three states: solid, liquid, and gas. These different states are caused by differences in the distances and angles between molecules or atoms, which result in differences in the energy that binds them. **Solid** structures are rigid or nearly rigid and have strong bonds. Molecules or atoms of **liquids** move around and have weak bonds, although they are not weak enough to readily break. Molecules or atoms of **gases** move almost independently of each other, are typically far apart, and do not form bonds. The current definition of matter describes it as having four states. The fourth is **plasma**, which is an ionized gas that has some electrons that are described as free because they are not bound to an atom or molecule. However, the HESI A2 will only be concerned with solids, liquids, and gases.

The table below outlines the characteristic properties of the three states of matter:

State of matter	Volume/shape	Density	Compressibility	Molecular motion
Gas	Assumes volume and shape of its container	Low	High	Very free motion
Liquid	Volume remains constant but it assumes shape of its container	High	Virtually none	Move past each other freely
Solid	Definite volume and shape	High	Virtually none	Vibrate around fixed positions

The three states of matter can be traversed by the addition or removal of **heat**. For example, when a solid is heated to its melting point, it can begin to form a liquid. However, in order to transition from solid to liquid, additional heat must be added at the melting point to overcome the **latent heat of fusion**. Upon further heating to its boiling point, the liquid can begin to form a gas, but again, additional heat must be added at the boiling point to overcome the **latent heat of vaporization**.

In the solid state, water is less dense than in the liquid state. This can be observed quite simply by noting that an ice cube floats at the surface of a glass of water. Were this not the case, ice would not form on the surface of lakes and rivers in those regions of the world where the climate produces temperatures below the freezing point. If water behaved as other substances do, lakes and rivers would freeze from the bottom up, which would be detrimental to many forms of aquatic life.

The lower density of ice occurs because of a combination of the unique structure of the water molecule and hydrogen bonding. In the case of ice, each oxygen atom is bound to four hydrogen atoms, two covalently and two by hydrogen bonds. This forms an ordered roughly **tetrahedral** structure that prevents the molecules from getting close to each other. As such, there are empty spaces in the structure that account for the low density of ice.

Review Video: States of Matter
Visit mometrix.com/academy and enter code: 742449

Review Video: States of Matter [Advanced]
Visit mometrix.com/academy and enter code: 298130

Changes in States of Matter

A substance that is undergoing a change from a solid to a liquid is said to be **melting**. If this change occurs in the opposite direction, from liquid to solid, this change is called **freezing**. A liquid which is being converted to a gas is undergoing **vaporization**. The reverse of this process is known as **condensation**. Direct transitions from gas to solid and solid to gas are much less common in everyday life, but they can occur given the proper conditions. Solid to gas conversion is known as **sublimation**, while the reverse is called **deposition**.

Evaporation: Evaporation is the change of state in a substance from a liquid to a gaseous form at a temperature below its boiling point (the temperature at which all of the molecules in a liquid are changed to gas through vaporization). Some of the molecules at the surface of a liquid always maintain enough **heat energy** to escape the cohesive forces exerted on them by neighboring molecules. At higher temperatures, the molecules in a substance move more rapidly, increasing their number with enough energy to break out of the liquid form. The rate of evaporation is higher when more of the surface area of a liquid is exposed (as in a large water body, such as an ocean). The amount of moisture already in the air also affects the rate of evaporation—if there is a significant amount of water vapor in the air around a liquid, some evaporated molecules will return to the liquid. The speed of the evaporation process is also decreased by increased **atmospheric pressure**.

Condensation: Condensation is the phase change in a substance from a gaseous to liquid form; it is the opposite of evaporation or vaporization. When temperatures decrease in a gas, such as water vapor, the material's component molecules move more slowly. The decreased motion of the molecules enables **intermolecular cohesive forces** to pull the molecules closer together and, in water, establish hydrogen bonds. Condensation can also be caused by an increase in the pressure exerted on a gas, which results in a decrease in the substance's volume (it reduces the distance between particles). In the **hydrologic cycle**, this process is initiated when warm air containing water vapor rises and then cools. This occurs due to convection in the air, meteorological fronts, or lifting over high land formations.

Chemical Reactions

Chemical reactions measured in human time can take place quickly or slowly. They can take a fraction of a second or billions of years. The **rates** of chemical reactions are determined by how frequently reacting atoms and molecules interact. Rates are also influenced by the temperature and various properties (such as shape) of the reacting materials. **Catalysts** accelerate chemical reactions, while **inhibitors** decrease reaction rates. Some types of reactions release energy in the form of heat and light. Some types of reactions involve the transfer of either electrons or hydrogen ions between reacting ions, molecules, or atoms. In other reactions, chemical bonds are broken down by heat or light to form **reactive radicals** with electrons that will readily form new bonds. Processes such as the formation of ozone and greenhouse gases in the atmosphere and the burning and processing of fossil fuels are controlled by radical reactions.

Review Video: Understanding Chemical Reactions
Visit mometrix.com/academy and enter code: 579876

Reading and Balancing Chemical Equations

Chemical equations describe chemical reactions. The reactants are on the left side before the arrow. The products are on the right side after the arrow. The arrow is the mark that points to the reaction or change. The coefficient is the number before the element. This gives the ratio of reactants to products in terms of moles.

The equation for making water from hydrogen and oxygen is $2H_{2(g)} + O_{2(g)} \rightarrow 2H_2O_{(l)}$. The number 2 before hydrogen and water is the coefficient. This means that there are 2 moles of hydrogen and 2 of water. There is 1 mole of oxygen. This does not need to have the number 1 before the symbol for the element. For additional information, the following subscripts are often included to indicate the state of the substance: (g) stands for gas, (l) stands for liquid, (s) stands for solid, and (aq) stands for aqueous. Aqueous means the substance is dissolved in water. Charges are shown by superscript for individual ions, not for ionic compounds. Polyatomic ions are separated by parentheses. This is done so the kind of ion will not be confused with the number of ions.

An unbalanced equation does not follow the law of conservation of mass. This law says that matter can only be changed, not created. If an equation is unbalanced, the numbers of atoms shown by the coefficients on each side of the arrow will not be equal.

To balance a chemical equation, you start by writing the formulas for each element or compound in the reaction. Next, count the atoms on each side and decide if the number is equal. Coefficients must be whole numbers. Fractional amounts (e.g., half a molecule) are not possible. Equations can be balanced by multiplying the coefficients by a constant that will make the smallest possible whole number coefficient. $H_2 + O_2 \rightarrow H_2O$ is an example of an unbalanced equation. The balanced equation is $2H_2 + O_2 \rightarrow 2H_2O$. This equation shows that it takes two moles of hydrogen and one of oxygen to make two moles of water.

Review Video: How Do You Balance Chemical Equations?
Visit mometrix.com/academy and enter code: 341228

Law of Conservation of Mass

The Law of Conservation of Mass in a chemical reaction is commonly stated as follows:

In a chemical reaction, matter is neither created nor destroyed.

What this means is that there will always be the same **total mass** of material after a reaction as before. This allows for predicting how molecules will combine by balanced equations in which the number of each type of atom is the same on either side of the equation. For example, two hydrogen molecules combine with one oxygen molecule to form water. This is a balanced chemical equation because the number of each type of atom is the same on both sides of the arrow. It has to balance because the reaction obeys the Law of Conservation of Mass.

Mechanism of Reactions

Chemical reactions normally occur when electrons are transferred from one atom or molecule to another. Reactions and reactivity depend on the **octet rule**, which describes the tendency of atoms to gain or lose electrons until their outer energy levels contain eight. The changes in a reaction may be in **composition** or **configuration** of a compound or substance, and result in one or more products being generated which were not present in isolation before the reaction occurred. For instance, when oxygen reacts with methane (CH_4), water and carbon dioxide are the products; one set of substances ($CH_4 + O$) was transformed into a new set of substances ($CO_2 + H_2O$).

Reactions depend on the presence of a **reactant**, or substance undergoing change, a **reagent**, or partner in the reaction less transformed than the reactant (such as a catalyst), and **products**, or the final result of the reaction. **Reaction conditions**, or environmental factors, are also important components in reactions. These include conditions such as temperature, pressure, concentration, whether the reaction occurs in solution, the type of solution, and presence or absence of catalysts. Chemical reactions are usually written in the following format: Reactants → Products.

Five Types of Reactions

Combination Reactions

Combination reactions: In a combination reaction, two or more reactants combine to make one product. This can be seen in the equation $A + B \rightarrow AB$. These reactions are also known as synthesis or addition reactions. An example is burning hydrogen in air to produce water. The equation is $2H_2 (g) + O_2 (g) \rightarrow 2H_2O (l)$. Another example is when water and sulfur trioxide react to form sulfuric acid. The equation is $H_2O + SO_3 \rightarrow H_2SO_4$.

Decomposition Reactions

Decomposition (or *desynthesis, decombination, or deconstruction*) reactions are considered chemical reactions whereby a reactant is broken down into two or more products. This can be seen in the equation $AB \rightarrow A + B$. These reactions are also called analysis reactions. When a compound or substance separates into these simpler substances, the byproducts are often substances that are different from the original. Decomposition can be viewed as the *opposite* of combination reactions. These reactions are also called analysis reactions. Most decomposition reactions are **endothermic**. Heat needs to be added for the chemical reaction to occur. **Thermal decomposition** is caused by heat. **Electrolytic decomposition** is due to electricity. An example of this type of reaction is the decomposition of water into hydrogen and oxygen gas. The equation is $2H_2O \rightarrow 2H_2 + O_2$. Separation processes can be **mechanical** or **chemical**, and usually involve reorganizing a mixture of substances without changing their chemical nature. The separated products may differ from the original mixture in terms of chemical or physical properties. Types of separation processes include **filtration**, **crystallization**, **distillation**, and **chromatography**. Basically, decomposition *breaks down* one compound into two or more compounds or substances that are different from the original; separation *sorts* the substances from the original mixture into like substances.

SINGLE REPLACEMENT REACTIONS

Single substitution, displacement, or replacement reactions occur when one reactant is displaced by another to form the final product (A + BC → B + AC). Single substitution reactions can be **cationic** or **anionic**. When a piece of copper (Cu) is placed into a solution of silver nitrate ($AgNO_3$), the solution turns blue. The copper appears to be replaced with a silvery-white material. The equation is $2AgNO_3 + Cu \rightarrow Cu(NO_3)_2 + 2Ag$. When this reaction takes place, the copper dissolves and the silver in the silver nitrate solution precipitates (becomes a solid), thus resulting in copper nitrate and silver. Copper and silver have switched places in the nitrate.

Review Video: What is a Single-Replacement Reaction?
Visit mometrix.com/academy and enter code: 442975

DOUBLE REPLACEMENT REACTIONS

Double displacement, double replacement, substitution, metathesis, or ion exchange reactions occur when ions or bonds are exchanged by two compounds to form different compounds (AC + BD → AD + BC). An example of this is that silver nitrate and sodium chloride form two different products (silver chloride and sodium nitrate) when they react. The formula for this reaction is $AgNO_3 + NaCl \rightarrow AgCl + NaNO_3$.

Double replacement reactions are metathesis reactions. In a **double replacement reaction**, the chemical reactants exchange ions. However, the oxidation state stays the same. One of the signs of this is the building of a solid precipitate. In acid/base reactions, an acid is a compound that can donate a proton. A base is a compound that can accept a proton. In these types of reactions, the acid and base react to make salt and water. When the proton is donated, the base becomes water. So, the remaining ions make a salt. One way to know if a reaction is a redox or a metathesis reaction is to note the oxidation number of atoms in the reaction. It does not change during a metathesis reaction.

COMBUSTION REACTIONS

Combustion, or burning, is a sequence of chemical reactions involving **fuel** and an **oxidant** that produces heat and sometimes light. There are many types of combustion, such as rapid, slow, complete, turbulent, microgravity, and incomplete. Fuels and oxidants determine the **compounds** formed by a combustion reaction. For example, when rocket fuel consisting of hydrogen and oxygen combusts, it results in the formation of water vapor. When air and wood burn, resulting compounds include nitrogen, unburned carbon, and carbon compounds. Combustion is an **exothermic** process, meaning it releases energy. Exothermic energy is commonly released as heat, but can take other forms, such as light, electricity, or sound.

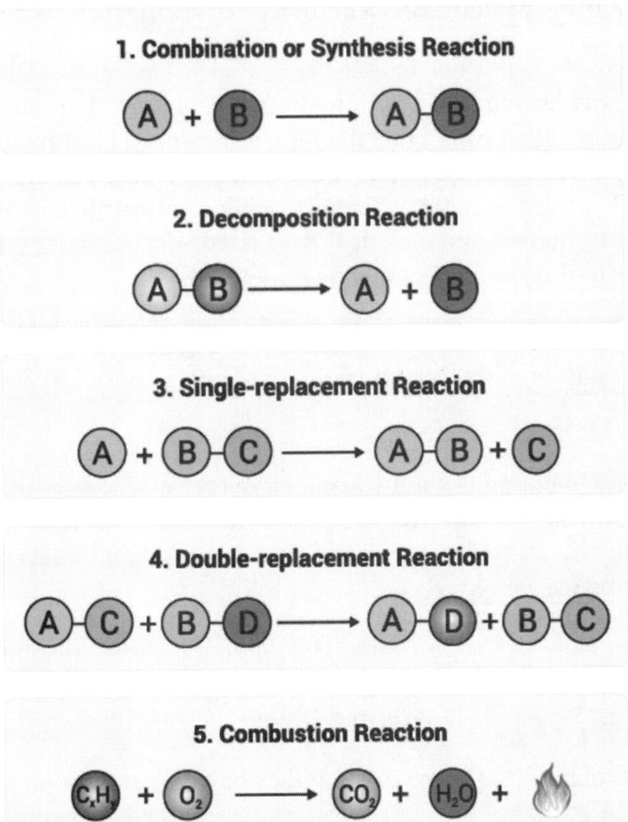

Review Video: Combustion
Visit mometrix.com/academy and enter code: 592219

Catalysts

Catalysts, substances that help *change the rate of reaction* without changing their form, can increase reaction rate by decreasing the number of steps it takes to form products. The **mass** of the catalyst should be the same at the beginning of the reaction as it is at the end. The **activation energy** is the minimum amount required to get a reaction started. Activation energy causes particles to collide with sufficient energy to start the reaction. A **catalyst** enables more particles to react, which lowers the activation energy. Examples of catalysts in reactions are manganese oxide (MnO_2) in the decomposition of hydrogen peroxide, iron in the manufacture of ammonia using the Haber process, and concentrate of sulfuric acid in the nitration of benzene.

Review Video: Catalysts
Visit mometrix.com/academy and enter code: 288189

Acids, Bases, and Salts

pH

The **potential of hydrogen** (pH) is a measurement of the *concentration of hydrogen ions* in a substance in terms of the number of moles of H^+ per liter of solution. All substances fall between 0 and 14 on the pH scale. A lower pH indicates a higher H^+ concentration, while a higher pH indicates a lower H^+ concentration.

Pure water has a **neutral pH**, which is 7. Anything with a pH lower than pure water (<7) is considered **acidic**. Anything with a pH higher than pure water (>7) is a **base**. Drain cleaner, soap, baking soda, ammonia, egg whites, and sea water are common bases. Urine, stomach acid, citric acid, vinegar, hydrochloric acid, and battery acid are acids. A **pH indicator** is a substance that acts as a detector of hydrogen or hydronium ions. It is **halochromic**, meaning it changes color to indicate that hydrogen or hydronium ions have been detected.

Review Video: Overview of pH Levels
Visit mometrix.com/academy and enter code: 187395

Bases

Basic chemicals are usually in aqueous solution and have the following traits: a bitter taste; a soapy or slippery texture to the touch; the capacity to restore the blue color of litmus paper which had previously been turned red by an acid; the ability to produce salts in reaction with acids. The word **alkaline** is used to describe bases.

In contrast to acids, which yield **hydrogen ions** (H^+) when dissolved in solution, bases yield **hydroxide ions** (OH^-); the same models used to describe acids can be inverted and used to describe bases—Arrhenius, Bronsted-Lowry, and Lewis.

Some **nonmetal oxides** (such as Na_2O) are classified as bases even though they do not contain hydroxides in their molecular form. However, these substances easily produce hydroxide ions when reacted with water, which is why they are classified as bases.

Acids

Acids are a unique class of compounds characterized by consistent properties. The most significant property of an acid is not readily observable and is what gives acids their unique behaviors: the **ionization of H atoms**, or their tendency to dissociate from their parent molecules and take on an electrical charge. **Carboxylic acids** are also characterized by ionization, but of the O atoms. Some other properties of acids are easy to observe without any experimental apparatus. These properties include the following:

- They have a sour taste
- They change the color of litmus paper to red
- They produce gaseous H_2 in reaction with some metals
- They produce salt precipitates in reaction with bases

Other properties, while no more complex, are less easily observed. For instance, most inorganic acids are easily soluble in water and have high boiling points.

Strong or Weak Acids and Bases

The characteristic properties of acids and bases derive from the tendency of atoms to **ionize** by donating or accepting charged particles. The strength of an acid or base is a reflection of the degree to which its atoms ionize in solution. For example, if all of the atoms in an acid ionize, the acid is said to be **strong**. When only a few of the atoms ionize, the acid is **weak**. Acetic acid ($HC_2H_3O_2$) is a weak acid because only its O_2 atoms ionize in solution. Another way to think of the strength of an acid or base is to consider its **reactivity**. Highly reactive acids and bases are strong because they tend to form and break bonds quickly and most of their atoms ionize in the process.

Review Video: Strong and Weak Acids and Bases
Visit mometrix.com/academy and enter code: 268930

Salts

Some properties of **salts** are that they are formed from acid base reactions, are ionic compounds consisting of metallic and nonmetallic ions, dissociate in water, and are comprised of tightly bonded ions. Some common salts are sodium chloride (NaCl), sodium bisulfate, potassium dichromate ($K_2Cr_2O_7$), and calcium chloride ($CaCl_2$). Calcium chloride is used as a drying agent, and may be used to absorb moisture when freezing mixtures. Potassium nitrate (KNO_3) is used to make fertilizer and in the manufacture of explosives. Sodium nitrate ($NaNO_3$) is also used in the making of fertilizer. Baking soda (sodium bicarbonate) is a salt, as are Epsom salts [magnesium sulfate ($MgSO_4$)]. Salt and water can react to form a base and an acid. This is called a **hydrolysis reaction**.

Biochemistry

CARBOHYDRATES

The simple sugars can be grouped into **monosaccharides** (glucose, fructose, and galactose) and **disaccharides.** These are both types of **carbohydrates.** Monosaccharides have one monomer of sugar and disaccharides have two. **Monosaccharides** (CH_2O) have one carbon for every water molecule. Aldose and ketose are monosaccharides with a carbonyl (=O, double bonded oxygen to carbon) functional group. The difference between aldose and ketose is that the carbonyl group in aldose is connected at an end carbon and the carbonyl group in ketose is connected at a middle carbon. Glucose is a monosaccharide containing six carbons, making it a hexose and an aldose. A **disaccharide** is formed from two monosaccharides with a glycosidic link. Examples include two glucoses forming a maltose, a glucose and a galactose forming a lactose, and a glucose and a fructose forming a sucrose. A starch is a polysaccharide consisting only of glucose monomers. Examples are amylose, amylopectin, and glycogen.

Review Video: Carbohydrates
Visit mometrix.com/academy and enter code: 601714

In **glycolysis**, glucose is converted into **pyruvate** and energy stored in ATP bonds is released. Glycolysis can involve various pathways. Various intermediates are produced that are used in other processes, and the pyruvic acid produced by glycolysis can be further used for respiration by the Krebs cycle or in fermentation. Glycolysis occurs in both aerobic and anaerobic organisms. Oxidation of molecules produces reduced **coenzymes**, such as NADH. The coenzymes relocate hydrogens to the electron transport chain. The proton is transported through the cell membrane and the electron is transported down the chain by proteins. At the end of the chain, water is formed when the final acceptor releases two electrons that combine with oxygen. The protons are pumped back into the cell or organelle by the **ATP synthase enzyme**, which uses energy produced to add a phosphate to ADP to form ATP. The **proton motive force** is produced by the protons being moved across the membrane.

Glycolysis can involve different metabolic pathways. The following 10 steps are based on the **Embden-Meyerhof pathway**, in which glucose is the starting product and pyruvic acid is the final product. Two molecules of ATP and two of NADH are the products of this process. To start, enzymes utilize ATP to form glucose-6-phosphate. The glucose-6 is converted to fructose-6-phosphate. Another ATP molecule and an enzyme are used to convert fructose-6-phosphate to fructose-1,6-disphosphate. Both dihydroxyacetone phosphate (DHAP) and glyceraldehyde-3-phosphate are formed from fructose-1,6-disphosphate. It is during the preceding reactions that energy is conserved or gained. NAD conversions to NADH molecules and phosphate influx result in 1,3-diphosphoglceric acid. Then, two ADP molecules are phosphorylated into ATP molecules, resulting in 3-phosphoglyceric acid, which reforms into 2-phosphoglyceric acid. At this point, water is produced as a product and phosphoenolpyruvic acid is formed. Another set of ADP molecules are phosphorylated into ATP molecules. **Pyruvic acid** is the end result.

Review Video: Glycolysis
Visit mometrix.com/academy and enter code: 466815

Glycolysis is a general term for the conversion of glucose into pyruvate.

Embden-Meyerhof pathway: This is a type of glycolysis in which one molecule of glucose becomes two ATP and two NADH molecules. Pyruvic acid (two pyruvate molecules) is the end product.

Entner-Doudoroff pathway: This is a type of glycolysis in which one glucose molecule forms into one molecule of ATP and two of NADPH, which are used for other reactions. The end product is two pyruvate molecules.

Pentose Phosphate pathway: Also known as the hexose monophosphate shunt, this is a type of glycolysis in which one glucose molecule produces one ATP and two NADPH molecules. Five carbon sugars are metabolized during this reaction. Glucose is broken down into ribose, ribulose, and xylose, which are used during glycolysis and during the Calvin (or Calvin-Benson) cycle to create nucleotides, nucleic acids, and amino acids.

PROTEINS

Proteins are macromolecules formed from amino acids. They are **polypeptides**, which consist of many (10 to 100) peptides linked together. The peptide connections are the result of condensation reactions. A **condensation reaction** results in a loss of water when two molecules are joined together. A **hydrolysis reaction** is the opposite of a condensation reaction. During hydrolysis, water is added. -H is added to one of the smaller molecules and OH is added to another molecule being formed. A **peptide** is a compound of two or more amino acids. **Amino acids** are formed by the partial hydrolysis of protein, which forms an amide bond. This partial hydrolysis involves an amine group and a carboxylic acid. In the carbon chain of amino acids, there is a carboxylic acid group (-COOH), an amine group ($-NH_2$), a central carbon atom between them with an attached hydrogen, and an attached "R" group (side chain), which is different for different amino acids. It is the "R" group that determines the properties of the protein.

Review Video: Proteins
Visit mometrix.com/academy and enter code: 903713

Alkyl: This is a nonpolar group that forms hydrophobic amino acids. Amino acids include glycine with a single hydrogen atom R group, alanine with a methyl R group, and valine with an isopropyl R group. Leucine and isoleucine also have alkyl side chains.

Hydroxyl: This is a polar group that forms hydrophilic amino acids such as serine and threonine.

Sulfur: Amino acids in this group include cysteine and methionine.

Carboxylic acid: In this group, a second carboxylic acid group is attached as the R group. This acid group is polar and can be negatively charged when the acidic proton attaches to a water molecule, which leaves a negatively charged carboxylate ion. Amino acids that belong to this group include aspartic acid and glutamic acid.

Amide: The formula for amides is $-CONH_2$. Amino acids belonging to this group include glutamine and asparagine.

Amino: This group includes lysine, arginine, and histidine. The double-bonded nitrogen atom can take a proton to become positively charged.

Aromatic: This group has a ring structure, and includes the amino acids phenylalanine, tyrosine, and tryptophan. Tyrosine is polar, while tryptophan and phenylalanine are nonpolar.

Looped: This group includes proline. Because it is nonpolar, it forms a ring rather than a chain.

LIPIDS

Carbohydrates, proteins, and nucleic acids are groups of macromolecules that are polymers. **Lipids** are molecules that are soluble in nonpolar solvents, but they are **hydrophobic**, meaning they do not bond well with water or mix well with water solutions. Lipids have numerous C-H bonds. In this way, they are similar to hydrocarbons (substances consisting only of carbon and hydrogen).The major roles of lipids include energy storage and structural functions. Examples of lipids include fats, phospholipids, steroids, and waxes. **Fats** (which are **triglycerides**) are made of long chains of fatty acids (three fatty acids bound to a glycerol). **Fatty acids** are chains with reduced carbon at one end and a carboxylic acid group at the other. An example is soap, which contains the sodium salts of free fatty acids. **Phospholipids** are lipids that have a phosphate group rather than a fatty acid. **Glycerides** are another type of lipid. Examples of glycerides are fat and oil. Glycerides are formed from fatty acids and glycerol (a type of alcohol).

Review Video: Lipids
Visit mometrix.com/academy and enter code: 269746

NUCLEIC ACIDS

Nucleic acids are macromolecules that are composed of nucleotides. **Hydrolysis** is a reaction in which water is broken down into hydrogen cations (H or H^+) and hydroxide anions (OH or OH^-). This is part of the process by which nucleic acids are broken down by enzymes to produce shorter strings of RNA and DNA (**oligonucleotides**). Oligonucleotides are broken down into smaller sugar nitrogenous units called nucleosides. These can be digested by cells since the sugar is divided from the nitrogenous base. This, in turn, leads to the formation of the five types of nitrogenous bases, sugars, and the preliminary substances involved in the synthesis of new RNA and DNA. DNA and RNA have a double helix shape.

Review Video: Nucleic Acids
Visit mometrix.com/academy and enter code: 503931

Macromolecular nucleic acid polymers, such as RNA and DNA, are formed from nucleotides, which are monomeric units joined by phosphodiester bonds. Cells require energy in the form of **ATP** to synthesize proteins from amino acids and replicate DNA. **Nitrogen fixation** is used to synthesize nucleotides for DNA and amino acids for proteins. Nitrogen fixation uses the enzyme **nitrogenase** in the reduction of dinitrogen gas (N_2) to ammonia (NH_3). Nucleic acids store information and energy and are also important catalysts. It is the RNA that catalyzes the transfer of DNA genetic information into protein-coded information. ATP is an RNA nucleotide. **Nucleotides** are used to form the nucleic acids. Nucleotides are made of a five-carbon sugar, such as ribose or deoxyribose, a nitrogenous base, and one or more phosphates. Nucleotides consisting of more than one phosphate can also store energy in their bonds.

Chapter Quiz

Ready to see how well you retained what you just read? Scan the QR code to go directly to the chapter quiz interface for this study guide. If you're using a computer, simply visit the bonus page at **mometrix.com/bonus948/hesia2** and click the Chapter Quizzes link.

Anatomy and Physiology

Transform passive reading into active learning! After immersing yourself in this chapter, put your comprehension to the test by taking a quiz. The insights you gained will stay with you longer this way. Scan the QR code to go directly to the chapter quiz interface for this study guide. If you're using a computer, simply visit the bonus page at **mometrix.com/bonus948/hesia2** and click the Chapter Quizzes link.

The Anatomy and Physiology section of the HESI A^2 exam consists of 25 questions. **This section may or may not be included on your specific test**, depending on the requirements where you are applying.

General Anatomy and Physiology

Cell

The cell is the basic *organizational unit* of all living things. Each piece within a cell has a function that helps organisms grow and survive. There are many different types of cells, but cells are unique to each type of organism. The one thing that all cells have in common is a **membrane**, which is comparable to a semi-permeable plastic bag. The membrane is composed of **phospholipids**. There are also some **transport holes**, which are proteins that help certain molecules and ions move in and out of the cell. The cell is filled with a fluid called **cytoplasm** or cytosol.

Within the cell are a variety of **organelles**, groups of complex molecules that help a cell survive, each with its own unique membrane that has a different chemical makeup from the cell membrane. The larger the cell, the more organelles it will need to live.

All organisms, whether plants, animals, fungi, protists, or bacteria, exhibit structural organization on the cellular and organism level. All cells contain **DNA** and **RNA** and can synthesize proteins. All organisms have a highly organized cellular structure. Each cell consists of **nucleic acids**, **cytoplasm**, and a **cell membrane**. Specialized organelles such as **mitochondria** and **chloroplasts** have specific functions within the cell. In single-celled organisms, that single cell contains all of the components necessary for life. In multicellular organisms, cells can become specialized. Different types of cells can have different functions. Life begins as a single cell whether by **asexual** or **sexual reproduction**. Cells are grouped together in **tissues**. Tissues are grouped together in **organs**. Organs are grouped together in **systems**. An **organism** is a complete individual.

Review Video: Cell Structure
Visit mometrix.com/academy and enter code: 591293

Cell Structure

Ribosomes: Ribosomes are involved in *synthesizing proteins from amino acids*. They are numerous, making up about one quarter of the cell. Some cells contain thousands of ribosomes. Some are mobile and some are embedded in the rough **endoplasmic reticulum**.

Golgi complex (Golgi apparatus): This is involved in *synthesizing materials* such as proteins that are transported out of the cell. It is located near the nucleus and consists of layers of **membranes**.

Vacuoles: These are sacs used for *storage, digestion, and waste removal.* There is one large vacuole in plant cells. Animal cells have small, sometimes numerous vacuoles.

Vesicle: This is a small organelle within a cell. It has a membrane and performs varying functions, including *moving materials within a cell.*

Cytoskeleton: This consists of **microtubules** that help *shape and support the cell.*

Microtubules: These are part of the **cytoskeleton** and help *support the cell.* They are made of protein.

Cytosol: This is the *liquid material in the cell.* It is mostly water, but also contains some floating molecules.

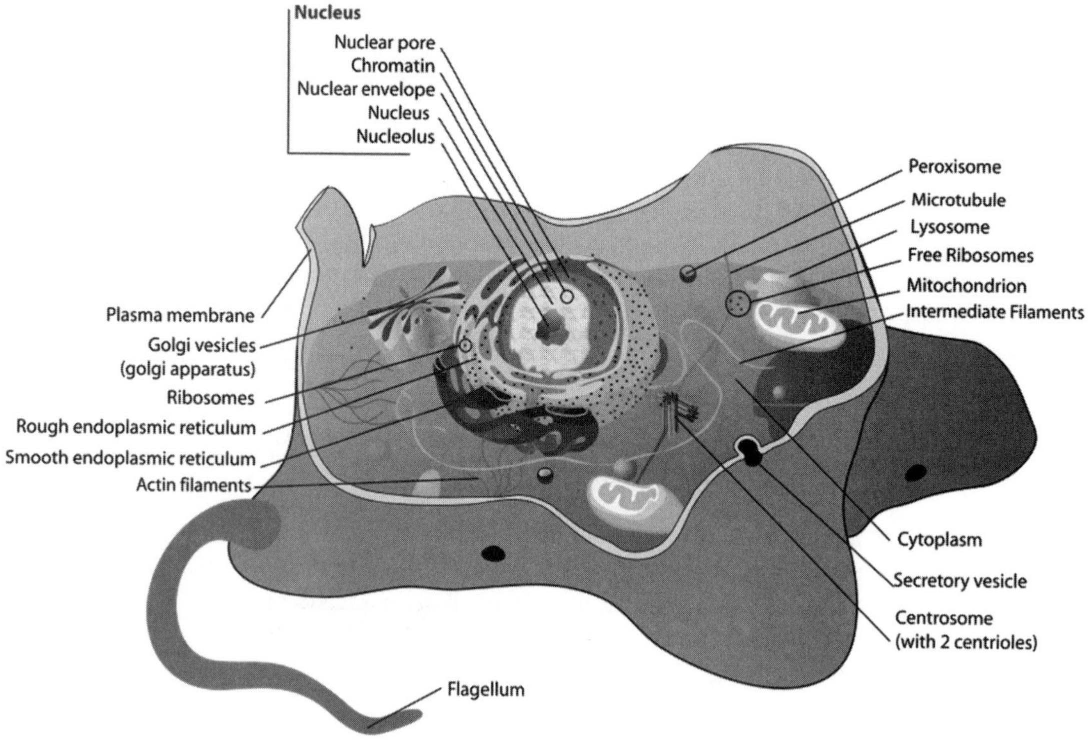

Cytoplasm: This is a general term that refers to cytosol and the substructures (organelles) found *within the plasma membrane*, but not within the nucleus.

Cell membrane (plasma membrane): This defines the cell by acting as a *barrier.* It helps keeps cytoplasm in and substances located outside the cell out. It also determines what is allowed to enter and exit the cell.

Endoplasmic reticulum: The two types of endoplasmic reticulum are **rough** (has ribosomes on the surface) and **smooth** (does not have ribosomes on the surface). It is a tubular network that comprises the *transport system of a cell.* It is fused to the nuclear membrane and extends through the cytoplasm to the cell membrane.

Mitochondrion (pl. mitochondria): These cell structures vary in terms of size and quantity. Some cells may have one mitochondrion, while others have thousands. This structure performs various functions such as *generating ATP*, and is also involved in *cell growth and death*. Mitochondria contain their own DNA that is separate from that contained in the nucleus.

Mitochondria Functions

Four functions of mitochondria are: the production of **cell energy**, **cell signaling** (how communications are carried out within a cell, **cellular differentiation** (the process whereby a non-differentiated cell becomes transformed into a cell with a more specialized purpose), and **cell cycle and growth regulation** (the process whereby the cell gets ready to reproduce and reproduces). Mitochondria are numerous in eukaryotic cells. There may be hundreds or even thousands of mitochondria in a single cell. Mitochondria can be involved in many functions, their main one being *supplying the cell with energy*. Mitochondria consist of an inner and outer membrane. The inner membrane encloses the **matrix**, which contains the **mitochondrial DNA** (mtDNA) and ribosomes. Between the inner and outer membranes are **folds** (cristae). Chemical reactions occur here that release energy, control water levels in cells, and recycle and create proteins and fats. **Aerobic respiration** also occurs in the mitochondria.

Review Video: Mitochondria
Visit mometrix.com/academy and enter code: 444287

Animal Cell Structure

Centrosome: This is comprised of the pair of **centrioles** located at right angles to each other and surrounded by protein. The centrosome is involved in *mitosis and the cell cycle.*

Centrioles: These are cylinder-shaped structures near the nucleus that are involved in *cellular division*. Each cylinder consists of nine groups of three **microtubules**. Centrioles occur in pairs.

Lysosome: This *digests proteins, lipids, and carbohydrates*, and also *transports undigested substances* to the cell membrane so they can be removed. The shape of a lysosome depends on the material being transported.

Cilia (singular: cilium): These are appendages extending from the surface of the cell, the movement of which *causes the cell to move*. They can also result in fluid being moved by the cell.

Flagella: These are tail-like structures on cells that use whip-like movements to *help the cell move*. They are similar to cilia, but are usually longer and not as numerous. A cell usually only has one or a few flagella.

Nuclear Parts of a Cell

- **Nucleus** (pl. nuclei): This is a small structure that contains the **chromosomes** and regulates the **DNA** of a cell. The nucleus is the defining structure of **eukaryotic cells**, and all eukaryotic cells have a nucleus. The nucleus is responsible for the passing on of genetic traits between generations. The nucleus contains a *nuclear envelope, nucleoplasm, a nucleolus, nuclear pores, chromatin, and ribosomes.*
- **Chromosomes**: These are highly condensed, threadlike rods of **DNA**. Short for **deoxyribonucleic acid**, DNA is the genetic material that *stores information about the plant or animal.*
- **Chromatin**: This consists of the DNA and protein that make up **chromosomes**.
- **Nucleolus**: This structure contained within the nucleus consists of protein. It is small, round, does not have a membrane, is involved in **protein synthesis**, and synthesizes and stores **RNA** (**ribonucleic acid**).

- **Nuclear envelope**: This encloses the structures of the nucleus. It consists of inner and outer membranes made of **lipids**.
- **Nuclear pores**: These are involved in the exchange of material between the nucleus and the **cytoplasm**.
- **Nucleoplasm**: This is the liquid within the nucleus, and is similar to cytoplasm.

CELL MEMBRANES

The cell membrane, also referred to as the **plasma membrane**, is a thin semipermeable membrane of lipids and proteins. The cell membrane isolates the cell from its external environment while still enabling the cell to communicate with that outside environment. It consists of a **phospholipid bilayer**, or double layer, with the **hydrophilic ends** of the outer layer facing the external environment, the inner layer facing the inside of the cell, and the **hydrophobic ends** facing each other. **Cholesterol** in the cell membrane adds stiffness and flexibility. **Glycolipids** help the cell to recognize other cells of the organisms. The **proteins** in the cell membrane help give the cells shape. Special proteins help the cell communicate with its external environment. Other proteins transport molecules across the cell membrane.

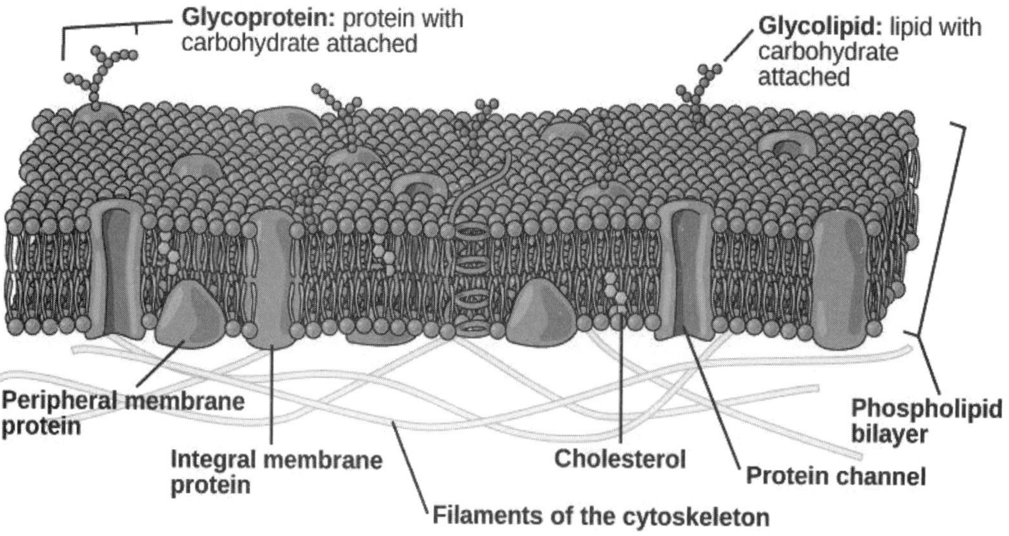

SELECTIVE PERMEABILITY

The cell membrane, or plasma membrane, has **selective permeability** with regard to size, charge, and solubility. With regard to molecule size, the cell membrane allows only small molecules to diffuse through it. **Oxygen** and **water** molecules are small and typically can pass through the cell membrane. The charge of the **ions** on the cell's surface also either attracts or repels ions. Ions with like charges are repelled, and ions with opposite charges are attracted to the cell's surface. Molecules that are soluble in **phospholipids** can usually pass through the cell membrane. Many molecules are not able to diffuse the cell membrane, and, if needed, those molecules must be moved through by active transport and **vesicles**.

CELL CYCLE

The term cell cycle refers to the process by which a cell **reproduces**, which involves *cell growth, the duplication of genetic material, and cell division*. Complex organisms with many cells use the cell cycle to replace cells as they lose their functionality and wear out. The entire cell cycle in animal cells can take 24 hours. The time required varies among different cell types. Human skin cells, for example, are constantly reproducing. Some other cells only divide infrequently. Once neurons are mature, they do not grow or divide. The two ways that cells can reproduce are through meiosis and mitosis. When cells replicate through **mitosis**, the "daughter cell" is an *exact replica* of the parent cell. When cells divide through **meiosis**, the daughter cells have *different genetic coding* than the parent cell. Meiosis only happens in specialized reproductive cells called **gametes**.

Cell Differentiation

The human body is filled with many different types of cells. The process that helps to determine the cell type for each cell is known as **differentiation**. Another way to say this is when *a less-specialized cell becomes a more-specialized cell*. This process is controlled by the genes of each cell among a group of cells known as a **zygote**. Following the directions of the genes, a cell builds certain proteins and other pieces that set it apart as a specific type of cell.

An example occurs with **gastrulation**—an early phase in the embryonic development of most animals. During gastrulation, the cells are organized into three primary germ layers: **ectoderm**, **mesoderm**, and **endoderm**. Then, the cells in these layers differentiate into special tissues and organs. For example, the *nervous system* develops from the ectoderm. The *muscular system* develops from the mesoderm. Much of the *digestive system* develops from the endoderm.

Mitosis

The primary events that occur during mitosis are:

- **Interphase**: The cell prepares for division by replicating its genetic and cytoplasmic material. Interphase can be further divided into G_1, S, and G_2.
- **Prophase**: The **chromatin** thickens into chromosomes and the **nuclear membrane** begins to disintegrate. Pairs of **centrioles** move to opposite sides of the cell and spindle fibers begin to form. The **mitotic spindle**, formed from cytoskeleton parts, moves chromosomes around within the cell.
- **Metaphase**: The spindle moves to the center of the cell and chromosome pairs align along the center of the spindle structure.
- **Anaphase**: The pairs of chromosomes, called sisters, begin to pull apart, and may bend. When they are separated, they are called **daughter chromosomes**. Grooves appear in the cell membrane.
- **Telophase**: The spindle disintegrates, the nuclear membranes reform, and the chromosomes revert to chromatin. In animal cells, the membrane is pinched. In plant cells, a new cell wall begins to form.
- **Cytokinesis**: This is the physical splitting of the cell (including the cytoplasm) into two cells. Some believe this occurs following telophase. Others say it occurs from anaphase, as the cell begins to furrow, through telophase, when the cell actually splits into two.

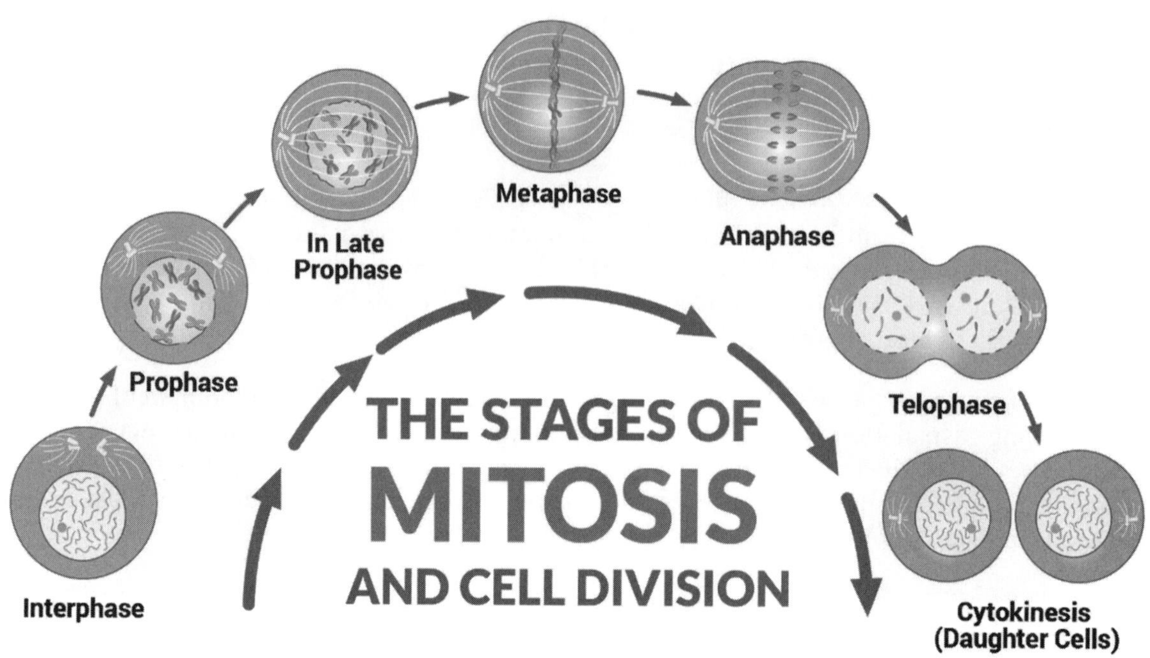

Review Video: Mitosis
Visit mometrix.com/academy and enter code: 849894

Meiosis

Meiosis has the same phases as mitosis, but they happen twice. In addition, different events occur during some phases of meiosis than mitosis. The events that occur during the first phase of meiosis are interphase (I), prophase (I), metaphase (I), anaphase (I), telophase (I), and cytokinesis (I). During this first phase of meiosis, *chromosomes cross over, genetic material is exchanged, and tetrads of four chromatids are formed*. The nuclear membrane dissolves. Homologous pairs of chromatids are separated and travel to different poles. At this point, there has been one cell division resulting in two cells. Each cell goes through a second cell division, which consists of prophase (II), metaphase (II), anaphase (II), telophase (II), and cytokinesis (II). The result is *four daughter cells* with different sets of chromosomes. The daughter cells are **haploid**, which means they contain half the genetic material of the parent cell. The second phase of meiosis is similar to the process of mitosis. Meiosis encourages genetic diversity.

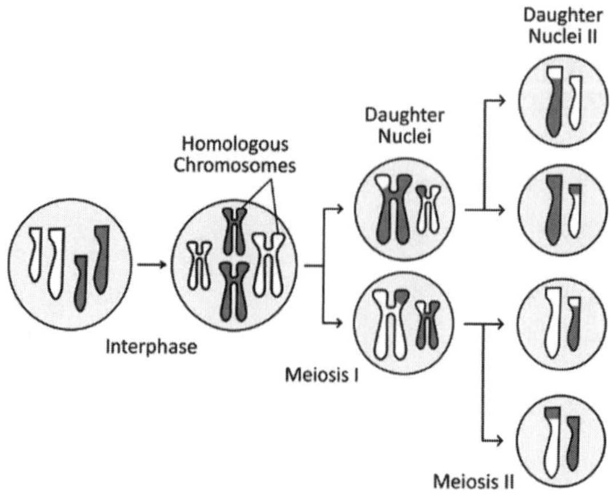

Tissues

Tissues are groups of cells that work together to perform a specific function. Tissues are divided into broad categories based on their function. Animal tissues may be divided into seven categories:

- **Epithelial** – Tissue in which cells are joined together tightly. *Skin* tissue is an example.
- **Connective** – Connective tissue may be dense, loose, or fatty. It protects and binds body parts. Connective tissues include *bone tissue, cartilage, tendons, ligaments, fat, blood, and lymph.*
- **Cartilage** – Cushions and provides structural support for body parts. It has a jelly-like base and is fibrous.
- **Blood** – Blood transports oxygen to cells and removes wastes. It also carries hormones and defends against disease.
- **Bone** – Bone is a hard tissue that supports and protects softer tissues and organs. Its marrow produces red blood cells.
- **Muscle** – Muscle tissue helps support and move the body. The three types of muscle tissue are *smooth, cardiac, and skeletal.*
- **Nervous** – Nerve tissue is located in the *brain, spinal cord, and nerves.* Cells called neurons form a network through the body that controls responses to changes in the external and internal environment. Some send signals to muscles and glands to trigger responses.

Organs

Organs are groups of tissues that work together to perform specific functions. Complex animals have several organs that are grouped together in multiple **systems**. For example, the **heart** is specifically designed to pump blood throughout an organism's body. The heart is composed mostly of muscle tissue in the myocardium, but it also contains connective tissue in the blood and membranes, nervous tissue that controls the heart rate, and epithelial tissue in the membranes. Gills in fish and lungs in reptiles, birds, and mammals are specifically designed to exchange gases. In birds, crops are designed to store food and gizzards are designed to grind food.

Organ systems are groups of organs that work together to perform specific functions. In mammals, there are 11 major organ systems: **integumentary system**, **respiratory system**, **cardiovascular system**, **endocrine system**, **nervous system**, **immune system**, **digestive system**, **excretory system**, **muscular system**, **skeletal system**, and **reproductive system**.

Terms of Direction

Medial means *nearer to the midline* of the body. In anatomical position, the little finger is medial to the thumb.

Lateral is the opposite of medial. It refers to structures *further away from the body's midline*, at the sides. In anatomical position, the thumb is lateral to the little finger.

Proximal refers to structures *closer to the center* of the body. The hip is proximal to the knee.

Distal refers to structures *further away from the center* of the body. The knee is distal to the hip.

Anterior refers to structures in *front.*

Posterior refers to structures *behind.*

Cephalad and **cephalic** are adverbs meaning towards the *head.* **Cranial** is the adjective, meaning of the *skull.*

Caudad is an adverb meaning towards the *tail* or posterior. **Caudal** is the adjective, meaning of the *hindquarters.*

Superior means *above*, or closer to the head.

Inferior means *below*, or closer to the feet.

THE THREE PRIMARY BODY PLANES

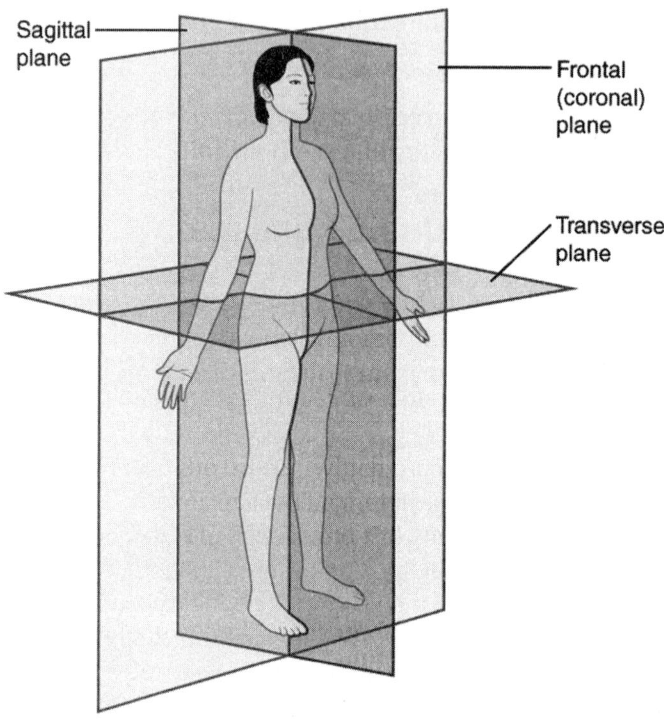

The **transverse (or horizontal) plane** divides the patient's body into imaginary upper (*superior*) and lower (*inferior or caudal*) halves.

The **sagittal plane** divides the body, or any body part, vertically into right and left sections. The sagittal plane runs parallel to the midline of the body.

The **coronal (or frontal) plane** divides the body, or any body structure, vertically into front and back (*anterior* and *posterior*) sections. The coronal plane runs vertically through the body at right angles to the midline.

Respiratory System

Structure of the Respiratory System

The respiratory system can be divided into the upper and lower respiratory system. The **upper respiratory system** includes the nose, nasal cavity, mouth, pharynx, and larynx. The **lower respiratory system** includes the trachea, lungs, and bronchial tree. Alternatively, the components of the respiratory system can be categorized as part of the airway, the lungs, or the respiratory muscles. The **airway** includes the nose, nasal cavity, mouth, pharynx (throat), larynx (voice box), trachea (windpipe), bronchi, and bronchial network. The airway is lined with **cilia** that trap microbes and debris and sweep them back toward the mouth. The **lungs** are structures that house the **bronchi** and bronchial network, which extend into the lungs and terminate in millions of **alveoli** (air sacs). The walls of the alveoli are only one cell thick, allowing for the exchange of gases with the blood capillaries that surround them. The right lung has three lobes. The left lung has only two lobes, leaving room for the heart on the left side of the body. The lungs are surrounded by a **pleural membrane**, which reduces friction between the lungs and walls of the thoracic cavity when breathing. The respiratory muscles include the **diaphragm** and the **intercostal muscles**. The diaphragm is a dome-shaped muscle that separates the thoracic and abdominal cavities; as it contracts, it expands the thoracic cavity which draws air into the lungs. The intercostal muscles are located between the ribs.

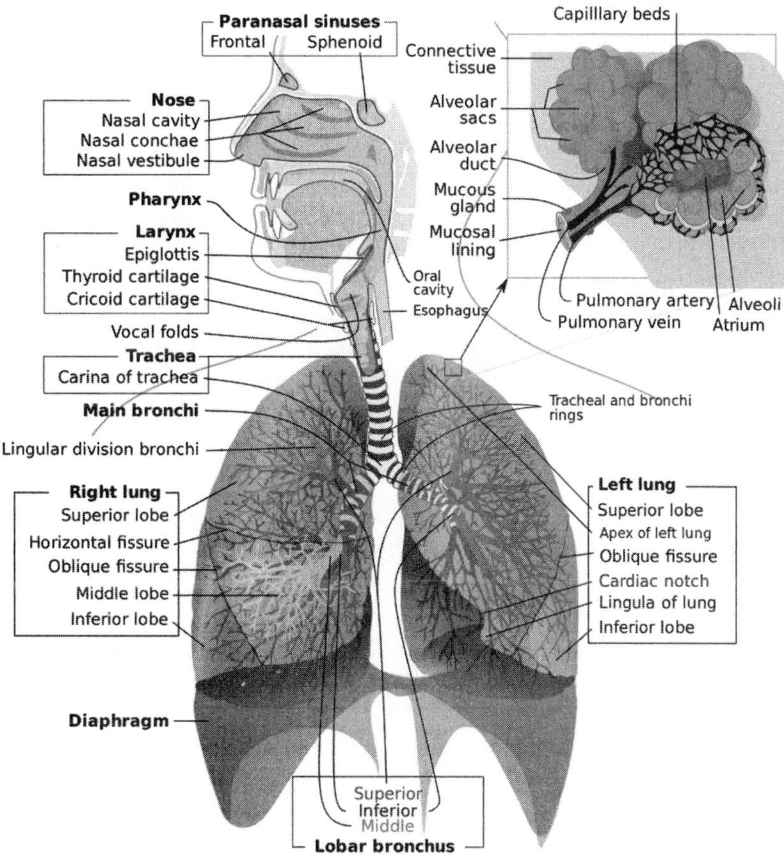

Functions of the Respiratory System

The main function of the respiratory system is to supply the body with **oxygen** and rid the body of **carbon dioxide**. This exchange of gases occurs in millions of tiny **alveoli**, which are surrounded by blood capillaries.

The respiratory system also filters air. Air is warmed, moistened, and filtered as it passes through the nasal passages before it reaches the lungs.

The respiratory system is responsible for speech. As air passes through the throat, it moves through the **larynx** (voice box), which vibrates and produces sound, before it enters the **trachea** (windpipe). The respiratory system is vital in cough production. Foreign particles entering the nasal passages or airways are expelled from the body by the respiratory system.

The respiratory system functions in the sense of smell. **Chemoreceptors** that are located in the nasal cavity respond to airborne chemicals. The respiratory system also helps the body maintain acid-base **homeostasis**. Hyperventilation can increase blood pH during **acidosis** (low pH). Slowing breathing during **alkalosis** (high pH) helps to lower blood pH.

Review Video: Respiratory System
Visit mometrix.com/academy and enter code: 783075

Breathing Process

During the breathing process, the **diaphragm** and the **intercostal muscles** contract to expand the lungs.

During **inspiration** or inhalation, the diaphragm contracts and moves down, increasing the size of the chest cavity. The intercostal muscles contract and the ribs expand, increasing the size of the **chest cavity**. As the volume of the chest cavity increases, the pressure inside the chest cavity decreases. Because the outside air is under a greater amount of pressure than the air inside the lungs, air rushes into the lungs.

When the diaphragm and intercostal muscles relax, the size of the chest cavity decreases, forcing air out of the lungs (**expiration** or exhalation). The breathing process is controlled by the portion of the brain stem called the **medulla oblongata**. The medulla oblongata monitors the level of carbon dioxide in the blood and signals the breathing rate to increase when these levels are too high.

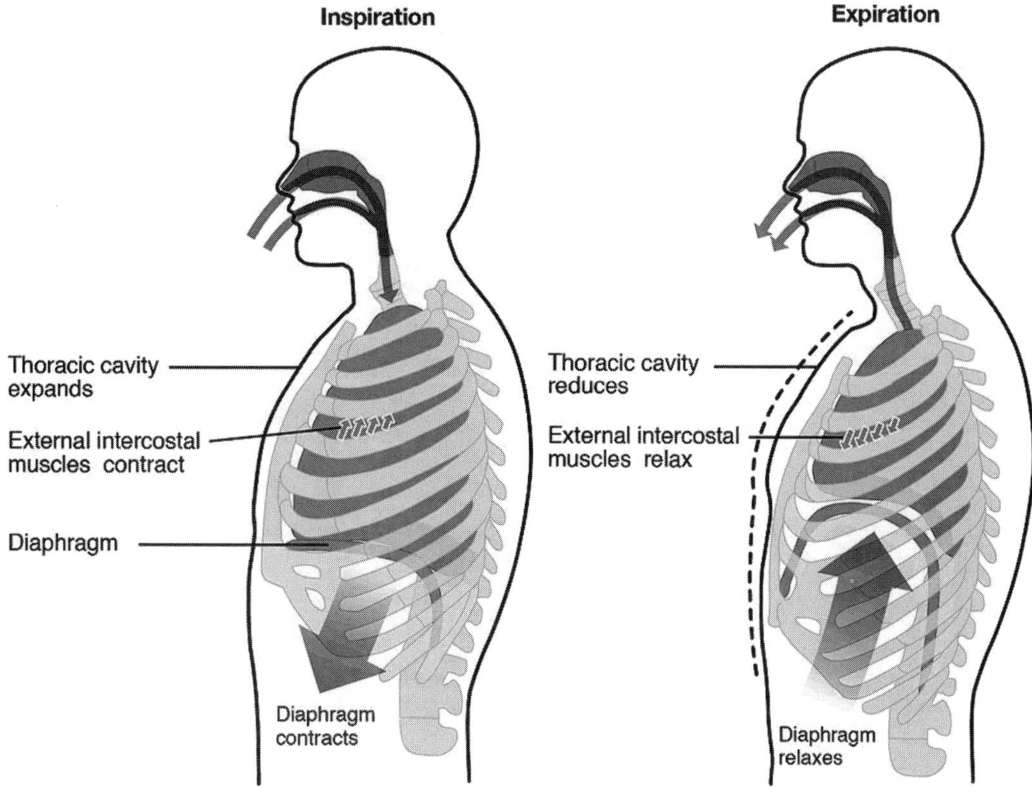

Cardiovascular System

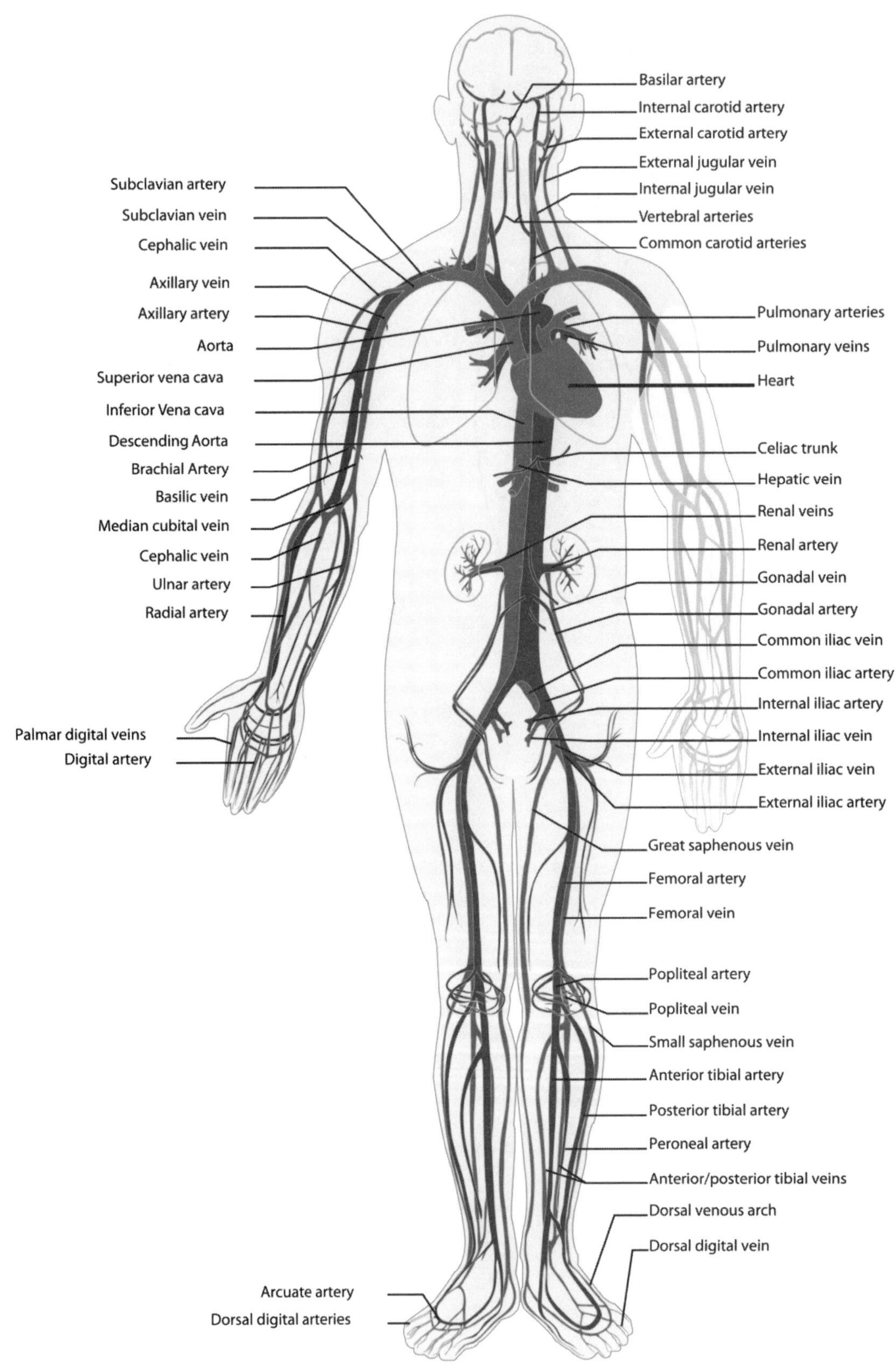

The **circulatory system** is responsible for the internal transport of substances to and from the cells. The circulatory system consists of the following parts:

- **Blood**: Blood is composed of water, solutes, and other elements in a fluid connective tissue.
- **Blood vessels**: Vessels are tubules of different sizes that transport blood in a closed system to tissues throughout the body.
- **Heart**: The heart is a muscular pump providing the pressure necessary to keep blood flowing throughout the circulatory system.

As the blood moves through the system from larger tubules through smaller ones, the rate slows. The flow of blood in the **capillary beds**, the smallest tubules, is quite slow.

A supplementary system, the **lymph vascular system**, cleans excess fluids and proteins and returns them to the circulatory system.

Review Video: Functions of the Circulatory System
Visit mometrix.com/academy and enter code: 376581

Arterial and Venous Systems (Arteries, Arterioles, Venules, Veins)

The walls of all blood vessels (except the capillaries) consist of three layers: the innermost **tunica intima**, the **tunica media** consisting of smooth muscle cells and elastic fibers, and the outer **tunica adventitia**.

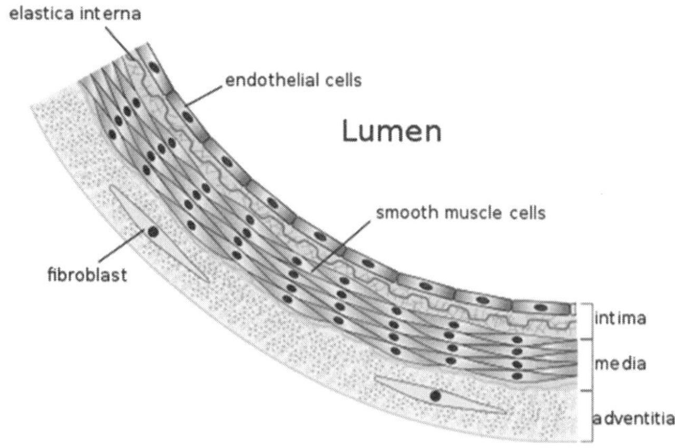

Vessel	Structure	Function
Elastic arteries	Includes the aorta and major branches Tunica media has more elastin than any other vessels Largest vessels in the arterial system	Stretch when blood is forced out of the heart, and recoil under low pressure
Muscular arteries	Includes the arteries that branch off of the elastic arteries Tunica media has a higher proportion of smooth muscle cells, and fewer elastic fibers as compared to elastic arteries	Regulate blood flow by vasoconstriction / vasodilation
Arterioles	Tiny vessels that lead to the capillary beds Tunica media is thin, but composed almost entirely smooth muscle cells	Primary vessels involved in vasoconstriction / vasodilation Control blood flow to capillaries
Venules	Tiny vessels that exit the capillary beds Thin, porous walls; few muscle cells and elastic fibers	Empty blood into larger veins

Vessel	Structure	Function
Veins	Thin tunica media and tunica intima Wide lumen Valves prevent backflow of blood	Carry blood back to the heart

Blood

Blood helps maintain a healthy internal environment in animals by carrying raw materials to cells and removing waste products. It helps stabilize internal pH and hosts cells of the immune system.

An adult human has about five quarts of blood. Blood is composed of **red blood cells, white blood cells**, **platelets**, and **plasma**. Plasma constitutes more than half of the blood volume. It is mostly water and serves as a solvent. Plasma contains plasma proteins, ions, glucose, amino acids, hormones, and dissolved gases. **Platelets** are fragments of stem cells and serve an important function in blood clotting.

Red blood cells transport **oxygen** to cells. Red blood cells form in the bone marrow and can live for about four months. These cells are constantly being replaced by fresh ones, keeping the total number relatively stable. They lack a nucleus.

Part of the immune system, white blood cells defend the body against **infection** and remove wastes. The types of white blood cells include lymphocytes, neutrophils, monocytes, eosinophils, and basophils.

Heart

The **heart** is a muscular pump made of cardiac muscle tissue. Heart chamber contraction and relaxation is coordinated by electrical signals from the self-exciting **sinoatrial node** and the **atrioventricular node**. **Atrial contraction** fills the ventricles and **ventricular contraction** forces blood into arteries leaving the heart. This sequence is called the **cardiac cycle**. Valves keep blood moving through the heart in a single direction and prevent any backwash as it flows through its four chambers.

Deoxygenated blood from the body flows through the heart in this order:

1. The **superior vena cava** brings blood from the upper body; the **inferior vena cava** brings blood from the lower body.
2. Right atrium
3. Tricuspid valve (right atrioventricular [AV] valve)
4. Right ventricle
5. Pulmonary valve
6. Left and right pulmonary artery (note: these arteries carry deoxygenated blood)
7. Lungs (where gas exchange occurs)

Oxygenated blood returns to the body through:

1. Left and right pulmonary veins (note: these veins carry oxygenated blood)
2. Left atrium
3. Mitral valve (left atrioventricular [AV] valve)
4. Left ventricle
5. Aortic valve
6. Aortic arch
7. Aorta

The left and right sides of the heart are separated by the septum. The heart has its own circulatory system with its own **coronary arteries**.

Cardiac Cycle

The **first phase** of the cardiac cycle is the ventricular filling phase. During this phase, the pressure in the ventricle is lower than the pressure in the atrium which forces open the atrioventricular valve and allows blood to pass from the atrium to the ventricle. Also, during the time, the pressure in the blood vessels leading from the ventricle (the aorta or pulmonary artery) is greater than ventricular pressure that forces the semilunar valves closed. The **second phase** of the cardiac cycle is ventricular contraction. The ventricle contracts during this phase, increasing the pressure within the ventricle. The atrial pressure is now lower than ventricular pressure, which pushes the atrioventricular valves closed. Initially, the semilunar valves are also closed. When the pressure in the ventricle rises above pressure in the blood vessel leading away from the heart (the aorta or the pulmonary artery), the semilunar valves are forced open and ventricular ejection begins. The **third phase** of the cardiac cycle is ventricular relaxation. Ventricular pressure decreases when blood is ejected from the ventricles into blood vessels leading away from the heart. When the pressure falls below the pressure in the blood vessel (the aorta or the pulmonary artery), the semilunar valves are forced closed. When the ventricle relaxes and the pressure falls below the pressure in the atrium, the atrioventricular valves are opened and the period of ventricular filling begins again.

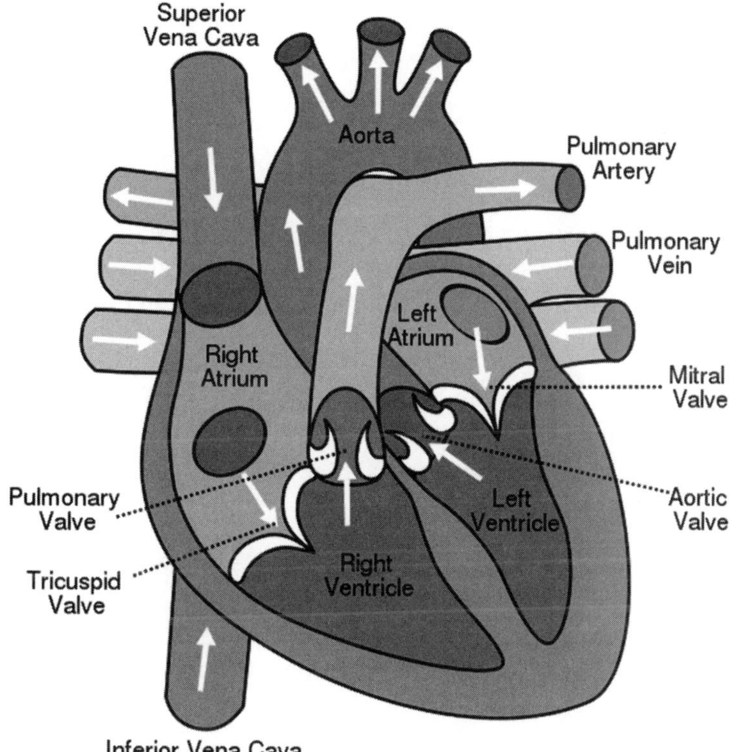

Types of Circulation

The **circulatory system** includes coronary circulation, pulmonary circulation, and systemic circulation. **Coronary circulation** is the flow of blood to the heart tissue. Blood enters the **coronary arteries**, which branch off the aorta, supplying major arteries, which enter the heart with oxygenated blood. The deoxygenated blood returns to the right atrium through the **cardiac veins**, which empty into the **coronary sinus**. **Pulmonary circulation** is the flow of blood between the heart and the lungs. Deoxygenated blood flows from the right ventricle to the lungs through **pulmonary arteries**. Oxygenated blood flows back to the left atrium through the **pulmonary veins**. **Systemic circulation** is the flow of blood to the entire body with the exception of coronary circulation and pulmonary circulation. Blood exits the left ventricle through the aorta, which branches into the *carotid arteries, subclavian arteries, common iliac arteries, and the renal artery.* Blood returns to the heart through the *jugular veins, subclavian veins, common iliac veins, and renal veins*, which empty into the **superior** and **inferior venae cavae**. Included in systemic circulation is **portal circulation**, which is the flow of blood from the digestive system to the liver and then to the heart, and **renal circulation**, which is the flow of blood between the heart and the kidneys.

Blood Pressure

Blood pressure is the fluid pressure generated by the cardiac cycle.

Arterial blood pressure functions by transporting oxygen-poor blood into the lungs and oxygen-rich blood to the body tissues. **Arteries** branch into smaller arterioles which contract and expand based on signals from the body. **Arterioles** are where adjustments are made in blood delivery to specific areas based on complex communication from body systems.

Capillary beds are diffusion sites for exchanges between blood and interstitial fluid. A capillary has the thinnest wall of any blood vessel, consisting of a single layer of **endothelial cells**.

Capillaries merge into venules, which in turn merge with larger diameter tubules called **veins**. Veins transport blood from body tissues *back to the heart.* Valves inside the veins facilitate this transport. The walls of veins are thin and contain smooth muscle and also function as blood volume reserves.

Lymphatic System

The main function of the **lymphatic system** is to *return excess tissue fluid to the bloodstream*. This system consists of transport vessels and lymphoid organs. The lymph vascular system consists of **lymph capillaries**, **lymph vessels**, and **lymph ducts**. The major functions of the lymph vascular system are:

- The return of excess fluid to the blood.
- The return of protein from the capillaries.
- The transport of fats from the digestive tract.
- The disposal of debris and cellular waste.

Lymphoid organs include the lymph nodes, spleen, appendix, adenoids, thymus, tonsils, and small patches of tissue in the small intestine. **Lymph nodes** are located at intervals throughout the lymph vessel system. Each node contains **lymphocytes** and **plasma cells**. The **spleen** filters blood stores of red blood cells and macrophages. The **thymus** secretes hormones and is the major site of lymphocyte production.

Spleen

The spleen is in the upper left of the abdomen. It is located behind the stomach and immediately below the diaphragm. It is about the size of a thick paperback book and weighs just over half a pound. It is made up of **lymphoid tissue**. The blood vessels are connected to the spleen by **splenic sinuses** (modified capillaries). The following **peritoneal ligaments** support the spleen:

- The **gastrolienal ligament** connects the stomach to the spleen.
- The **lienorenal ligament** connects the kidney to the spleen.
- The middle section of the **phrenicocolic ligament** (connects the left colic flexure to the thoracic diaphragm).

The main functions of the spleen are to *filter unwanted materials* from the blood (including old red blood cells) and to help *fight infections*. Up to ten percent of the population has one or more accessory spleens that tend to form at the **hilum** of the original spleen.

Gastrointestinal System

The digestive system function by the following means:

- **Movement** – Movement mixes and passes nutrients through the system and eliminates waste.
- **Secretion** – Enzymes, hormones, and other substances necessary for digestion are secreted into the digestive tract.
- **Digestion** – Includes the chemical breakdown of nutrients into smaller units that enter the internal environment.
- **Absorption** – The passage of nutrients through plasma membranes into the blood or lymph and then to the body.

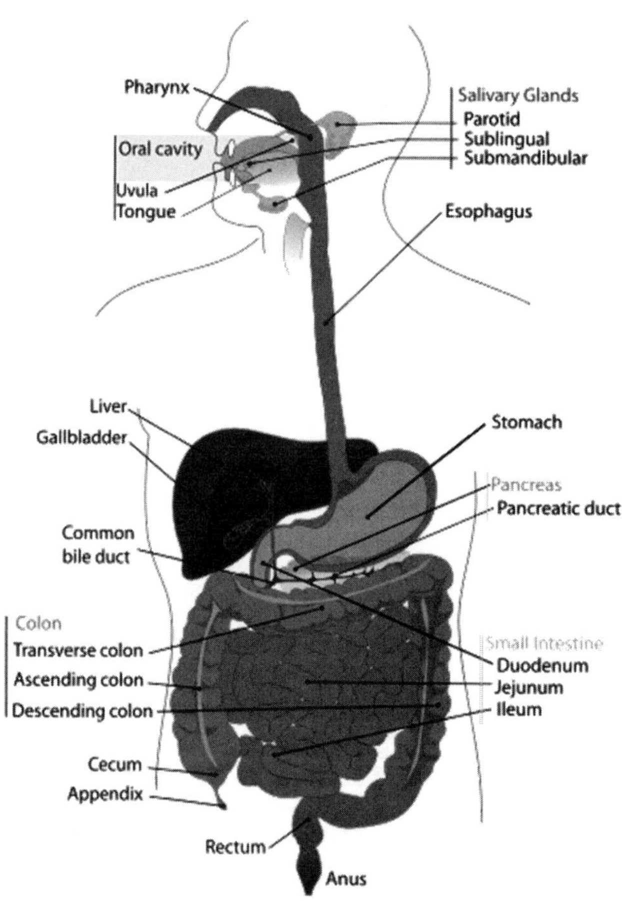

Review Video: Gastrointestinal System
Visit mometrix.com/academy and enter code: 378740

Mouth and Stomach

Digestion begins in the mouth with the chewing and mixing of nutrients with **saliva**. Only humans and other mammals actually chew their food. **Salivary glands** are stimulated and secrete saliva. Saliva contains **enzymes** that initiate the breakdown of starch in digestion. Once swallowed, the food moves down the **pharynx** into the **esophagus** en route to the stomach.

The **stomach** is a flexible, muscular sac. It has three main functions:

- Mixing and storing food
- Dissolving and degrading food via secretions
- Controlling passage of food into the small intestine

Protein digestion begins in the stomach. Stomach acidity helps break down the food and make nutrients available for absorption. Smooth muscle moves the food by **peristalsis**, contracting and relaxing to move nutrients along. Smooth muscle contractions move nutrients into the small intestine where the **absorption** process begins.

LIVER

The liver is the largest solid organ of the body. It is also the largest gland. It weighs about three pounds in an adult and is located below the diaphragm on the right side of the abdomen. The liver is made up of four **lobes**: right, left, quadrate, and caudate lobes. The liver is secured to the diaphragm and abdominal walls by five **ligaments**. They are called the falciform (which forms a membrane-like barrier between the right and left lobes), coronary, right triangular, left triangular, and round ligaments.

The liver processes blood once it has received nutrients from the intestines via the **hepatic portal vein**. The **hepatic artery** supplies oxygen-rich blood from the abdominal aorta so that the organ can function. Blood leaves the liver through the **hepatic veins**. The liver's functional units are called **lobules** (made up of layers of liver cells). Blood enters the lobules through branches of the portal vein and hepatic artery. The blood then flows through small channels called **sinusoids**.

The liver is responsible for performing many vital functions in the body including:

- Production of **bile**
- Production of certain **blood plasma proteins**
- Production of **cholesterol** (and certain proteins needed to carry fats)
- Storage of excess glucose in the form of **glycogen** (that can be converted back to glucose when needed)
- Regulation of **amino acids**
- Processing of **hemoglobin** (to store iron)
- Conversion of ammonia (that is poisonous to the body) to **urea** (a waste product excreted in urine)
- **Purification** of the blood (clears out drugs and other toxins)
- Regulation of **blood clotting**
- Controlling infections by boosting **immune factors** and removing bacteria.

The nutrients (and drugs) that pass through the liver are converted into forms that are appropriate for the body to use.

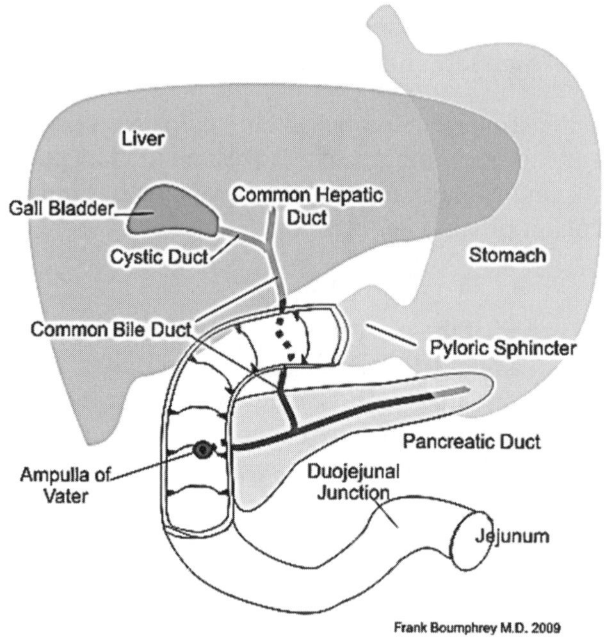

PANCREAS

The pancreas is six to ten inches long and located at the back of the abdomen behind the stomach. It is a long, tapered organ. The wider (right) side is called the **head** and the narrower (left) side is called the **tail**. The head lies near the **duodenum** (the first part of the small intestine) and the tail ends near the **spleen**. The body of the pancreas lies between the head and the tail. The pancreas is made up of exocrine and endocrine tissues. The **exocrine tissue** secretes digestive enzymes from a series of ducts that collectively form the main pancreatic duct (that runs the length of the pancreas). The **main pancreatic duct** connects to the common bile duct near the duodenum. The **endocrine tissue** secretes hormones (such as insulin) into the bloodstream. Blood is supplied to the pancreas from the *splenic artery, gastroduodenal artery, and the superior mesenteric artery*.

DIGESTIVE ROLE OF PANCREAS

The pancreas assists in the digestion of foods by secreting **enzymes** (to the small intestine) that help to break down many foods, especially fats and proteins.

The precursors to these enzymes (called **zymogens**) are produced by groups of exocrine cells (called **acini**). They are converted, through a chemical reaction in the gut, to the active enzymes (such as **pancreatic lipase** and **amylase**) once they enter the small intestine. The pancreas also secretes large amounts of **sodium bicarbonate** to neutralize the stomach acid that reaches the small intestine.

The **exocrine** functions of the pancreas are controlled by hormones released by the stomach and small intestine (duodenum) when food is present. The exocrine secretions of the pancreas flow into the main pancreatic duct (**Wirsung's duct**) and are delivered to the duodenum through the pancreatic duct.

Small Intestine

In the digestive process, most nutrients are absorbed in the **small intestine**. Enzymes from the pancreas, liver, and stomach are transported to the small intestine to aid digestion. These enzymes act on *fats, carbohydrates, nucleic acids, and proteins.* **Bile** is a secretion of the liver and is particularly useful in breaking down fats. It is stored in the **gall bladder** between meals.

By the time food reaches the lining of the small intestine, it has been reduced to small molecules. The lining of the small intestine is covered with **villi**, tiny absorptive structures that greatly increase the surface area for interaction with chyme (the semi-liquid mass of partially digested food). Epithelial cells at the surface of the villi, called **microvilli**, further increase the ability of the small intestine to serve as the *main absorption organ* of the digestive tract.

Large Intestine

Also called the **colon**, the large intestine concentrates, mixes, and stores waste material. A little over a meter in length, the colon ascends on the right side of the abdominal cavity, cuts across transversely to the left side, then descends and attaches to the **rectum**, a short tube for waste disposal.

When the rectal wall is distended by waste material, the nervous system triggers an impulse in the body to expel the waste from the rectum. A muscle **sphincter** at the end of the **anus** is stimulated to facilitate the expelling of waste matter.

The speed at which waste moves through the colon is influenced by the volume of fiber and other undigested material present. Without adequate bulk in the diet, it takes longer to move waste along, sometimes with negative effects. Lack of bulk in the diet has been linked to a number of disorders.

Nervous System

The human nervous system senses, interprets, and issues commands as a response to conditions in the body's environment. This process is made possible by a complex communication system of cells called **neurons**.

Messages are sent across the plasma membrane of neurons through a process called **action potential**. These messages occur when a neuron is stimulated past a necessary threshold. These stimulations occur in a sequence from the stimulation point of one neuron to its contact with another neuron. At the point of contact, called a **chemical synapse**, a substance is released that stimulates or inhibits the action of the adjoining cell. A network of nerves composed of neurons fans out across the body and forms the framework for the nervous system. The direction the information flows depends on the specific organizations of nerve circuits and pathways.

Review Video: What is the Function of the Nervous System
Visit mometrix.com/academy and enter code: 708428

The Somatic Nervous System and the Reflex Arc

The somatic nervous system (**SNS**) controls the five senses and the voluntary movement of skeletal muscle. So, this system has all of the neurons that are connected to sense organs. Efferent (motor) and afferent (sensory) nerves help the somatic nervous system operate the senses and the movement of skeletal muscle. **Efferent nerves** bring signals from the central nervous system to the sensory organs and the muscles. **Afferent nerves** bring signals from the sensory organs and the muscles to the central nervous system. The somatic nervous system also performs involuntary movements which are known as reflex arcs.

A **reflex**, the simplest act of the nervous system, is an automatic response without any conscious thought to a stimulus via the reflex arc. The **reflex arc** is the simplest nerve pathway, which bypasses the brain and is controlled by the spinal cord. For example, in the classic knee-jerk response (patellar tendon reflex), the stimulus is the reflex hammer hitting the tendon, and the response is the muscle contracting, which jerks the foot upward. The stimulus is detected by sensory receptors, and a message is sent along a **sensory** (afferent) neuron to one or more **interneurons** in the spinal cord. The interneuron(s) transmit this message to a **motor** (efferent) neuron, which carries the message to the correct **effector** (muscle).

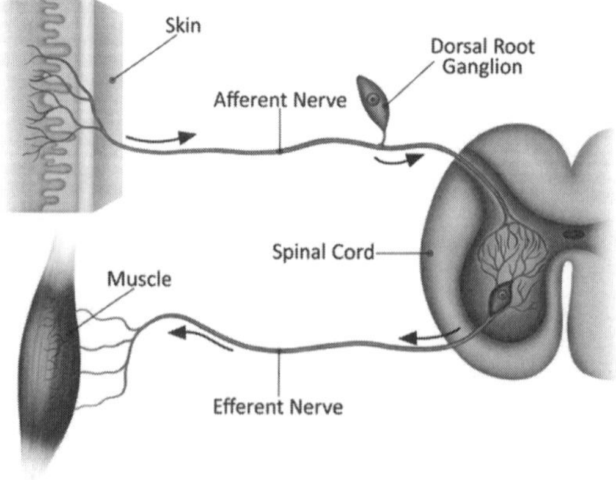

Muscular System

There are three types of muscle tissue: **skeletal**, **cardiac**, and **smooth**. There are more than 600 muscles in the human body. All muscles have these three properties in common:

- **Excitability**: All muscle tissues have an electric gradient that can reverse when stimulated.
- **Contraction**: All muscle tissues have the ability to contract, or shorten.
- **Elongate**: All muscle tissues share the capacity to elongate, or relax.

Review Video: Muscular System
Visit mometrix.com/academy and enter code: 967216

Types of Muscular Tissue

The three types of muscular tissue are skeletal muscle, smooth muscle, and cardiac muscle.

Skeletal muscles are *voluntary* muscles that work in pairs to move various parts of the skeleton. Skeletal muscles are composed of **muscle fibers** (cells) that are bound together in parallel **bundles**. Skeletal muscles are also known as **striated muscle** due to their striped appearance under a microscope.

Smooth muscle tissues are *involuntary* muscles that are found in the walls of internal organs such as the stomach, intestines, and blood vessels. Smooth muscle tissues or **visceral tissue** is nonstriated. Smooth muscle cells are shorter and wider than skeletal muscle fibers. Smooth muscle tissue is also found in sphincters or valves that control various openings throughout the body.

Cardiac muscle tissue is *involuntary* muscle that is found only in the heart. Like skeletal muscle cells, cardiac muscle cells are also striated.

Only skeletal muscle interacts with the skeleton to move the body. When they contract, the muscles transmit **force** to the attached bones. Working together, the muscles and bones act as a system of levers which move around the joints. A small contraction of a muscle can produce a large movement. A limb can be extended and rotated around a joint due to the way the muscles are arranged.

Skeletal Muscle Contraction

Skeletal muscles consist of numerous muscle fibers. Each muscle fiber contains a bundle of **myofibrils**, which are composed of multiple repeating contractile units called **sarcomeres**.

Myofibrils contain two protein **microfilaments**: a thick filament and a thin filament. The thick filament is composed of the protein **myosin**. The thin filament is composed of the protein **actin**. The dark bands (**striations**) in skeletal muscles are formed when thick and thin filaments overlap. Light bands occur where the thin filament is overlapped. Skeletal muscle attraction occurs when the thin filaments slide over the thick filaments, shortening the sarcomere.

When an **action potential** (electrical signal) reaches a muscle fiber, **calcium ions** are released. According to the sliding filament model of muscle contraction, these calcium ions bind to the myosin and actin, which assists in the binding of the **myosin heads** of the thick filaments to the

actin molecules of the thin filaments. **Adenosine triphosphate** released from glucose provides the energy necessary for the contraction.

Structure of a Skeletal Muscle

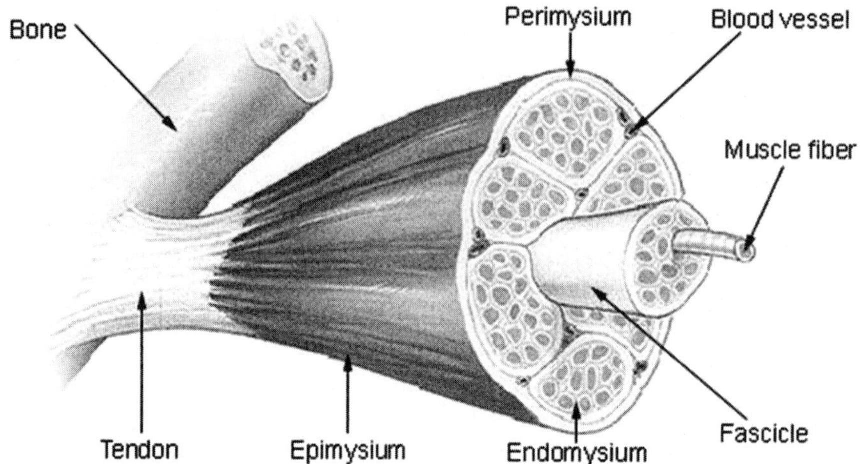

Major Muscles of the Body

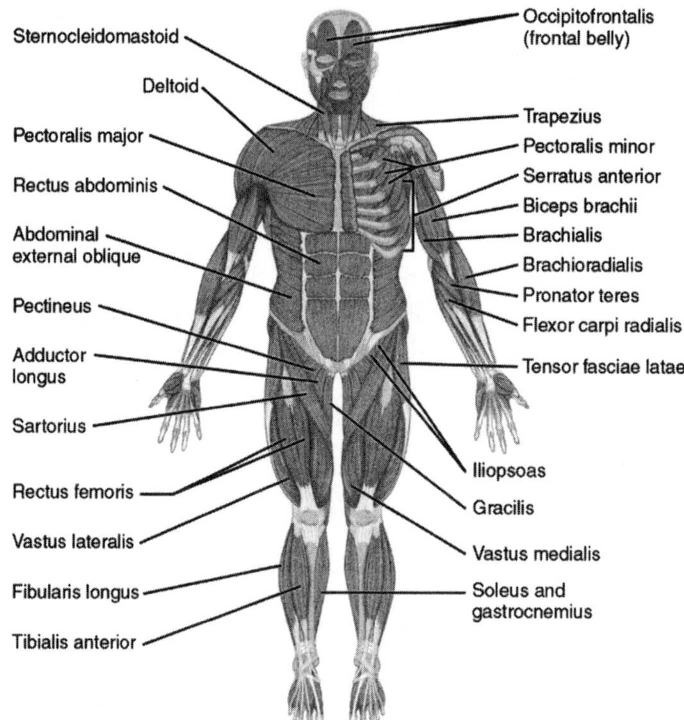

Major muscles of the body.
Right side: superficial; left side: deep (anterior view)

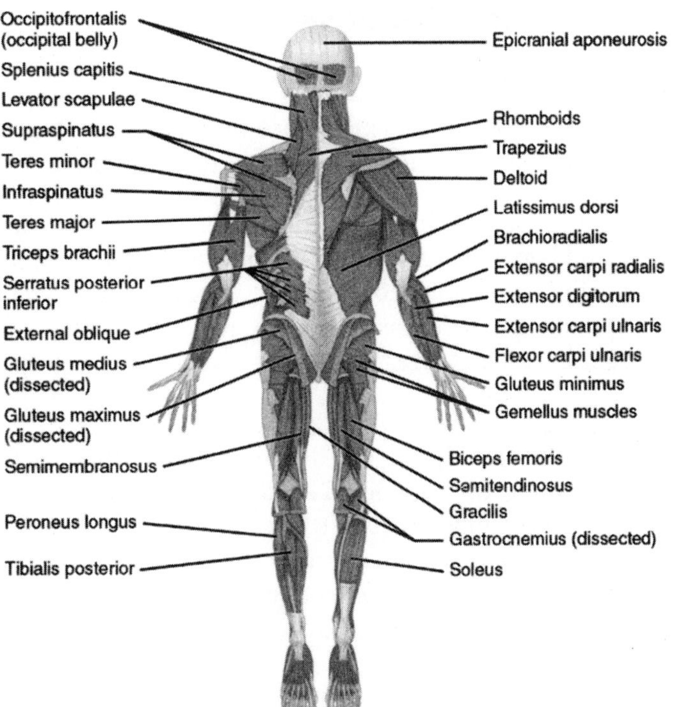

Major muscles of the body.
Right side: superficial; left side:
deep (posterior view)

Reproductive System

Male Reproductive System

The functions of the male reproductive system are to produce, maintain, and transfer **sperm** and **semen** into the female reproductive tract and to produce and secrete **male hormones**.

The external structure includes the penis, scrotum, and testes. The **penis**, which contains the **urethra**, can fill with blood and become erect, enabling the deposition of semen and sperm into the female reproductive tract during sexual intercourse. The **scrotum** is a sack of skin and smooth muscle that houses the testes and keeps the testes outside the body wall at a cooler, proper temperature for **spermatogenesis**. The **testes**, or testicles, are the male gonads, which produce sperm and testosterone.

The internal structure includes the epididymis, vas deferens, ejaculatory ducts, urethra, seminal vesicles, prostate gland, and bulbourethral glands. The **epididymis** stores the sperm as it matures. Mature sperm moves from the epididymis through the **vas deferens** to the **ejaculatory duct**. The **seminal vesicles** secrete alkaline fluids with proteins and mucus into the ejaculatory duct also. The **prostate gland** secretes a milky white fluid with proteins and enzymes as part of the semen. The **bulbourethral**, or Cowper's, glands secrete a fluid into the urethra to neutralize the acidity in the urethra, which would damage sperm.

Additionally, the hormones associated with the male reproductive system include **follicle-stimulating hormone (FSH)**, which stimulates spermatogenesis; **luteinizing hormone (LH)**, which stimulates testosterone production; and **testosterone**, which is responsible for the male sex characteristics. FSH and LH are gonadotropins, which stimulate the gonads (male testes and female ovaries).

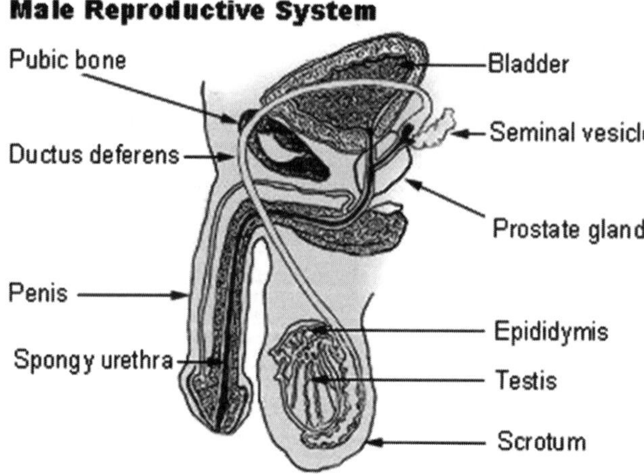

Female Reproductive System

The functions of the female reproductive system are to produce **ova** (oocytes or egg cells), transfer the ova to the **fallopian tubes** for fertilization, receive the sperm from the male, and provide a protective, nourishing environment for the developing **embryo**.

The external portion of the female reproductive system includes the labia majora, labia minora, Bartholin's glands, and clitoris. The **labia majora** and the **labia minora** enclose and protect the vagina. The **Bartholin's glands** secrete a lubricating fluid. The **clitoris** contains erectile tissue and nerve endings for sensual pleasure.

The internal portion of the female reproductive system includes the ovaries, fallopian tubes, uterus, and vagina. The **ovaries**, which are the female gonads, produce the ova and secrete **estrogen** and **progesterone**. The **fallopian tubes** carry the mature egg toward the uterus. Fertilization typically occurs in the fallopian tubes. If fertilized, the egg travels to the **uterus**, where it implants in the uterine wall. The uterus protects and nourishes the developing embryo until birth. The **vagina** is a muscular tube that extends from the **cervix** of the uterus to the outside of the body. The vagina receives the semen and sperm during sexual intercourse and provides a birth canal when needed.

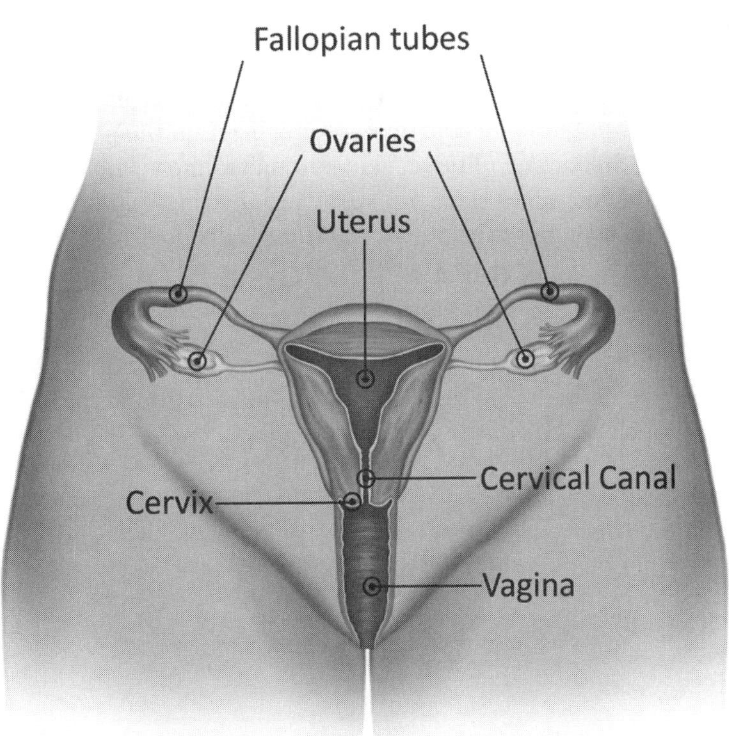

Female Reproductive Cycle

The female reproductive cycle is characterized by changes in both the ovaries and the uterine lining (endometrium).

The ovarian cycle has three phases: the follicular phase, ovulation, and the luteal phase. During the **follicular phase**, FSH stimulates the maturation of the follicle, which then secretes estrogen. Estrogen helps to regenerate the uterine lining that was shed during menstruation. **Ovulation**, the release of a secondary oocyte from the ovary, is induced by a surge in LH. The **luteal phase** begins with the formation of the corpus luteum from the remnants of the follicle. The corpus luteum secretes progesterone and estrogen, which inhibit FSH and LH. Progesterone also maintains the thickness of the endometrium. Without the implantation of a fertilized egg, the corpus luteum begins to regress, and the levels of estrogen and progesterone drop. FSH and LH are no longer inhibited, and the cycle renews.

The uterine cycle also consists of three phases: the proliferative phase, secretory phase, and menstrual phase. The **proliferative phase** is characterized by the regeneration of the uterine lining. During the **secretory phase**, the endometrium becomes increasingly vascular, and nutrients are secreted to prepare for implantation. Without implantation, the endometrium is shed during **menstruation**.

PREGNANCY, PARTURITION, LACTATION

Pregnancy: When a blastocyst implants in the uterine lining, it releases hCG. This hormone prevents the corpus luteum from degrading, and it continues to produce estrogen and progesterone. These hormones are necessary to maintain the uterine lining. By the second trimester, the placenta secretes enough of its own estrogen and progesterone to sustain pregnancy and the levels continue to increase throughout pregnancy, while hCG hormone levels decrease.

Parturition: The precise mechanism for the initiation of parturition (birth) is unclear. Birth is preceded by increased levels of fetal glucocorticoids, which act on the placenta to increase estrogen and decrease progesterone. Stretching of the cervix stimulates the release of oxytocin from the posterior pituitary gland. Oxytocin and estrogen stimulate the release of prostaglandins, and prostaglandins and oxytocin increase uterine contractions. This positive feedback mechanism results in the birth of the fetus.

Lactation: During pregnancy, levels of the hormone prolactin increase, but its effect on the mammary glands is inhibited by estrogen and progesterone. After parturition, the levels of these hormones decrease, and prolactin is able to stimulate the production of milk. Suckling stimulates the release of oxytocin, which results in the ejection of milk.

Integumentary System

The integumentary system, which consists of the skin including the sebaceous glands, sweat glands, hair, and nails, serves a variety of functions associated with protection, secretion, and communication. In the functions associated with protection, the integumentary system protects the body from **pathogens** including bacteria, viruses, and various chemicals. In the functions associated with secretion, **sebaceous glands** secrete **sebum** (oil) that waterproofs the skin, and **sweat glands** are associated with the body's homeostatic relationship of **thermoregulation**. Sweat glands also serve as excretory organs and help rid the body of metabolic wastes. In the functions associated with communication, **sensory receptors** distributed throughout the skin send information to the brain regarding pain, touch, pressure, and temperature. In addition to protection, secretion, and communication, the skin manufactures **vitamin D** and can absorb certain chemicals such as specific medications.

Review Video: Integumentary System
Visit mometrix.com/academy and enter code: 655980

Layers of the Skin

The layers of the skin from the surface of the skin inward are the epidermis and dermis. The subcutaneous layer lying below the dermis is also part of the integumentary system. The **epidermis** is the most superficial layer of the skin. The epidermis, which consists entirely of **epithelial cells**, does not contain any blood vessels. The deepest portion of the epidermis is the **stratum basale**, which is a single layer of cells that continually undergo division. As more and more cells are produced, older cells are pushed toward the surface. Most epidermal cells are keratinized. **Keratin** is a waxy protein that helps to waterproof the skin. As the cells die, they are sloughed off. The **dermis** lies directly beneath the epidermis. The dermis consists mostly of connective tissue. The dermis contains blood vessels, sensory receptors, hair follicles, sebaceous glands, and sweat glands. The dermis also contains **elastin** and **collagen fibers**. The **subcutaneous layer** or **hypodermis** is actually not a layer of the skin. The subcutaneous layer consists of connective tissue, which binds the skin to the underlying muscles. Fat deposits in the subcutaneous layer help to cushion and insulate the body.

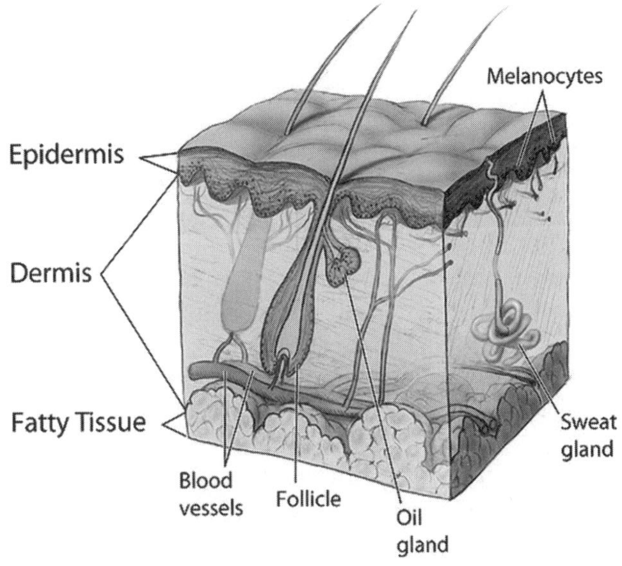

The types of cells found in the epidermis and dermis:

Cell Type	Location	Description
Keratinocytes	Epidermis	The most common type of cell in the epidermis. Arise from stem cells in the stratum basale They flatten and die as they move toward the surface of the skin Produce keratin - a fibrous protein that hardens the cell and helps make the skin water resistant
Melanocytes	Epidermis	Produces melanin - a pigment that gives skin its color and protects against UV radiation
Langerhans cells	Epidermis	Antigen-presenting cells of the immune system (phagocytes) More common in stratum spinosum than other layers of epidermis
Merkel cells	Epidermis	Cutaneous receptors, detect light touch. Located in stratum basale
Fibroblasts	Dermis	Secrete collagen, elastin, glycosaminoglycans, and other components of the extracellular matrix
Adipocytes	Dermis	Fat cells
Macrophages	Dermis	Phagocytic cells that engulf potential pathogens
Mast cells	Dermis	Antigen-presenting cells that play a role in the inflammatory response (release histamine)

Skin's Involvement in Temperature Homeostasis

The skin is involved in **temperature homeostasis** or thermoregulation through the activation of the sweat glands. By **thermoregulation**, the body maintains a stable body temperature as one component of a stable internal environment. The temperature of the body is controlled by a negative feedback system consisting of a receptor, control center, and effector. The **receptors** are sensory cells located in the dermis of the skin. The **control center** is the **hypothalamus**, which is located in the brain. The **effectors** include the *sweat glands, blood vessels, and muscles* (shivering). The evaporation of sweat across the surface of the skin cools the body to maintain its tolerance range. **Vasodilation** of the blood vessels near the surface of the skin also releases heat into the environment to lower body temperature. Shivering is associated with the muscular system.

Sebaceous Glands vs. Sweat Glands

Sebaceous glands and sweat glands are exocrine glands found in the skin. **Exocrine glands** secrete substances into **ducts**. In this case, the secretions are through the ducts to the surface of the skin.

Sebaceous glands are **holocrine glands**, which secrete sebum. **Sebum** is an oily mixture of lipids and proteins. Sebaceous glands are connected to hair follicles and secrete sebum through the hair pore. Sebum inhibits water loss from the skin and protects against bacterial and fungal infections.

Sweat glands are either eccrine glands or apocrine glands. **Eccrine glands** are not connected to hair follicles. They are activated by elevated body temperature. Eccrine glands are located throughout the body and can be found on the forehead, neck, and back. Eccrine glands secrete a salty solution of electrolytes and water containing sodium chloride, potassium, bicarbonate, glucose, and antimicrobial peptides.

Eccrine glands are activated as part of the body's thermoregulation. **Apocrine glands** secrete an oily solution containing fatty acids, triglycerides, and proteins. Apocrine glands are located in the armpits, groin, palms, and soles of the feet. Apocrine glands secrete this oily sweat when a person experiences stress or anxiety. Bacteria feed on apocrine sweat and expel aromatic fatty acids, producing body odor.

Endocrine System

The endocrine system is responsible for secreting the **hormones** and other molecules that help regulate the entire body in both the short and the long term. There is a close working relationship between the endocrine system and the nervous system. The **hypothalamus** and the **pituitary gland** coordinate to serve as a **neuroendocrine control center**.

Hormone secretion is triggered by a variety of signals, including hormonal signs, chemical reactions, and environmental cues. Only cells with particular **receptors** can benefit from hormonal influence. This is the "key in the lock" model for hormonal action. **Steroid hormones** trigger gene activation and protein synthesis in some target cells. **Protein hormones** change the activity of existing enzymes in target cells. Hormones such as **insulin** work quickly when the body signals an urgent need. Slower acting hormones afford longer, gradual, and sometimes permanent changes in the body.

Endocrine glands are intimately involved in a myriad of reactions, functions, and secretions that are crucial to the well-being of the body. The eight major endocrine glands and their functions include the following:

- **Adrenal cortex**: Monitors blood sugar level; helps in lipid and protein metabolism
- **Adrenal medulla**: Controls cardiac function; raises blood sugar and controls the size of blood vessels
- **Thyroid gland**: Helps regulate metabolism and functions in growth and development
- **Parathyroid**: Regulates calcium levels in the blood
- **Pancreas islets**: Raises and lowers blood sugar; active in carbohydrate metabolism
- **Thymus gland**: Plays a role in immune responses
- **Pineal gland**: Has an influence on daily biorhythms and sexual activity
- **Pituitary gland**: Plays an important role in growth and development

Review Video: Endocrine System
Visit mometrix.com/academy and enter code: 678939

Hormones of the Hypothalamus and Pituitary

The **hypothalamus** is the link between the nervous system and the endocrine system. It is located in the brain, superior to the pituitary and inferior to the thalamus. The hypothalamus communicates with the pituitary by secreting "releasing hormones" (RH) and "inhibiting hormones" (IH). Hormones of the hypothalamus include:

Hormone	Action
GnRH - gonadotropin RH	Stimulates anterior pituitary to release LH and FSH
GHRH - growth hormone RH	Stimulates anterior pituitary to release GH
GHIH - growth hormone IH (somatostatin)	Inhibits the release of GH from the anterior pituitary
TRH - thyrotropin RH	Stimulates anterior pituitary to release thyrotropin (TSH)
PRH - prolactin RH	Stimulates anterior pituitary to release prolactin
PIH - prolactin IH (dopamine)	Inhibits the release of prolactin from the anterior pituitary
CRH - corticotropin RH	Stimulates anterior pituitary to release ACTH

Hormone	Action
Oxytocin	Targets the uterus - stimulates contractions. Targets the mammary glands - milk secretion
ADH - antidiuretic hormone (vasopressin)	Targets the kidneys and blood vessels - increases water retention

The **pituitary** is nicknamed the "master gland" because many of the hormones it secretes act on other endocrine glands. It is located within the sella turcica of the sphenoid bone, beneath the hypothalamus. This pea-sized gland hangs from a thin stalk called the infundibulum, and it consists of an anterior and posterior lobe - each with a different function.

Source	Hormone	Action
Pituitary gland (anterior)	TSH - thyroid stimulating hormone (thyrotropin)	Targets the thyroid - stimulates the secretion of thyroid hormones
	ACTH - adrenocorticotropic hormone	Targets the adrenal cortex - stimulates the release of glucocorticoids and mineralocorticoids
	GH - growth hormone	Targets muscle and bone - stimulates growth
	FSH - follicle stimulating hormone	Targets the gonads - stimulates the maturation of sperm cells and ovarian follicles
	LH - luteinizing hormone	Targets the gonads - stimulates the production of sex hormones; surge stimulates ovulation in females
	PRL - prolactin	Targets the mammary glands - stimulates production of milk
Pituitary gland (posterior)	Oxytocin (produced in hypothalamus; stored and released by posterior pituitary)	Targets the uterus - stimulates contractions Targets the mammary glands - stimulates milk secretion
	ADH - antidiuretic hormone (vasopressin) (produced in hypothalamus; stored and released by posterior pituitary)	Targets the kidneys and blood vessels - increases water retention

HORMONE SOURCES OF THE HEAD AND NECK

Source/Description	Hormone	Action
Pineal gland Situated between the two hemispheres of the brain where the two halves of the thalamus join.	Melatonin	Targets the brain - regulates daily rhythm (wake and sleep)
Thyroid gland Butterfly-shaped gland; the point of attachment between the two lobes is called the isthmus. The isthmus is on the anterior portion of the trachea, with the lobes wrapping partially around the trachea.	T_3 - triiodothyronine	Targets most cells - stimulates cellular metabolism
	T_4 - thyroxine	Targets most cells - stimulates cellular metabolism
	Calcitonin	Targets bone and kidneys - lowers blood calcium

Source/Description	Hormone	Action
Parathyroid gland Four small glands that are embedded in the posterior aspect of the thyroid.	PTH - Parathyroid hormone	Targets bone and kidneys - raises blood calcium

HORMONE SOURCES OF THE ABDOMEN

Source/Description	Hormone	Action
Thymus gland Located between the sternum and the heart, embedded in the mediastinum. It slowly decreases in size after puberty.	Thymosin	Targets lymphatic tissues - stimulates the production of T-cells
Pancreas The head of the pancreas is situated in the curve of the duodenum and the tail points toward the left side of the body. The pancreas is mostly posterior to the stomach.	Insulin	Targets the liver, muscle, and adipose tissue - decreases blood glucose
	Glucagon	Targets the liver - increases blood glucose
	GHIH - growth hormone IH (somatostatin)	Inhibits the secretion of insulin and glucagon
Adrenal medulla Located on top of the kidneys. The adrenal medulla is the inner part of the gland.	Epinephrine and norepinephrine	Target heart, blood vessels, liver, and lungs - increase heart rate, increase blood sugar (fight or flight response)
Adrenal cortex The adrenal cortex is the outer portion of the adrenal gland.	Mineralocorticoids (aldosterone)	Target the kidneys - increase the retention of Na^+ and excretion of K^+
	Glucocorticoids	Target most tissues - released in response to long-term stressors, increase blood glucose (but not as quickly as glucagon)
	Androgens	Target most tissues - stimulate development of secondary sex characteristics
GI tract	Gastrin	Targets the stomach - stimulates the release of HCl
	Secretin	Targets the pancreas and liver - stimulates the release of digestive enzymes and bile
	CCK - cholecystokinin	Targets the pancreas and liver - stimulates the release of digestive enzymes and bile

Source/Description	Hormone	Action
Kidneys	Erythropoietin	Targets the bone marrow - stimulates the production of red blood cells
	Calcitriol	Targets the intestines - increases the reabsorption of Ca^{2+}
Heart	ANP - atrial natriuretic peptide	Targets the kidneys and adrenal cortex - reduces reabsorption of Na^{+}, lowers blood pressure
Adipose Tissue	Leptin	Targets the brain - suppresses appetite

Hormone Sources of the Reproductive System

Source/Description	Hormone	Action
Ovaries The ovaries rest in depressions in the pelvic cavity on each side of the uterus. (Note that ovaries produce testosterone in small amounts.)	Estrogen	Target the uterus, ovaries, mammary glands, brain, and other tissues - stimulate uterine lining growth, regulate menstrual cycle, facilitate the development of secondary sex characteristics
	Progesterone	Targets mainly the uterus and mammary glands - stimulates uterine lining growth, regulates menstrual cycle, required for maintenance of pregnancy
	Inhibin	Targets the anterior pituitary - inhibits the release of FSH
Placenta Attached to the wall of the uterus during pregnancy	Estrogen, progesterone, and inhibin	(See above)
	Human chorionic gonadotropin (hCG)	Targets the ovaries - stimulates the production of estrogen and progesterone
Testes Located within the scrotum, behind the penis.	Testosterone	Targets the testes and many other tissues - promotes spermatogenesis, secondary sex characteristics
	Inhibin	(See above)

Urinary System

The urinary system is capable of eliminating excess substances while preserving the substances needed by the body to function. The **urinary system** consists of the kidneys, urinary ducts, and bladder.

Components of the Urinary System

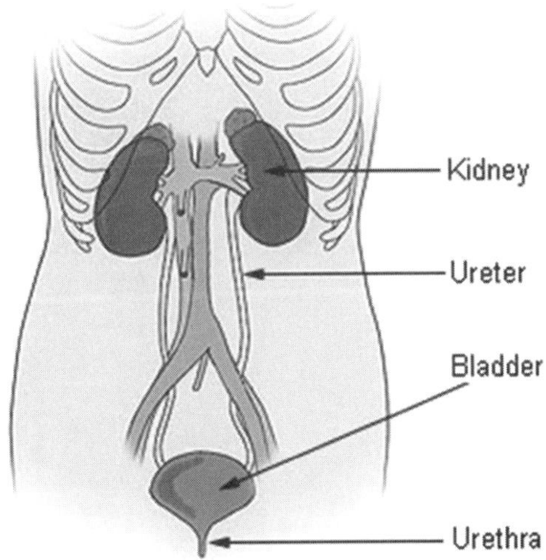

Review Video: Urinary System
Visit mometrix.com/academy and enter code: 601053

KIDNEYS

The kidneys are bean-shaped organs that are located at the back of the abdominal cavity just under the diaphragm. Each **kidney** (the labelled diagram on the left) consists of the renal cortex (outer layer), renal medulla (inner layer), and renal pelvis, which collects waste products from the nephrons and funnels them to the ureter.

The **renal cortex** (1) is composed of approximately one million **nephrons** (6 and the labelled diagram on the right), which are the tiny, individual filters of the kidneys. Each nephron contains a cluster of capillaries called a **glomerulus** (8) surrounded by the cup-shaped **Bowman's capsule** (9), which leads to a **tubule** (10).

The kidneys receive blood from the **renal arteries (3)**, which branch off the aorta. In general, the kidneys filter the blood (F), reabsorb needed materials (R), and secrete (S) and excrete (E) wastes and excess water in the urine. More specifically, blood flows from the renal arteries into **arterioles** (7) into the glomerulus, where it is filtered. The **glomerular filtrate** enters the **proximal convoluted tubule,** where water, glucose, ions, and other organic molecules are reabsorbed back into the bloodstream through the **renal vein** (4). Reabsorption and secretion occur between the tubules and the **peritubular capillaries** (12).

Additional substances such as urea and drugs are removed from the blood in the **distal convoluted tubule**. Also, the pH of the blood can be adjusted in the distal convoluted tubule by the secretion of **hydrogen ions**. Finally, the unabsorbed materials flow out from the collecting tubules located in the **renal medulla** (2) to the **renal pelvis** as urine. Urine is drained from the kidneys through the

ureters (5) to the **urinary bladder**, where it is stored until expulsion from the body through the **urethra**.

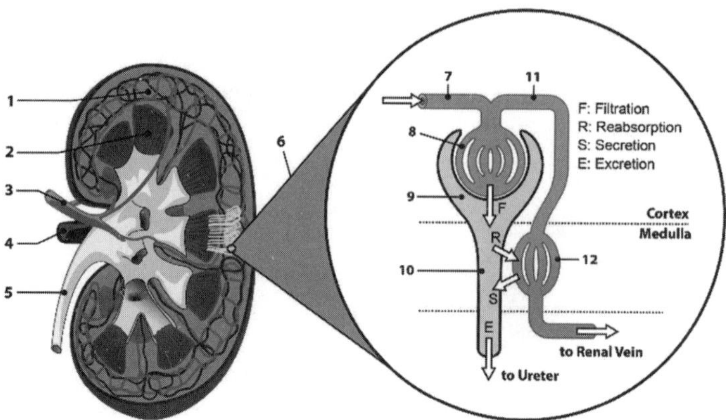

Immune System

The immune system protects the body against invading **pathogens** including bacteria, viruses, fungi, and protists. The immune system includes the **lymphatic system** (lymph, lymph capillaries, lymph vessel, and lymph nodes) as well as the **red bone marrow** and numerous **leukocytes**, or white blood cells. Tissue fluid enters the **lymph capillaries**, which combine to form **lymph vessels**. Skeletal muscle contractions move the lymph one way through the lymphatic system to lymphatic ducts, which dump back into the venous blood supply and the **lymph nodes**, which are situated along the lymph vessels, and filter the lymph of pathogens and other matter. The lymph nodes are concentrated in the neck, armpits, and groin areas. Outside the lymphatic vessel system lies the **lymphatic tissue,** including the tonsils, adenoids, thymus, spleen, and Peyer's patches. The **tonsils**, located in the pharynx, protect against pathogens entering the body through the mouth and throat. The **thymus** serves as a maturation chamber for immature T cells that are formed in the bone marrow. The **spleen** cleans the blood of dead cells and pathogens. **Peyer's patches**, which are located in the small intestine, protect the digestive system from pathogens.

Review Video: Immune System
Visit mometrix.com/academy and enter code: 622899

The body's general immune defenses include:

- **Skin** – An intact epidermis and dermis form a formidable barrier against bacteria.
- **Ciliated Mucous Membranes** – Cilia sweep pathogens out of the respiratory tract.
- **Glandular Secretions** – Secretions from exocrine glands destroy bacteria.
- **Gastric Secretions** – Gastric acid destroys pathogens.
- **Normal Bacterial Populations** – Compete with pathogens in the gut and vagina.

In addition, **phagocytes** and inflammation responses mobilize white blood cells and chemical reactions to stop infection. These responses include localized redness, tissue repair, and fluid-seeping healing agents. Additionally, **plasma proteins** act as the complement system to repel bacteria and pathogens.

Three types of white blood cells form the foundation of the body's immune system:

- **Macrophages** – Phagocytes that alert T cells to the presence of foreign substances.
- **T Lymphocytes** – These directly attack cells infected by viruses and bacteria.
- **B Lymphocytes** – These cells target specific bacteria for destruction.

Memory cells, **suppressor T cells**, and **helper T cells** also contribute to the body's defense. Immune responses can be **antibody-mediated** when the response is to an antigen, or **cell-mediated** when the response is to already infected cells. These responses are controlled and measured counterattacks that recede when the foreign agents are destroyed. Once an invader has attacked the body, if it returns it is immediately recognized and a secondary immune response occurs. This secondary response is rapid and powerful, much more so than the original response. These memory lymphocytes circulate throughout the body for years, alert to a possible new attack.

Types of Leukocytes

Leukocytes, or white blood cells, are produced in the red bone marrow. Leukocytes can be classified as **monocytes** (macrophages and dendritic cells), **granulocytes** (neutrophils, basophils, and eosinophils), **T lymphocytes**, **B lymphocytes**, or **natural killer cells**.

Macrophages found traveling in the lymph or fixed in lymphatic tissue are the largest, long-living phagocytes that engulf and destroy pathogens. **Dendritic cells** present antigens (foreign particles) to T cells. **Neutrophils** are short-living phagocytes that respond quickly to invaders. **Basophils** alert the body of invasion. **Eosinophils** are large, long-living phagocytes that defend against multicellular invaders.

T lymphocytes or T cells include helper T cells, killer T cells, suppressor T cells, and memory T cells. **Helper T cells** help the body fight infections by producing antibodies and other chemicals. **Killer T cells** destroy cells that are infected with a virus or pathogen and tumor cells. **Suppressor T cells** stop or "suppress" the other T cells when the battle is over. **Memory T cells** remain in the blood on alert in case the invader attacks again. **B lymphocytes**, or B cells, produce antibodies.

Antigen and Typical Immune Response

Antigens are substances that stimulate the **immune system**. Antigens are typically proteins on the surfaces of bacteria, viruses, and fungi.

Substances such as drugs, toxins, and foreign particles can also be antigens. The human body recognizes the antigens of its own cells, but it will attack cells or substances with unfamiliar antigens.

Specific **antibodies** are produced for each antigen that enters the body. In a typical immune response, when a pathogen or foreign substance enters the body, it is engulfed by a **macrophage**, which presents fragments of the antigen on its surface. A **helper T cell** joins the macrophage, and the killer (cytotoxic) T cells and B cells are activated. **Killer T cells** search out and destroy cells presenting the same antigens. **B cells** differentiate into plasma cells and memory cells.

Plasma cells produce antibodies specific to that pathogen or foreign substance. **Antibodies** bind to antigens on the surface of pathogens and mark them for destruction by other phagocytes. **Memory cells** remain in the blood stream to protect against future infections from the same pathogen.

Active and Passive Immunity

At birth, an **innate immune system** protects an individual from pathogens. When an individual encounters infection or has an immunization, the individual develops an **adaptive immunity** that reacts to pathogens. So, this adaptive immunity is acquired. Active and passive immunities can be acquired naturally or artificially.

A **naturally acquired active immunity** is natural because the individual is exposed and builds immunity to a pathogen *without an immunization*. An **artificially acquired active immunity** is artificial because the individual is exposed and builds immunity to a pathogen *by a vaccine*.

A **naturally acquired passive immunity** is natural because it happens *during pregnancy* as antibodies move from the mother's bloodstream to the bloodstream of the fetus. The antibodies can also be transferred from a mother's breast milk. During infancy, these antibodies provide temporary protection until childhood.

An **artificially acquired passive immunity** is an *immunization* that is given in recent outbreaks or emergency situations. This immunization provides quick and short-lived protection to disease by the use of antibodies that can come from another person or animal.

Skeletal System

AXIAL SKELETON AND THE APPENDICULAR SKELETON

The human skeletal system, which consists of 206 bones along with numerous tendons, ligaments, and cartilage, is divided into the axial skeleton and the appendicular skeleton.

The **axial skeleton** consists of 80 bones and includes the vertebral column, rib cage, sternum, skull, and hyoid bone. The **vertebral column** consists of 33 vertebrae classified as cervical vertebrae, thoracic vertebrae, lumbar vertebrae, and sacral vertebrae. The **rib cage** includes 12 paired ribs, 10 pairs of true ribs and two pairs of floating ribs, and the **sternum**, which consists of the manubrium, corpus sterni, and xiphoid process. The **skull** includes the cranium and facial bones. The **ossicles** are bones in the middle ear. The **hyoid bone** provides an attachment point for the tongue muscles. The axial skeleton protects vital organs including the brain, heart, and lungs.

The **appendicular skeleton** consists of 126 bones including the pectoral girdle, pelvic girdle, and appendages. The **pectoral girdle** consists of the scapulae (shoulder blades) and clavicles (collarbones). The **pelvic girdle** attaches to the sacrum at the sacroiliac joint. The upper appendages (arms) include the humerus, radius, ulna, carpals, metacarpals, and phalanges. The lower appendages (legs) include the femur, patella, fibula, tibia, tarsals, metatarsals, and phalanges.

Review Video: Skeletal System
Visit mometrix.com/academy and enter code: 256447

ADULT HUMAN SKELETON

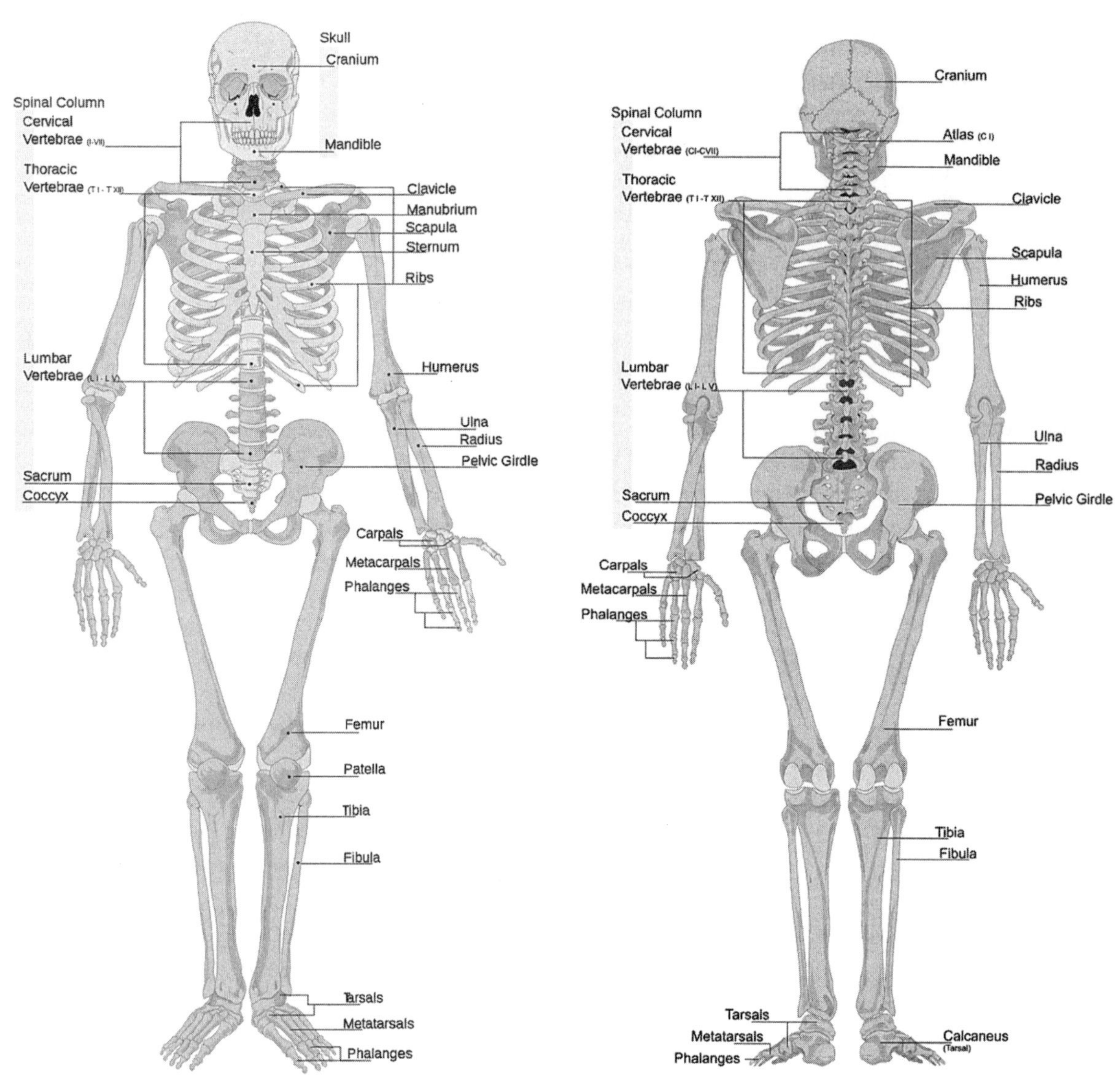

JOINT STRUCTURES

Joints are the locations where two or more elements of the skeleton connect. They can be classified according to range of motion, as well as the material that holds the joint together.

Functional classification

Class	Description	Range of Motion	Examples
Synarthrosis	Either fibrous or cartilaginous	Immovable	Skull sutures, teeth/mandible
Amphiarthrosis	Either fibrous or cartilaginous	Slight	Intervertebral discs, distal tibiofibular joint
Diarthrosis	Always synovial	Free movement	Wrist, knee, shoulder

Structural classification

Class	Description	Types, Range of Motion	Examples
Fibrous	Held together by fibrous connective tissue	**Suture**: immovable	skull
		Gomphosis: immovable	teeth/mandible
		Syndesmosis: slightly movable	distal tibiofibular joint
Cartilaginous	Held together by cartilage	**Synchondrosis**: hyaline cartilage, nearly immovable	first rib/sternum
		Symphysis: fibrocartilage, slightly movable	intervertebral discs, pubic symphysis
Synovial	The most common type of joint; characterized by a joint cavity filled with synovial fluid	**Pivot**: allows rotation	atlantoaxial joint
		Hinge: allows movement in one plane	knee
		Saddle: allows pivoting in two planes and axial rotation	first metacarpal/ trapezium
		Gliding: allows sliding	carpals
		Condyloid: allows pivoting in two planes but no axial rotation	radiocarpal joint
		Ball and socket: have the highest range of motion	hip

Functions of the Skeletal System

The skeletal system serves many functions including providing structural support, providing movement, providing protection, producing blood cells, and storing substances such as fat and minerals. The skeletal system provides the body with structure and support for the muscles and organs. The axial skeleton transfers the weight from the upper body to the lower appendages. The skeletal system provides movement with **joints** and the muscular system. Bones provide attachment points for muscles. Joints including **hinge joints**, **ball-and-socket joints**, **pivot joints**, **ellipsoid joints**, **gliding joints**, and **saddle joints**. Each muscle is attached to two bones: the origin and the insertion. The **origin** remains immobile, and the **insertion** is the bone that moves as the muscle contracts and relaxes. The skeletal system serves to protect the body. The **cranium** protects the brain. The **vertebrae** protect the spinal cord. The **rib cage** protects the heart and lungs. The **pelvis** protects the reproductive organs. The **red marrow** manufactures red and white blood cells. All bone marrow is red at birth, but adults have approximately one-half red bone marrow and one-half yellow bone marrow. **Yellow bone marrow** stores fat. Also, the skeletal system provides a reservoir to store the minerals **calcium** and **phosphorus**.

The skeletal system has an important role in the following body functions:

- **Movement** – The action of skeletal muscles on bones moves the body.
- **Mineral Storage** – Bones serve as storage facilities for essential mineral ions.
- **Support** – Bones act as a framework and support system for the organs.
- **Protection** – Bones surround and protect key organs in the body.
- **Blood Cell Formation** – Red blood cells are produced in the marrow of certain bones.

Bones are classified as long, short, flat, or irregular. They are a connective tissue with a base of pulp containing **collagen** and living cells. Bone tissue is constantly regenerating itself as the mineral composition changes. This allows for special needs during growth periods and maintains calcium levels for the body. Bone regeneration can deteriorate in old age, particularly among women, leading to **osteoporosis**.

The flexible and curved **backbone** is supported by muscles and ligaments. **Intervertebral discs** are stacked one above another and provide cushioning for the backbone. Trauma or shock may cause these discs to **herniate** and cause pain. The sensitive **spinal cord** is enclosed in a cavity which is well protected by the bones of the vertebrae.

Joints are areas of contact adjacent to bones. **Synovial joints** are the most common, and are freely moveable. These may be found at the shoulders and knees. **Cartilaginous joints** fill the spaces between some bones and restrict movement. Examples of cartilaginous joints are those between vertebrae. **Fibrous joints** have fibrous tissue connecting bones and no cavity is present.

Compact and Spongy Bone

Compact Bone & Spongy (Cancellous) Bone

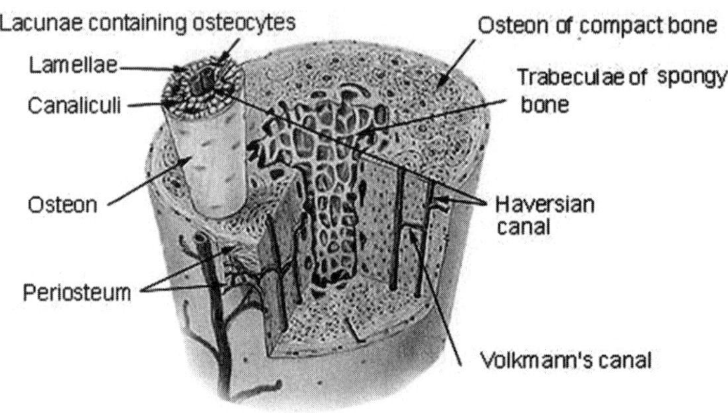

Two types of connective bone tissue include compact bone and spongy bone.

Compact, or **cortical**, bone, which consists of tightly packed cells, is strong, dense, and rigid. Running vertically throughout compact bone are the **Haversian canals**, which are surrounded by concentric circles of bone tissue called **lamellae**. The spaces between the lamellae are called the **lacunae**. These lamellae and canals along with their associated arteries, veins, lymph vessels, and nerve endings are referred to collectively as the **Haversian system**.

The Haversian system provides a reservoir for calcium and phosphorus for the blood. Also, bones have a thin outside layer of compact bone, which gives them their characteristic smooth, white appearance.

Spongy, or **cancellous**, bone consists of **trabeculae**, which are a network of girders with open spaces filled with red bone marrow.

Compared to compact bone, spongy bone is lightweight and porous, which helps reduce the bone's overall weight. The red marrow manufactures red and white blood cells. In long bones, the **diaphysis** consists of compact bone surrounding the marrow cavity and spongy bone containing red marrow in the **epiphyses**. Bones have varying amounts of compact bone and spongy bone depending on their classification.

Chapter Quiz

Ready to see how well you retained what you just read? Scan the QR code to go directly to the chapter quiz interface for this study guide. If you're using a computer, simply visit the bonus page at **mometrix.com/bonus948/hesia2** and click the Chapter Quizzes link.

Physics

Transform passive reading into active learning! After immersing yourself in this chapter, put your comprehension to the test by taking a quiz. The insights you gained will stay with you longer this way. Scan the QR code to go directly to the chapter quiz interface for this study guide. If you're using a computer, simply visit the bonus page at **mometrix.com/bonus948/hesia2** and click the Chapter Quizzes link.

Kinematics

To begin, we will look at the basics of physics. At its heart, physics is just a set of explanations for the ways in which matter and energy behave. There are three key concepts used to describe how matter moves:

1. Displacement
2. Velocity
3. Acceleration

Displacement

Concept: Where and how far an object has gone

Calculation: Final position – initial position

When something changes its location from one place to another, it is said to have undergone displacement. If a golf ball is hit across a sloped green into the hole, the displacement only takes into account the final and initial locations, not the path of the ball.

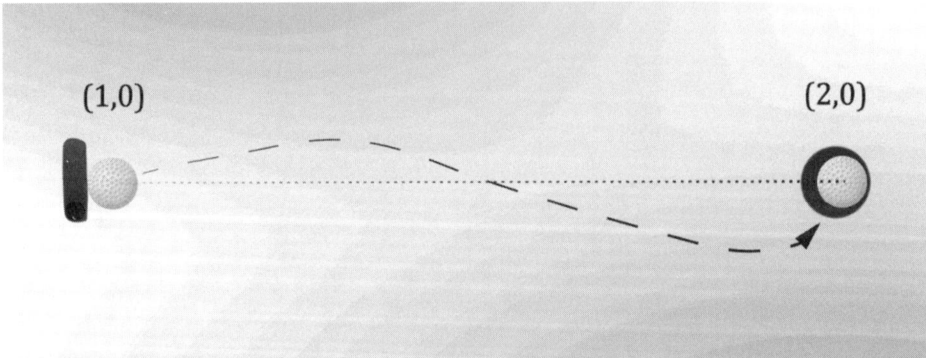

Displacement along a straight line is a very simple example of a vector quantity; it has both a magnitude and a direction. Direction is as important as magnitude in many measurements. If we can determine the original and final position of the object, then we can determine the total displacement with this simple equation:

$$\text{Displacement} = \text{final position} - \text{original position}$$

The hole (final position) is at the Cartesian coordinate location (2,0) and the ball is hit from the location (1,0). The displacement is:

$$\text{Displacement} = (2,0) - (1,0)$$

$$\text{Displacement} = (1,0)$$

The displacement has a magnitude of 1 and a direction of the positive x-direction.

Review Video: Displacement in Physics
Visit mometrix.com/academy and enter code: 236197

VELOCITY

Concept: The rate of moving from one position to another

Calculation: Change in position / change in time

Velocity answers the question, "How quickly is an object moving?" For example, if a car and a plane travel between two cities that are a hundred miles apart, but the car takes two hours and the plane takes one hour, the car has the same displacement as the plane but a smaller velocity.

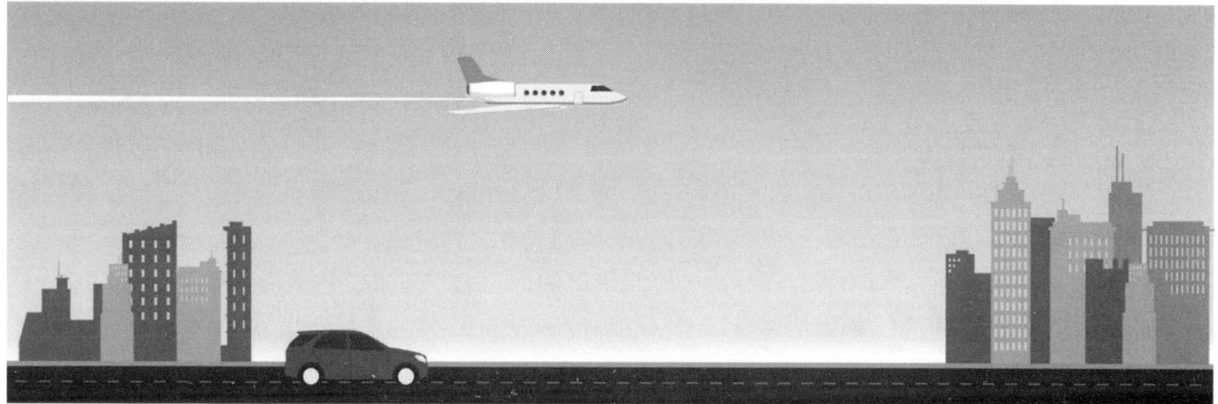

In order to solve some of the problems on the exam, you may need to assess the velocity of an object. If we want to calculate the average velocity of an object, we must know two things. First, we must know its displacement. Second, we must know the time it took to cover this distance. The formula for average velocity is quite simple:

$$\textbf{average velocity} = \frac{\textbf{displacement}}{\textbf{change in time}}$$

Or

$$\textbf{average velocity} = \frac{\textbf{final position} - \textbf{original position}}{\textbf{final time} - \textbf{original time}}$$

To complete the example, the velocity of the plane is calculated to be:

$$\text{plane average velocity} = \frac{100 \text{ miles}}{1 \text{ hour}} = 100 \text{ miles per hour}$$

The velocity of the car is less:

$$\text{car average velocity} = \frac{100 \text{ miles}}{2 \text{ hours}} = 50 \text{ miles per hour}$$

Often, people confuse the words *speed* and *velocity*. There is a significant difference. The average velocity is based on the amount of displacement, a vector. Alternately, the average speed is based on the distance covered or the path length. The equation for speed is:

$$\textbf{average speed} = \frac{\textbf{total distance traveled}}{\textbf{change in time}}$$

Notice that we used total distance and *not* change in position, because speed is path-dependent.

If the plane traveling between cities had needed to fly around a storm on its way, making the distance traveled 50 miles greater than the distance the car traveled, the plane would still have the same total displacement as the car.

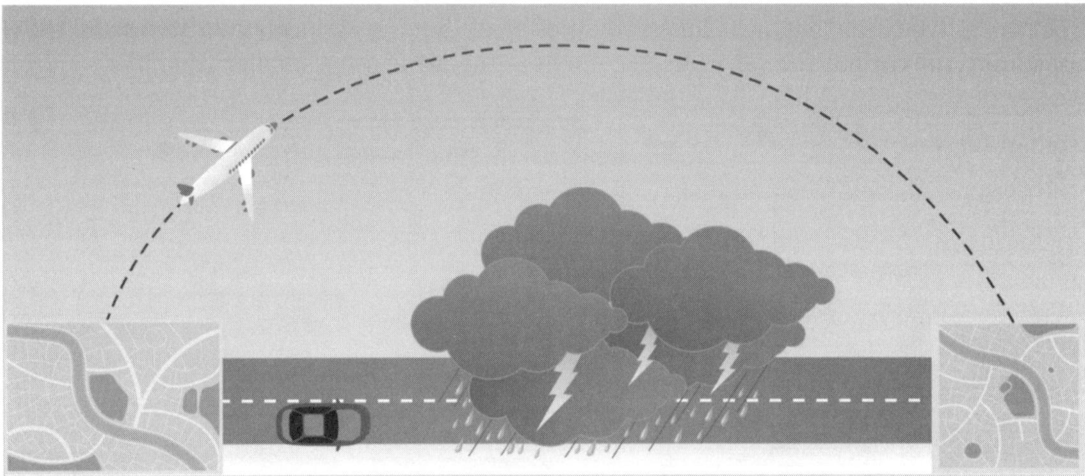

For this reason, the average speed can be calculated:

$$\text{plane average speed} = \frac{150 \text{ miles}}{1 \text{ hour}} = 150 \text{ miles per hour}$$

$$\text{car average speed} = \frac{100 \text{ miles}}{2 \text{ hours}} = 50 \text{ miles per hour}$$

ACCELERATION

Concept: How quickly something changes from one velocity to another

Calculation: Change in velocity / change in time

Acceleration is the rate of change of the velocity of an object. If a car accelerates from zero velocity to 60 miles per hour (88 feet per second) in two seconds, the car has an impressive acceleration.

But if a car performs the same change in velocity in eight seconds, the acceleration is much lower and not as impressive.

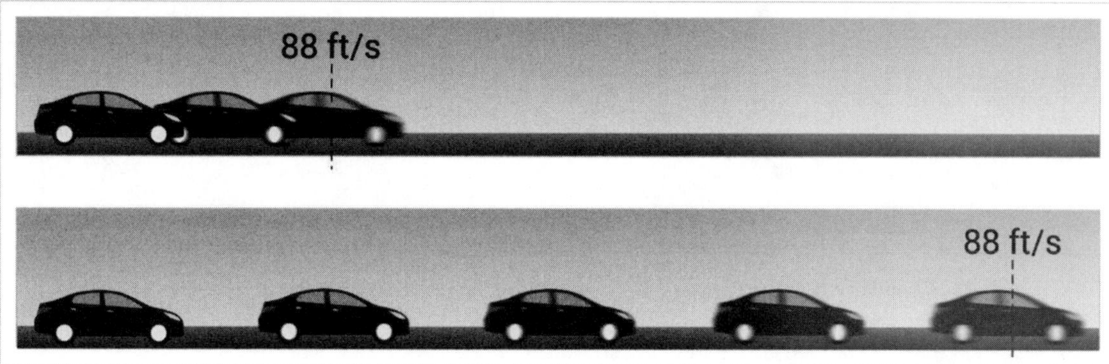

To calculate average acceleration, we may use the equation:

$$\textbf{average acceleration} = \frac{\textbf{change in velocity}}{\textbf{change in time}}$$

The acceleration of the cars is found to be:

$$\text{Car \#1 average acceleration} = \frac{88 \text{ feet per second}}{2 \text{ seconds}} = 44 \frac{\text{feet}}{\text{second}^2}$$

$$\text{Car \#2 average acceleration} = \frac{88 \text{ feet per second}}{8 \text{ seconds}} = 11 \frac{\text{feet}}{\text{second}^2}$$

Acceleration will be expressed in units of distance divided by time squared; for instance, meters per second squared or feet per second squared.

Review Video: Displacement, Velocity, and Acceleration
Visit mometrix.com/academy and enter code: 671849

Projectile Motion

A specific application of the study of motion is projectile motion. Simple projectile motion occurs when an object is in the air and experiencing only the force of gravity. We will disregard drag for this topic. Some common examples of projectile motion are thrown balls, flying bullets, and falling rocks. The characteristics of projectile motion are:

1. The horizontal component of velocity doesn't change
2. The vertical acceleration due to gravity affects the vertical component of velocity

Because gravity only acts downwards, objects in projectile motion only experience acceleration in the y-direction (vertical). The horizontal component of the object's velocity does not change in flight. This means that if a rock is thrown out off a cliff, the horizontal velocity (think of the shadow if the sun is directly overhead) will not change until the ball hits the ground.

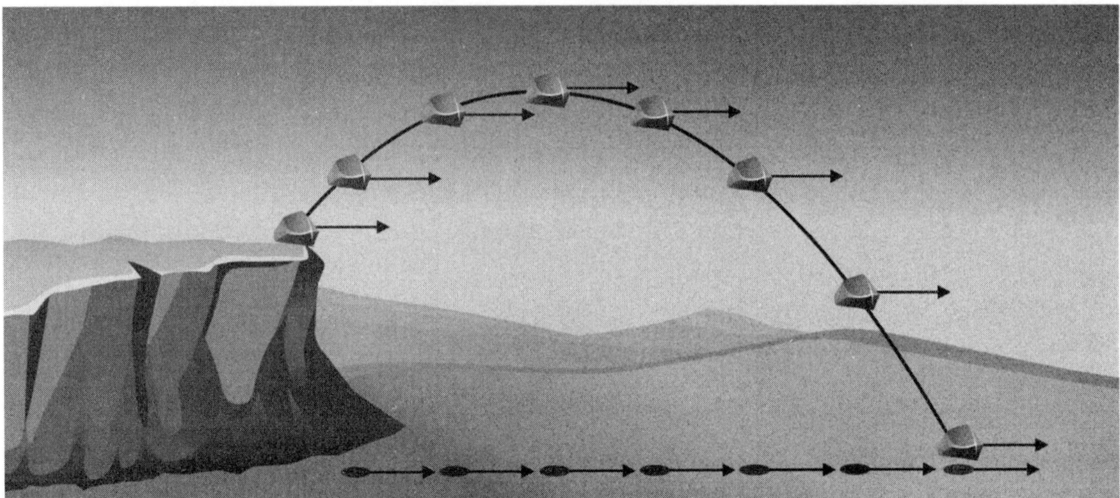

The velocity in the vertical direction is affected by gravity. Gravity imposes an acceleration of $g = 9.8\frac{\text{m}}{\text{s}^2}$ or $32\frac{\text{ft}}{\text{s}^2}$ downward on projectiles. The vertical component of velocity at any point is equal to:

$$\textbf{vertical velocity} = \textbf{original vertical velocity} - \textbf{g} \times \textbf{time}$$

When these characteristics are combined, there are three points of particular interest in a projectile's flight. At the beginning of a flight, the object has a horizontal component and a vertical component giving it a large speed. At the top of a projectile's flight, the vertical velocity equals zero, making the top the slowest part of travel. When the object passes the same height as the launch, the vertical velocity is opposite of the initial vertical velocity, making the speed equal to the initial speed.

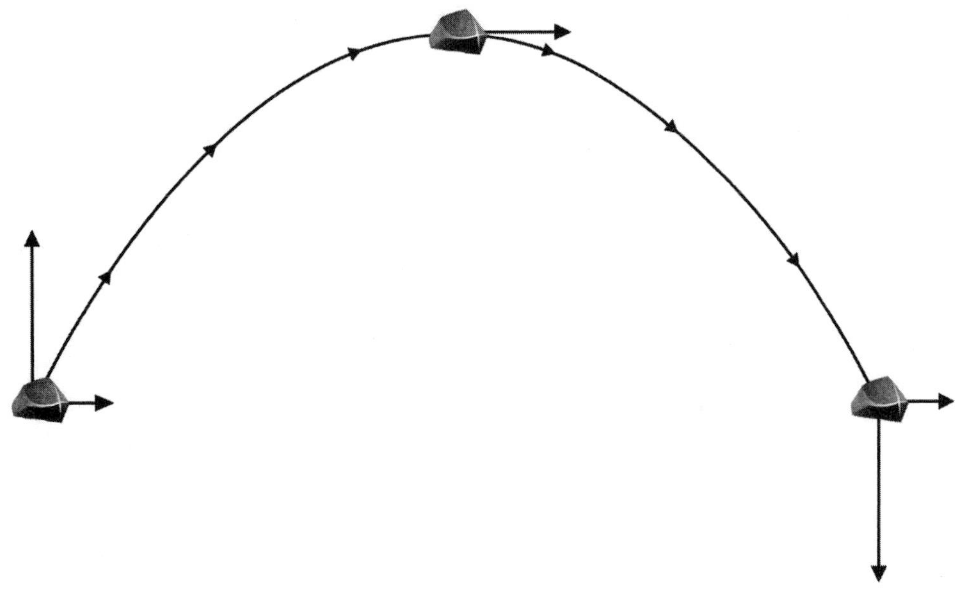

If the object continues falling below the initial height from which it was launched (e.g., it was launched from the edge of a cliff), it will have an even greater velocity than it did initially from that point until it hits the ground.

Review Video: Projectile Motion
Visit mometrix.com/academy and enter code: 719700

Newton's Three Laws of Mechanics

The questions on the exam may require you to demonstrate familiarity with the concepts expressed in Newton's three laws of motion which relate to the concept of force.

Newton's first law – A body at rest tends to remain at rest, while a body in motion tends to remain in motion, unless acted upon by an external force.

Newton's second law – The acceleration of an object is directly proportional to the force being exerted on it and inversely proportional to its mass.

Newton's third law – For every force, there is an equal and opposite force.

First Law

Concept: Unless something interferes, an object won't start or stop moving

Although intuition supports the idea that objects do not start moving until a force acts on them, the idea of an object continuing forever without any forces can seem odd. Before Newton formulated his laws of mechanics, general thought held that some force had to act on an object continuously in order for it to move at a constant velocity. This seems to make sense; when an object is briefly pushed, it will eventually come to a stop. Newton, however, determined that unless some other force acted on the object (most notably friction or air resistance), it would continue in the direction it was pushed at the same velocity forever.

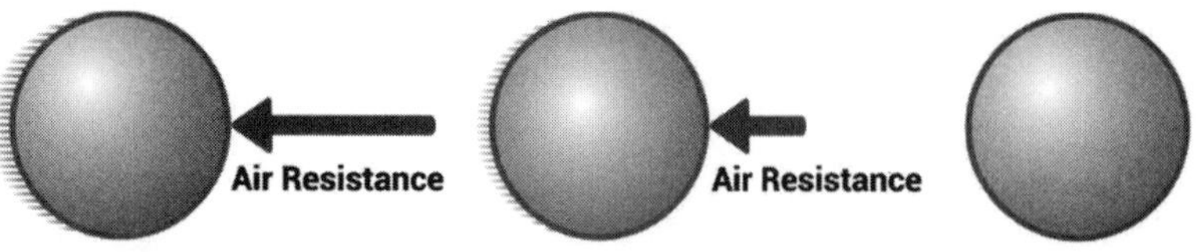

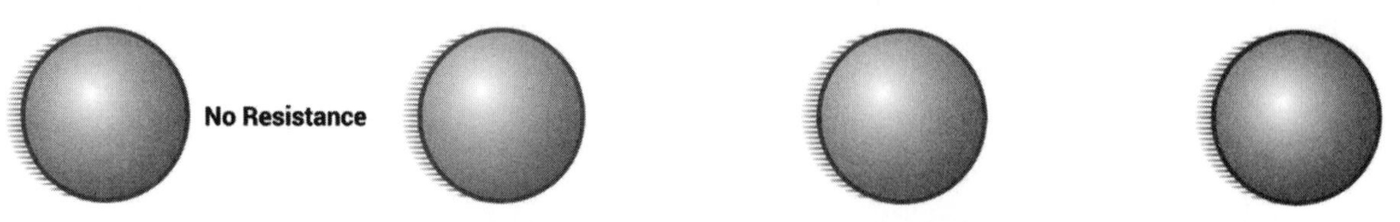

Review Video: Newton's First Law of Motion
Visit mometrix.com/academy and enter code: 590367

SECOND LAW

Concept: Acceleration increases linearly with force.

Although Newton's second law can be conceptually understood as a series of relationships describing how an increase in one factor will decrease another factor, the law can be understood best in equation format:

$$\textbf{Force} = \textbf{mass} \times \textbf{acceleration}$$

Or

$$\textbf{Acceleration} = \frac{\textbf{force}}{\textbf{mass}}$$

Or

$$\textbf{Mass} = \frac{\textbf{force}}{\textbf{acceleration}}$$

Each of the forms of this equation allows for a different look at the same relationships. To examine the relationships, change one factor and observe the result. If a steel ball with a diameter of 6.3 cm has a mass of 1 kg and an acceleration of 1 m/s^2, then the net force on the ball will be 1 Newton.

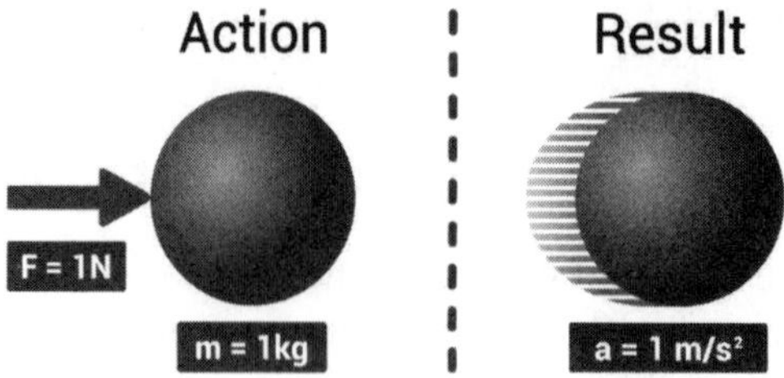

Review Video: Newton's Second Law of Motion
Visit mometrix.com/academy and enter code: 737975

THIRD LAW

Concept: Nothing can push or pull without being pushed or pulled in return.

When any object exerts a force on another object, the other object exerts the opposite force back on the original object. To observe this, consider two spring-based fruit scales, both tipped on their sides as shown with the weighing surfaces facing each other. If fruit scale #1 is pressing fruit scale #2 into the wall, it exerts a force on fruit scale #2, measurable by the reading on scale #2. However, because fruit scale #1 is exerting a force on scale #2, scale #2 is exerting a force on scale #1 with an opposite direction, but the same magnitude.

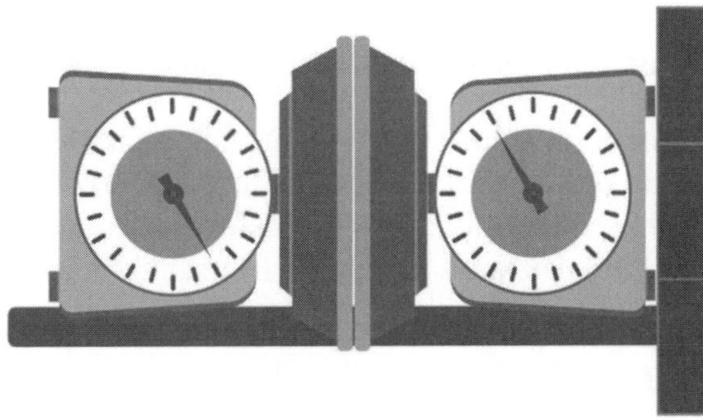

Review Video: Newton's Third Law of Motion
Visit mometrix.com/academy and enter code: 838401

FORCE

Concept: A push or pull on an object

Calculation: Force = mass × acceleration

A force is a vector that causes acceleration of a body. Force has both magnitude and direction. Furthermore, multiple forces acting on one object combine in vector addition. This can be demonstrated by considering an object placed at the origin of the coordinate plane. If it is pushed along the positive direction of the x-axis, it will move in this direction. If the force acting on it is in the positive direction of the y-axis, it will move in that direction.

However, if both forces are applied at the same time, then the object will move at an angle to both the x- and y-axes, an angle determined by the relative amount of force exerted in each direction. In this way, we may see that the resulting force is a vector sum; a net force that has both magnitude and direction.

Resultant vectors from applied forces:

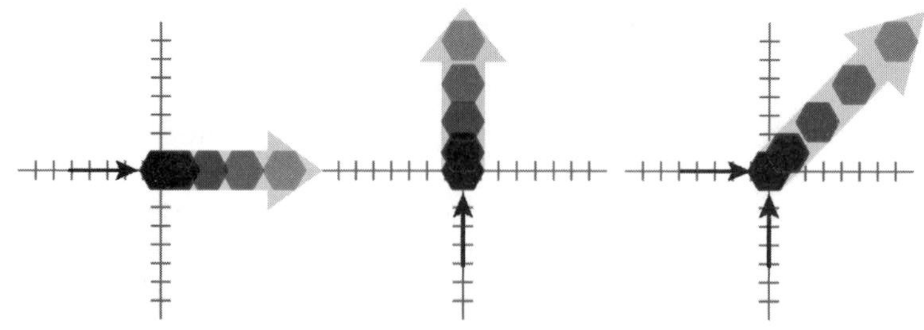

> **Review Video: Push and Pull Forces**
> Visit mometrix.com/academy and enter code: 104731

Friction

Concept: Friction is a resistance to motion between contacting surfaces

In order to illustrate the concept of friction, let us imagine a book resting on a table. As it sits, the force of its weight is equal to and opposite of the normal force. If, however, we were to exert a force on the book, attempting to push it to one side, a frictional force would arise, equal and opposite to our force. This kind of frictional force is known as static frictional force.

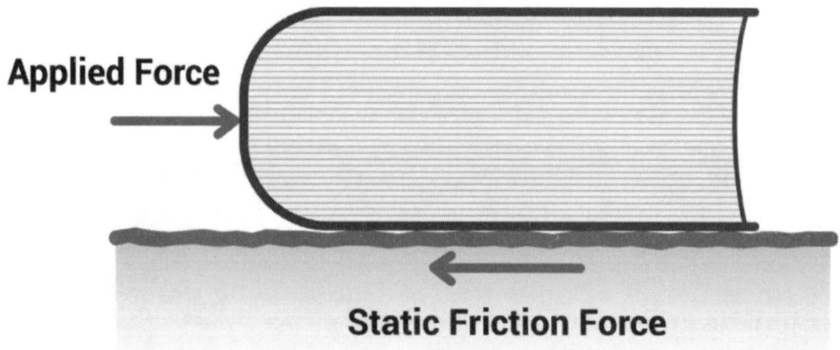

As we increase our force on the book, however, we will eventually cause it to accelerate in the direction of our force. At this point, the frictional force opposing us will be known as kinetic friction. For many combinations of surfaces, the magnitude of the kinetic frictional force is lower than that of the static frictional force, and consequently, the amount of force needed to maintain the movement of the book will be less than that needed to initiate the movement.

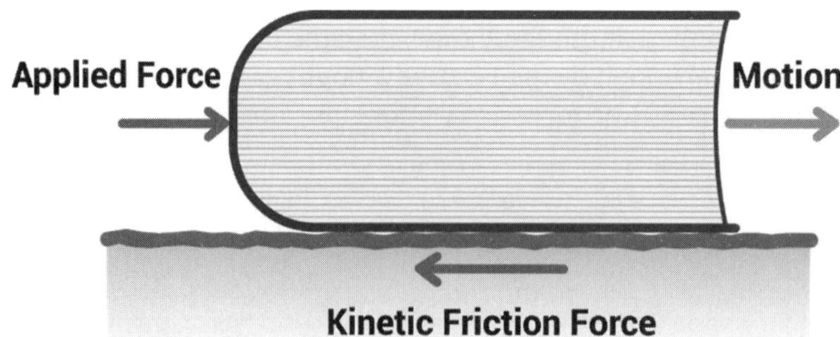

Review Video: Friction
Visit mometrix.com/academy and enter code: 716782

Rolling Friction

Occasionally, a question will ask you to consider the amount of friction generated by an object that is rolling. If a wheel is rolling at a constant speed, then the point at which it touches the ground will not slide, and there will be no friction between the ground and the wheel inhibiting movement. In fact, the friction at the point of contact between the wheel and the ground is static friction necessary to propel with wheels. When a vehicle accelerates, the static friction between the wheels and the ground allows the vehicle to achieve acceleration. Without this friction, the vehicle would spin its wheels and go nowhere.

Although the static friction does not impede movement for the wheels, a combination of frictional forces can resist rolling motion. One such frictional force is bearing friction. Bearing friction is the kinetic friction between the wheel and an object it rotates around, such as a stationary axle.

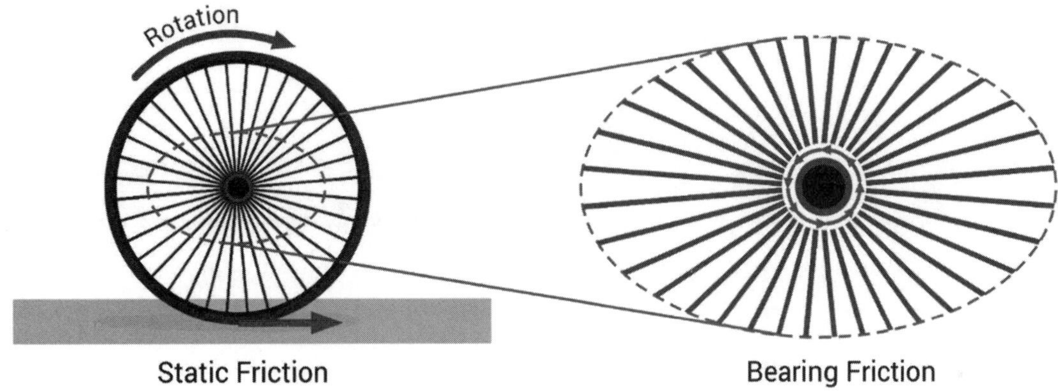

Rotation

Rotational Kinetics

Many equations and concepts in linear kinematics and kinetics transfer to rotation. For example, angular position is an angle. Angular velocity, like linear velocity, is the change in the position (angle) divided by the time. Angular acceleration is the change in angular velocity divided by time. Although most tests will not require you to perform angular calculations, they will expect you to understand the angular version of force: torque.

Concept: Torque is a twisting force on an object

Calculation: Torque = radius × force

Torque, like force, is a vector and has magnitude and direction. As with force, the sum of torques on an object will affect the angular acceleration of that object. The key to solving problems with torque is understanding the lever arm. A better description of the torque equation is:

Torque = force × the distance perpedicular to the force from the center of rotation

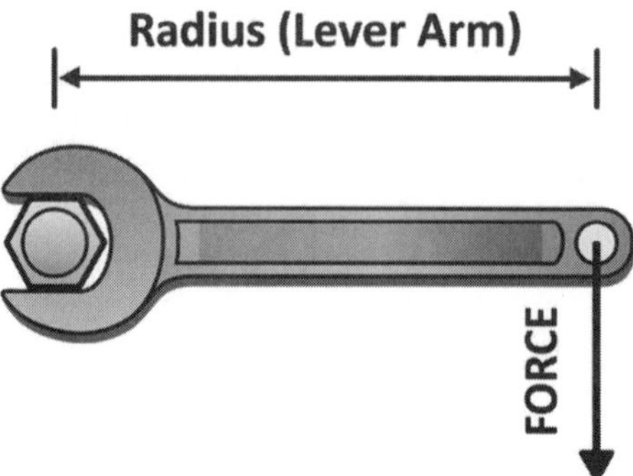

Because torque is directly proportional to the radius, or lever arm, a greater lever arm will result in a greater torque with the same amount of force. The wrench on the right has twice the radius and, as a result, twice the torque.

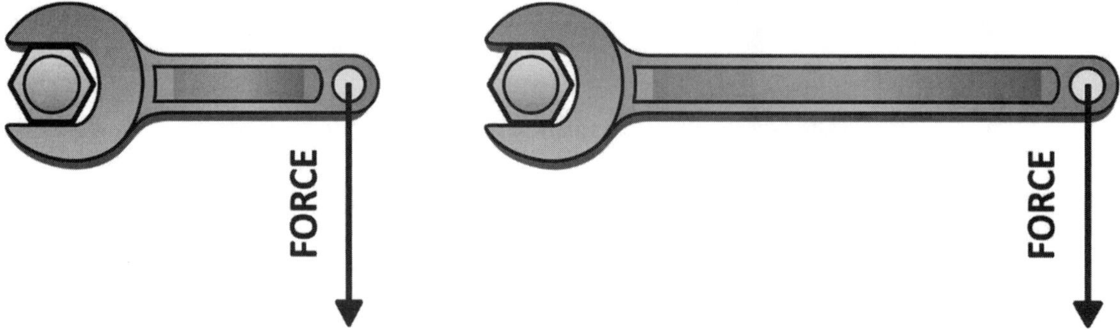

Alternatively, a greater force also increases torque. The wrench on the right has twice the force and twice the torque.

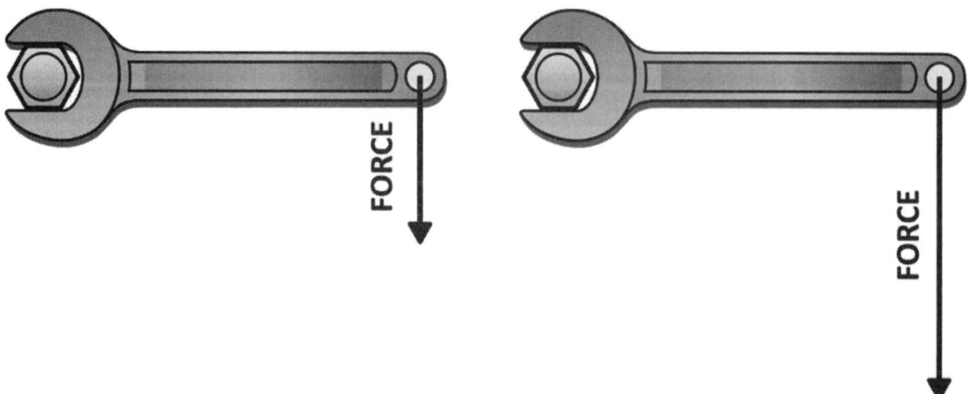

Rotational Kinematics

Concept: Increasing the radius increases the linear speed

Calculation: Linear speed = radius × rotational speed

Another interesting application of the study of motion is rotation. In practice, simple rotation is when an object rotates around a point at a constant speed. Most questions covering rotational kinematics will provide the distance from a rotating object to the center of rotation (radius) and ask about the linear speed of the object. A point will have a greater linear speed when it is farther from the center of rotation.

If a potter is spinning his wheel at a constant speed of one revolution per second, the clay six inches away from the center will be going faster than the clay three inches from the center. The clay directly in the center of the wheel will not have any linear velocity.

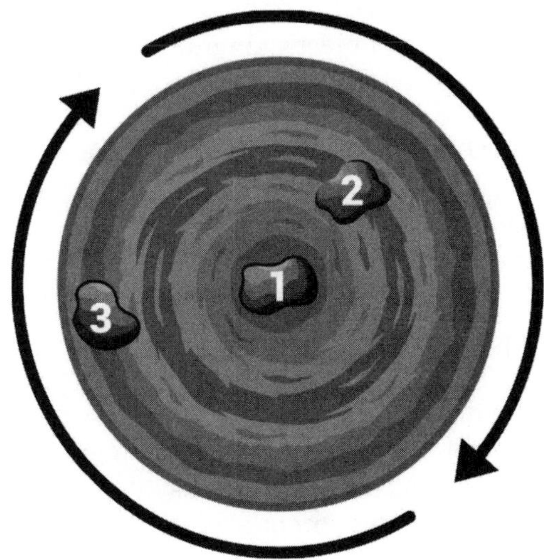

To find the linear speed of rotating objects using radians, we use the equation:

$$\textbf{linear speed} = (\textbf{rotational speed [in radians]}) \times (\textbf{radius})$$

Using degrees, the equation is:

$$\textbf{linear speed} = (\textbf{rotational speed [in degrees]}) \times \frac{\boldsymbol{\pi}\ \textbf{radians}}{\textbf{180 degrees}} \times (\textbf{radius})$$

To find the speed of the pieces of clay, we use the known values (rotational speed of 1 revolution per second, radii of 0 inches, 3 inches, and 6 inches) and the knowledge that one revolution = 2π.

$$\text{clay \#1 speed} = \left(2\pi \frac{\text{rad}}{\text{s}}\right) \times (0 \text{ inches}) = 0 \frac{\text{inches}}{\text{second}}$$

$$\text{clay \#2 speed} = \left(2\pi \frac{\text{rad}}{\text{s}}\right) \times (3 \text{ inches}) = 18.8 \frac{\text{inches}}{\text{second}}$$

$$\text{clay \#3 speed} = \left(2\pi \frac{\text{rad}}{\text{s}}\right) \times (6 \text{ inches}) = 37.7 \frac{\text{inches}}{\text{second}}$$

Review Video: Linear Speed
Visit mometrix.com/academy and enter code: 327101

Kinetic and Potential Energy

Energy

Concept: The ability of a body to do work on another object

Energy is a word that has developed several different meanings in the English language, but in physics, it refers to the measure of a body's ability to do work. In physics, energy may not have a million meanings, but it does have many forms. Each of these forms, such as chemical, electric, and nuclear, is the capability of an object to perform work. However, for the purpose of most tests, mechanical energy and mechanical work are the only forms of energy worth understanding in depth. Mechanical energy is the sum of an object's kinetic and potential energies. Although they will be introduced in greater detail, these are the forms of mechanical energy:

Kinetic Energy – energy an object has by virtue of its motion

Gravitational Potential Energy – energy by virtue of an object's height

Elastic Potential Energy – energy stored in compression or tension

Neglecting frictional forces, mechanical energy is conserved.

As an example, imagine a ball moving perpendicular to the surface of the earth, in other words straight up and down, with its weight being the only force acting on it. As the ball rises, the weight will be doing work on the ball, decreasing its speed and its kinetic energy and slowing it down until it momentarily stops. During this ascent, the potential energy of the ball will be rising. Once the ball begins to fall back down, it will lose potential energy as it gains kinetic energy. Mechanical energy is conserved throughout; the potential energy of the ball at its highest point is equal to the kinetic energy of the ball at its lowest point prior to impact.

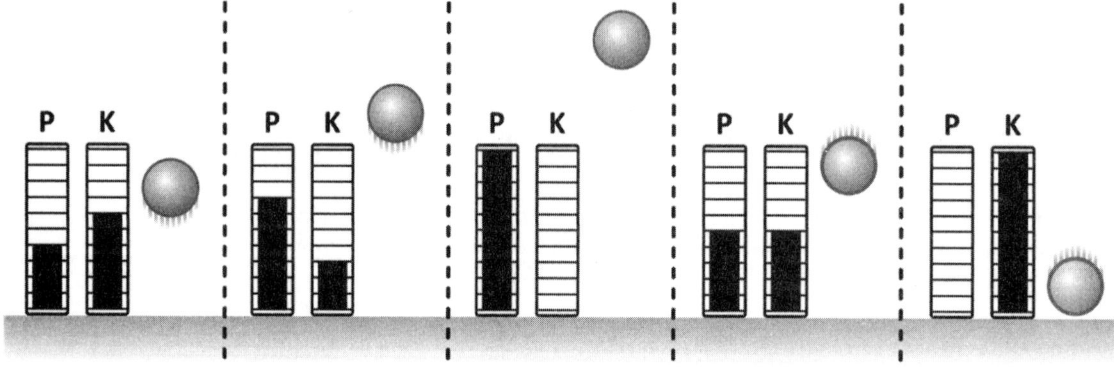

In systems where friction and air resistance are not negligible, we observe a different sort of result. For example, imagine a block sliding across the floor until it comes to a stop due to friction. Unlike a compressed spring or a ball flung into the air, there is no way for this block to regain its energy with a return trip. Therefore, we cannot say that the lost kinetic energy is being stored as potential energy. Instead, it has been dissipated and cannot be recovered. The total mechanical energy of the block-floor system has been not conserved in this case but rather reduced. The total energy of the system has not decreased, since the kinetic energy has been converted into thermal energy, but that energy is no longer useful for work.

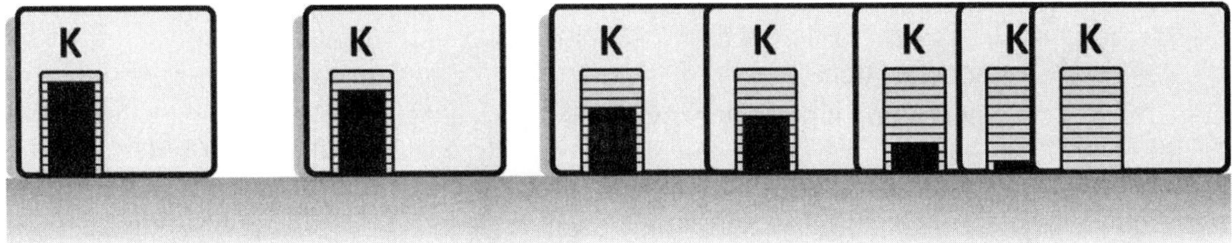

Energy, though it may change form, will be neither created nor destroyed during physical processes. However, if we construct a system and some external force performs work on it, the result may be slightly different. If the work is positive, then the overall store of energy is increased; if it is negative, however, we can say that the overall energy of the system has decreased.

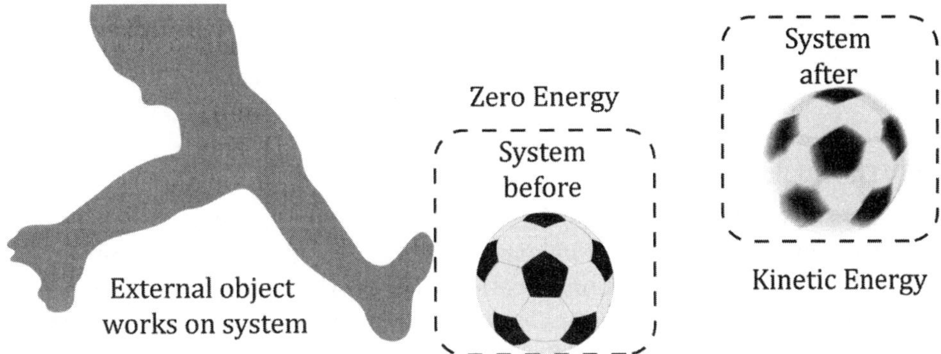

Kinetic Energy

The kinetic energy of an object is the amount of energy it possesses by reason of being in motion. Kinetic energy cannot be negative. Changes in kinetic energy will occur when a force does work on an object, such that the motion of the object is altered. This change in kinetic energy is equal to the amount of work that is done. This relationship is commonly referred to as the work-energy theorem.

One interesting application of the work-energy theorem is that of objects in a free fall. To begin with, let us assert that the force acting on such an object is its weight, which is equal to its mass times g (the force of gravity). The work done by this force will be positive, as the force is exerted in the direction in which the object is traveling. Kinetic energy will, therefore, increase, according to the work-kinetic energy theorem.

If the object is dropped from a great enough height, it eventually reaches its terminal velocity, where the drag force is equal to the weight, so the object is no longer accelerating and its kinetic energy remains constant.

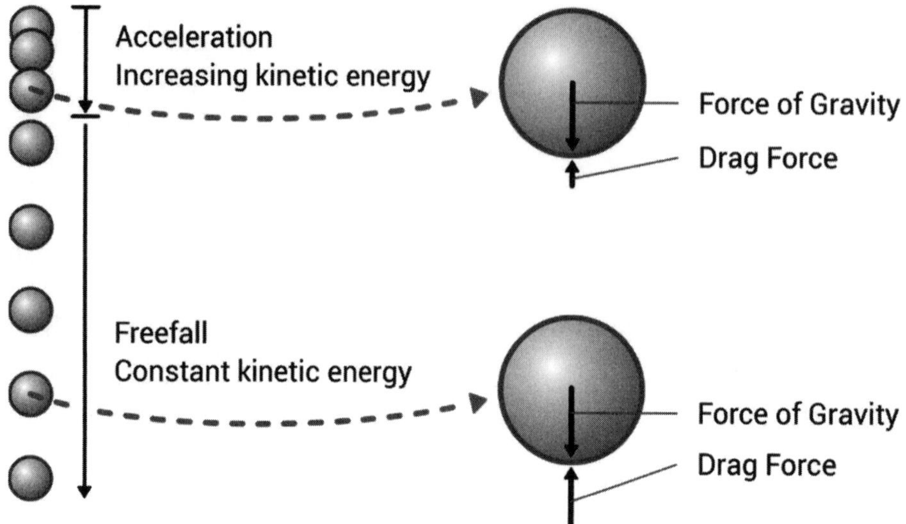

Gravitational Potential Energy

Gravitational potential energy is simply the potential for a certain amount of work to be done by one object on another using gravity. For objects on earth, the gravitational potential energy is equal to the amount of work which the earth can act on the object. The work which gravity performs on objects moving entirely or partially in the vertical direction is equal to the force exerted by the earth (weight) times the distance traveled in the direction of the force (height above the ground or reference point): Work from gravity = weight × height above the ground. Thus, the gravitational potential energy is the same as the potential work.

Gravitational Potential Energy = weight × height

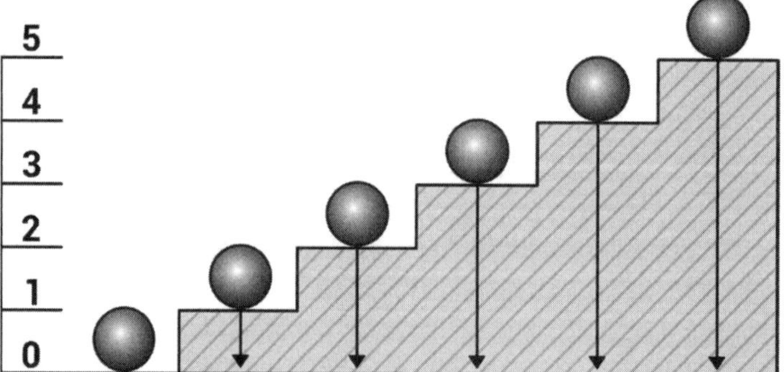

Elastic Potential Energy

Elastic potential energy is the potential for a certain amount of work to be done by one object on another using elastic compression or tension. The most common example is the spring. A spring will resist any compression or tension away from its equilibrium position (natural position). A small buggy is pressed into a large spring. The spring contains a large amount of elastic potential energy. If the buggy and spring are released, the spring will exert a force on the buggy, pushing it for a distance. This work will put kinetic energy into the buggy. The energy can be imagined as a liquid poured from one container into another. The spring pours its elastic energy into the buggy, which receives the energy as kinetic energy.

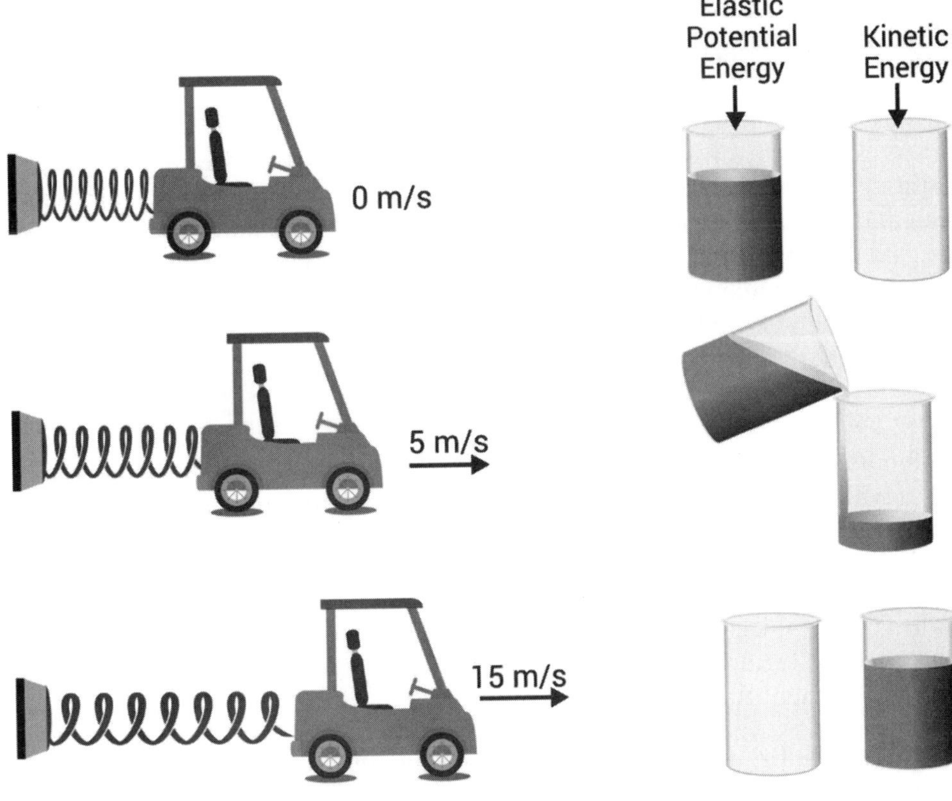

Review Video: Potential and Kinetic Energy
Visit mometrix.com/academy and enter code: 491502

POWER

Concept: The rate of work

Calculation: Work/time

On occasion, you may need to demonstrate an understanding of power as it is defined in applied physics. Power is the rate at which work is done. Power, like work and energy, is a scalar quantity. Power can be calculated by dividing the amount of work performed by the amount of time in which the work was performed: $\textbf{Power} = \frac{\textbf{work}}{\textbf{time}}$. If more work is performed in a shorter amount of time, more power has been exerted. Power can be expressed in a variety of units. The preferred metric expression is one of watts or joules per seconds. Engine power is often expressed in horsepower.

Linear Momentum and Impulse

Linear Momentum

Concept: How much a body will resist stopping

Calculation: Momentum = mass × velocity

In physics, linear momentum can be found by multiplying the mass and velocity of an object. Momentum and velocity will always be in the same direction. Newton's second law describes momentum, stating that the rate of change of momentum is proportional to the force exerted and is in the direction of the force. If we assume a closed and isolated system (one in which no objects leave or enter, and upon which the sum of external forces is zero), then we can assume that the momentum of the system will neither increase nor decrease. That is, we will find that the momentum is a constant. The law of conservation of linear momentum applies universally in physics, even in situations of extremely high velocity or with subatomic particles.

Collisions

This concept of momentum takes on new importance when we consider collisions. A collision is an isolated event in which a strong force acts between each of two or more colliding bodies for a brief period of time. However, a collision is more intuitively defined as one or more objects hitting each other.

When two bodies collide, each object exerts a force on the opposite member. These equal and opposite forces change the linear momentum of the objects. However, when both bodies are considered, the net momentum in collisions is conserved.

There are two types of collisions: elastic and inelastic. The difference between the two lies in whether kinetic energy is conserved. If the total kinetic energy of the system is conserved, the collision is elastic. Visually, elastic collisions are collisions in which objects bounce perfectly. If some of the kinetic energy is transformed into heat or another form of energy, the collision is inelastic. Visually, inelastic collisions are collisions in which the objects stick to each other or bounce but do not return to their original height.

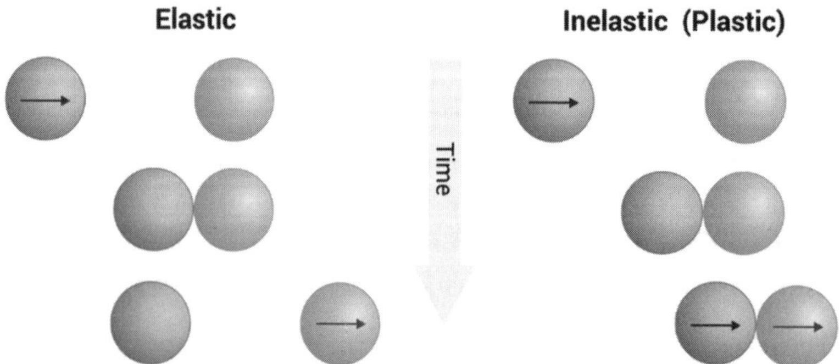

If the two bodies involved in an elastic collision have the same mass, then the body that was moving will stop completely, and the body that was at rest will begin moving at the same velocity as the projectile was moving before the collision.

Nature of Electricity

ELECTRIC CHARGE

Much like gravity, electricity is an everyday observable phenomenon which is very complex, but may be understood as a set of behaviors. As the gravitational force exists between objects with mass, the electric force exists between objects with electrical charge. In all atoms, the protons have a positive charge, while the electrons have a negative charge. An imbalance of electrons and protons in an object results in a net charge. Unlike gravity, which only pulls, electrical forces can push objects apart as well as pull them together.

Similar electric charges repel each other. Opposite charges attract each other.

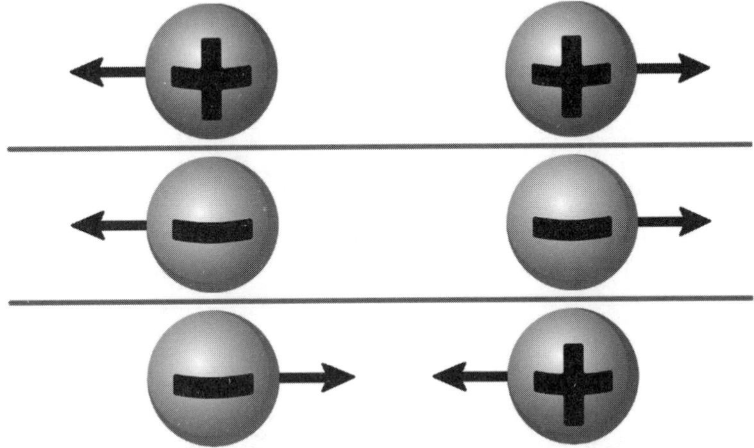

Review Video: Electric Charge
Visit mometrix.com/academy and enter code: 323587

CURRENT

Electrons (and electrical charge with it) move through conductive materials by switching quickly from one atom to another. This electrical flow can manipulate energy like mechanical systems.

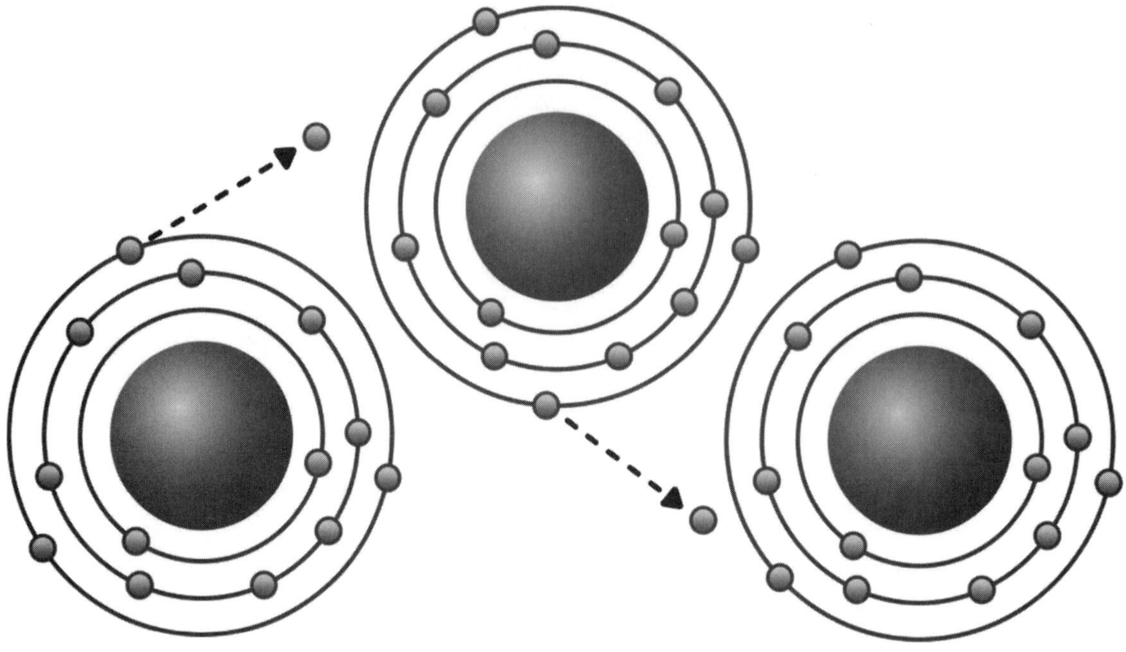

The term for the rate at which the charge flows through a conductive material is *current*. Because each electron carries a specific charge, current can be thought of as the number of electrons passing a point in a length of time. Current is measured in Amperes (A), each unit of which is approximately 6.24×10^{18} electrons per second.

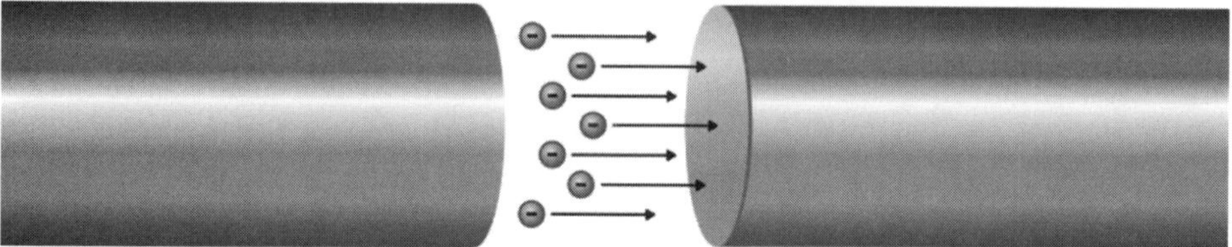

Electric current carries energy much like moving balls carry energy.

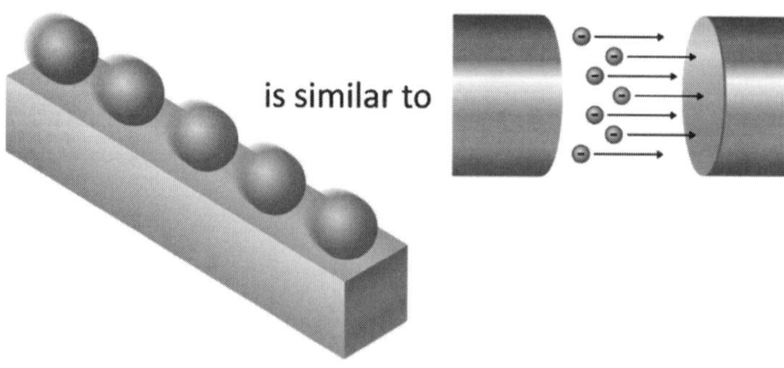

VOLTAGE

Voltage is the potential for electric work. It can also be thought of as the *push* behind electrical work. Voltage is similar to gravitational potential energy.

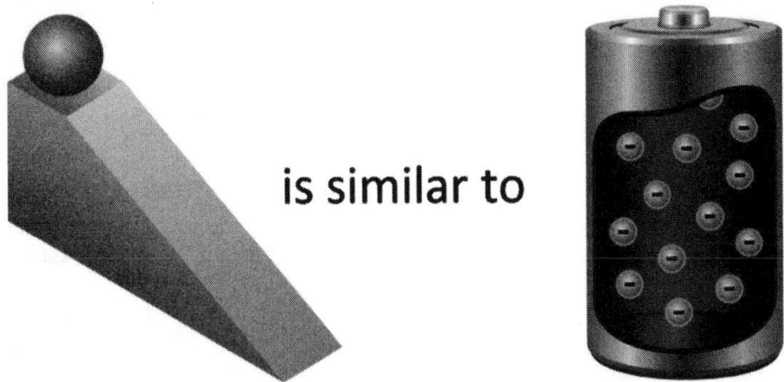

Anything used to generate a voltage, such as a battery or a generator, is called a voltage source. Voltage is conveniently measured in Volts (V).

RESISTANCE

Resistance is the amount something hinders the flow of electrical current. Electrical resistance is much like friction, resisting flow and dissipating energy.

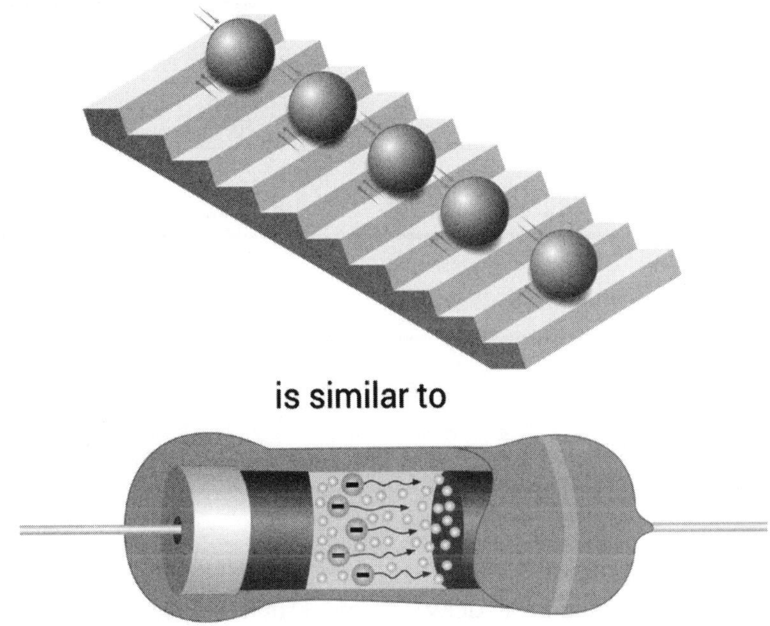

Different objects have different resistances. A resistor is an electrical component designed to have a specific resistance, measured in Ohms (Ω).

Review Video: Resistance of Electric Currents
Visit mometrix.com/academy and enter code: 668423

Basic Circuits

A circuit is a closed loop through which current can flow. A simple circuit contains a voltage source and a resistor. The current flows from the positive side of the voltage source through the resistor to the negative side of the voltage source.

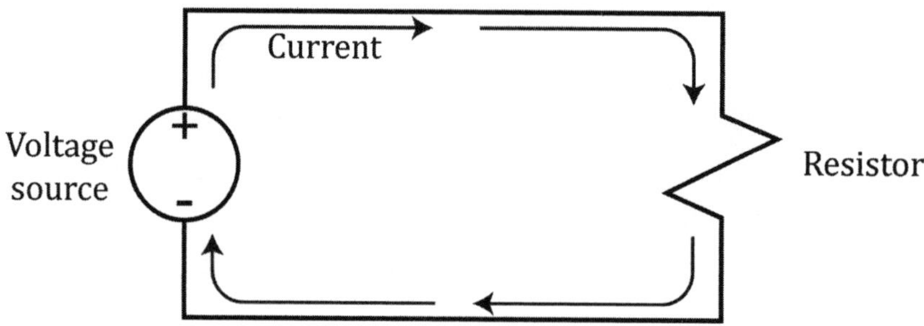

If we plot the voltage of a simple circuit, the similarities to gravitational potential energy appear.

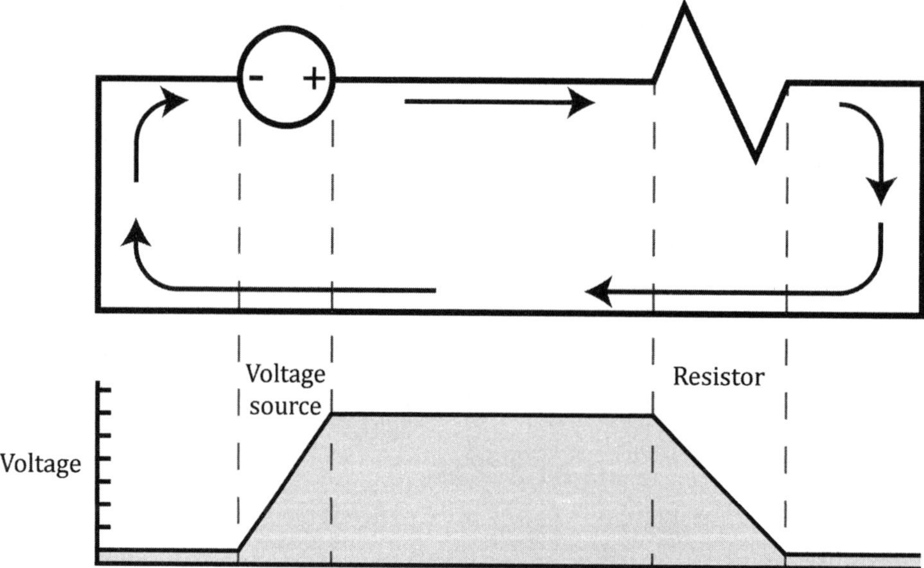

If we consider the circuit to be a track, the electrons would be balls, the voltage source would be a powered lift, and the resistor would be a sticky section of the track. The lift raises the balls, increasing their potential energy. This potential energy is expended as the balls roll down the sticky section of the track.

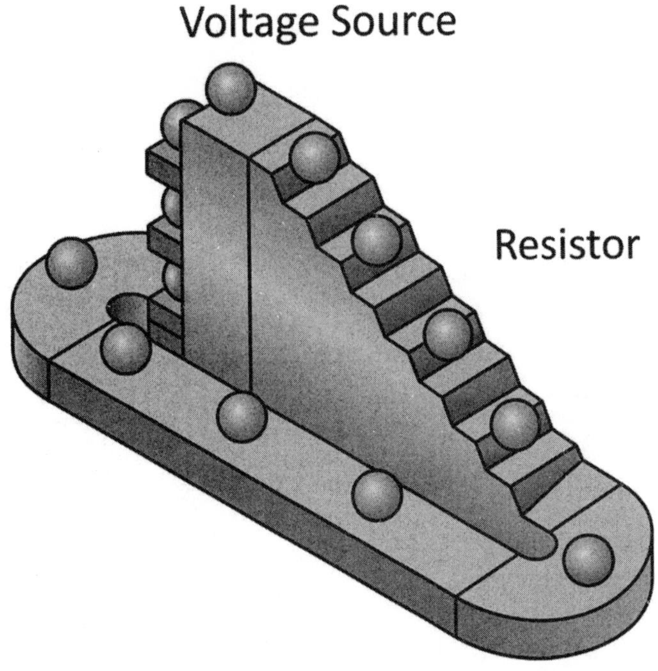

Magnetism

Magnetism is an attraction between opposite poles of magnetic materials and a repulsion between similar poles of magnetic materials. Magnetism can be natural or induced with the use of electric currents. Magnets almost always exist with two polar sides: north and south. A magnetic force exists between two poles on objects. Different poles attract each other. Like poles repel each other.

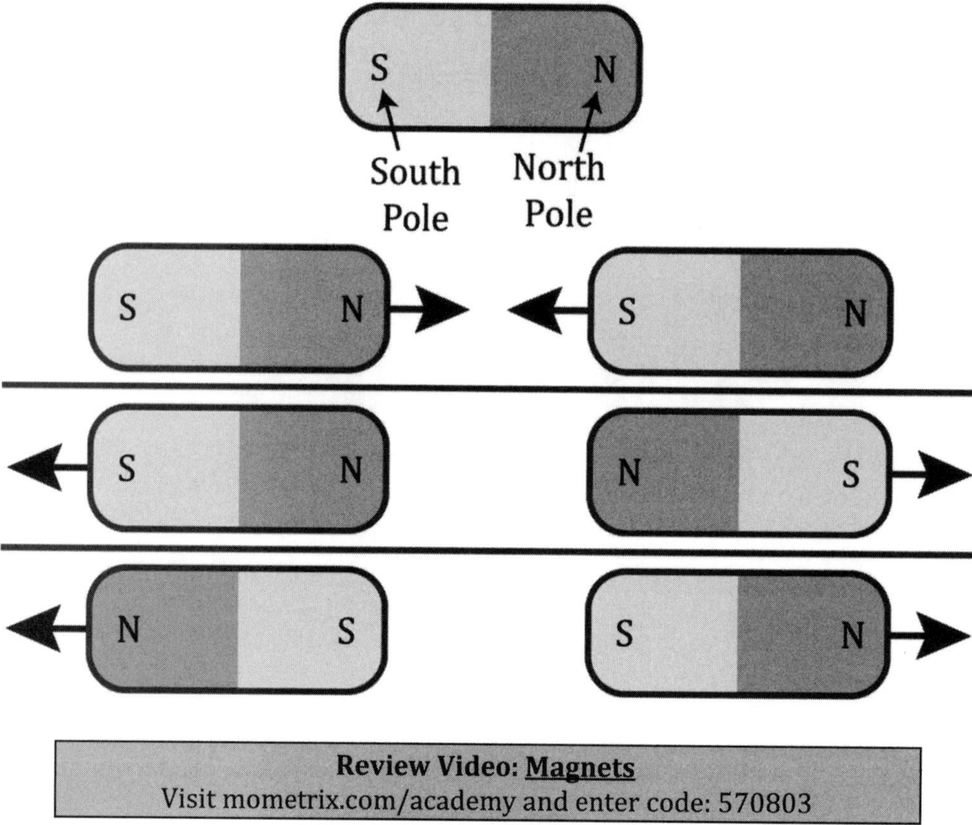

Review Video: Magnets
Visit mometrix.com/academy and enter code: 570803

Chapter Quiz

Ready to see how well you retained what you just read? Scan the QR code to go directly to the chapter quiz interface for this study guide. If you're using a computer, simply visit the bonus page at **mometrix.com/bonus948/hesia2** and click the Chapter Quizzes link.

Professional Practice

Practice Settings

Nurses can work in a variety of industries. The obvious locations where nurses can apply their skills are hospitals, clinics, and doctor's offices. Nurses also practice in community agencies, schools, businesses, military units, summer camps, vacation resorts, and cruise ships. Some nurses put their skills and knowledge to use by teaching others to become nurses in college courses or nursing schools. Nurses can work in nursing homes, retirement communities, ambulatory care agencies, volunteer organizations, private practices, hospices, occupational health facilities, and federal or state agencies.

Nurses' Roles

One of the most basic tasks that a nurse can perform is **patient care**. Nurses must constantly manage and care for patients. While caring for patients, nurses may perform many other roles, and sometimes they may fill multiple roles at once. Nurses can find themselves in the role of caregiver, comforter, teacher, counselor, role model, protector, advocate, decision maker, case manager, researcher, or communicator. Additionally, it is important to note that nurses do not work exclusively one-on-one with patients; nurses can actually work with groups of patients. In some cases, a nurse will work with a whole family or an entire community.

Career Opportunities

A nursing degree will allow you to pursue a variety of career options within the field. In general, the **career opportunities** for nurses increase as the education level of the nurse increases. In other words, more education can result in better job opportunities and higher pay. In addition to working as a general duty or staff nurse, a nurse may work as a private practice nurse, home health nurse, midwife, or anesthetist. Nurses can focus their careers on teaching others by becoming educators in nursing programs. They can work as clinical specialists, administrators, practitioners, or consultants. Nurses can also focus their career in the area of research. Nurses can actually pursue career paths that target their own special areas of interest. For example, midwives can visit expectant mothers and help them prepare for childbirth in the comfort of their own home.

Qualities of Successful Nurses

Successful nurses possess certain qualities that help them excel at their jobs. A good nurse is a **team player**. Nurses should be able to work well with their peers. The best nurses are honest, dependable, responsible, and accountable. They are capable of following directions and managing stressful situations. Nurses must understand that they are **responsible** for the well-being of others, and they should avoid abusing substances that could alter their decision-making ability. In other words, nurses should avoid drugs and alcohol. Nurses must be able to care for all patients, regardless of gender, race, religion, or other individual characteristics. Nurses must also be able to control their temper. Patients can be disagreeable and colleagues can be frustrating, but nurses must manage their **emotions** to perform their job effectively.

Nursing Technicians vs. Generalists

There are three types of programs that nursing candidates can choose to pursue: diploma programs, associate degree programs, and baccalaureate programs. Students who complete **diploma programs** or **associate degree programs** are considered **technicians**. These types of programs prepare students for the technical practice of nursing. In other words, these nurses will focus almost exclusively on patient care. Graduates of nursing **baccalaureate programs** are considered **generalists**. These nurses are equipped to work in a variety of health care environments. Nurses with a baccalaureate degree can fill many roles, including (but not limited to) caregivers, educators, and consultants. While technicians care for individual patients in a structured setting, a generalist may care for groups of patients in unstructured settings.

Graduate Education Options

Nurses who hold either a master's degree or doctoral degree will have more professional opportunity, as well as higher paying careers. The first step for nurses who wish to pursue higher education in nursing is to obtain a **baccalaureate degree**. Obtaining a **master's degree** prepares a nurse to become an educator in various nursing programs. A master's degree also allows a nurse to become a researcher, manager, nurse practitioner, or administrator. Doctoral training allows a nurse to earn degrees in education, nursing science, nursing, and philosophy. A nurse with a **doctoral degree** can become an educator in undergraduate or graduate nursing programs. He or she can become an advanced clinical researcher, consultant, or independent practitioner.

Nursing Programs

In the United States, there are three types of programs available for those who want to become a registered nurse. Each program has a unique curriculum, accreditation agency, and professional organization. The three programs are associate degree programs, diploma programs, and baccalaureate degree programs. **Associate degree programs** are the shortest—usually taking only two years to complete. **Diploma programs**, which take three years to complete, are generally affiliated with a hospital. **Baccalaureate programs** are the longest type of nursing program, lasting four years. These programs are typically offered at a college or university.

Admissions Departments

Nursing programs consider many factors when deciding which candidates will be accepted. In general, nursing programs will consider a candidate's GPA, SAT or ACT scores, writing ability, community service, interviews, references, and entrance exam scores. Nursing schools must often set high standards for admission because of the number of students attempting to join the program. Each program can only accept a certain number of students, making it a highly competitive field. High **GPAs** and **test scores** are all key factors in the selection process; they indicate that a candidate is studious and dedicated, and will do well in rigorous nursing courses. Candidates should also be able to provide a list of **references**—usually people to whom they are not related. References should be people with whom the candidates have worked, such as teachers and employers.

Financial Requirements

In addition to the time commitment required when entering a nursing program, there is a large **financial investment** involved. Baccalaureate programs are more expensive than other programs because they take longer to complete. Each student must decide how he or she will pay for his or her nursing education. Working while in school is an option, but nursing courses require many hours outside of the classroom. If obtaining **financial aid** is an option, students are advised to pursue it. Nursing school costs, in addition to the obvious tuition cost, can include many fees, room and board, daily meals at clinical sites, books, uniforms, and malpractice insurance. Students will also have to purchase nursing supplies, such as stethoscopes, bandage scissors, and thermometers. Students must also consider the cost of vehicle maintenance, personal health costs, and the costs of life outside of nursing school.

Financial Assistance Considerations

The first step for students pursuing financial aid is to consult with their nursing program's **financial aid department**. Before accepting financial aid, students must be sure to understand fully all of the terms of the loan. Financial aid may require students to maintain a certain grade-point average or number of credit hours. While student loans are usually associated with lower interest rates, they must be repaid upon graduation from the nursing program (earlier if the student fails or withdraws from the nursing program). Students who do not repay the loan can be impacted by a negative credit score and, in more severe cases, forfeiture of their license to practice nursing. In some cases, students may be eligible to receive grants or scholarships that do not require repayment.

Sociology

Sociology is the study of humans as they coexist in groups. One of the basic principles of sociology is that humans will behave in the same manner as those around them. **Sociologists** study the development of society and social behavior among humans, origins, organizations, and institutions. They may study one group or institution as a self-contained entity or as part of a greater whole. Sociology also concerns itself with the question of whether nature or nurture exerts greater influence on the existence of a human. It may be said that a sociologist studies the various processes that create and maintain a system of **social structure**.

Psychology

Psychology is the study of the mental processes and behavior of an individual. Psychologists may study the general characteristics of individuals or large groups. The field of psychology can be divided into applied and experimental areas. Certain psychologists examine **mental processes**. Other psychologists examine the elements of **consciousness**, such as mental activity, free will, and memory. The field of **social psychology** combines psychology and sociology. It is the study of the interactions that occur between individuals and groups. It also is the study of the effects of groups on the behaviors and attitudes of the individual.

Ethics

Ethical principles should be understood and used by nurses. When applied correctly, ethical principles can facilitate decision making in all facets of life. Nursing especially is a profession in which ethics play a large role. The patients trust that the nurses will always make decisions that are in the best interest of the patient. The study of science and medicine can equip an individual with the skills necessary to save or improve a person's life; however, ethics give the individual the ability to make decisions regarding matters of life and death. Nurses must always be aware of the impact their behavior and actions will have on their patients.

Ethical Principle of Beneficence

Beneficence is the practice of always helping other people. The definition of the word *beneficent* is *doing or producing good, especially through the acts of charity and kindness.* This principle is central to the role of health care providers that it is part of the **Hippocratic Oath** sworn by medical doctors. In the field of ethics, the term *beneficence* has an additional component that requires that no **intentional harm** be done to another person. In other words, **nonmaleficence** is an essential component of beneficence. There are three theories regarding beneficence: Humes' theory, utilitarian theory, and Kant's theory. **Hume's theory** claims that the motive behind an act of kindness determines the validity of the act. **Utilitarian theory** states that beneficence is simply the drive to create happiness through kindness or unhappiness through unkindness. **Kant's theory** states that beneficence is motivated by a sense of duty.

Ethical Principle of Justice

The ethical principle of justice centers on the fair and equal treatment of all individuals. Nurses must constantly evaluate their own motives when treating patients. Each patient should receive the same degree of attention, compassion, and care. Nurses must remember to speak confidentially about patients, as well as to maintain discretion about a patient's condition. In the health care field, questions of **ethical justice** often arise because of insurance and patient needs. Oftentimes, a patient will need a specific type of care but may not have the financial resources to pay for it. There is also the question of **compensatory justice**, in which one individual or group of individuals has been harmed by the actions of another.

Ethical Principle of Autonomy

In the most basic sense, the ethical principle of **autonomy** refers to a patient's right to choose a course of action and follow or change it as they see fit. In order for patients to choose freely, they must be provided with the appropriate information. Medical facilities often attempt to uphold the ethical principle of autonomy by providing patients with **informed consent documents**. Autonomy requires that patients be allowed to decide and act without pressure or coercion from another party. Medical professionals can aid in the freedom to choose by making sure that patients have adequate information about the choices available to them. Medical professionals can aid in the freedom to act by ensuring that the patient and the patient's family understand the importance of respecting the autonomy of the individual.

Mass Casualties

It seems that the increasing technological capabilities of the modern world are accompanied by the increasing threat of **mass devastation**. Entire cities can be built of towers that reach hundreds of stories in height. With all of this development comes an increase in the risk of mass injury. Imagine that you are a triage nurse working the emergency room when over 300 seriously injured patients are routed to your hospital. How do you decide who is treated first? Nurses must use the **utilitarian principle of ethics**, in which the greatest good must be done for the greatest number of people.

Bioethical Issues

The most intense bioethical issues faced by nurses involve the beginning and end of life. Modern technology has introduced in vitro fertilization, contraception, abortion, genetic modification, cloning, and surrogate mothers. All of these are useful tools, but each comes with its own set of **ethical dilemmas**. This is also the case with issues surrounding the end of life. Ethical concerns include euthanasia, the definition of death, death through outside intervention, and the handling of patients with diseases brought about by avoidable behaviors. For example, imagine that a hospital with a limited staff has two patients suffering from lung cancer. They are the same age with similar backgrounds. Now imagine one patient is a lifelong smoker, while the other has never smoked. If the hospital only has resources to treat one of those patients, which one should they choose?

Testing

CRITICAL THINKING SKILLS

Critical thinking is a skill that nurses must use on a regular basis. Critical thinking is a combination of **scientific knowledge** and the **logical application** of that knowledge. In the course of daily life, people are constantly faced with opportunities to use critical thinking skills. An individual may be presented with a problem for which they must find the best possible **solution**. In order to do so, the individual must consider a variety of possible solutions. They must understand the **consequences** associated with each solution and the manner in which the solution will resolve the problem. Students should carefully read and analyze each possible response for each test question. By understanding fully all of the options available, students can select the best solution.

STANDARDIZED TESTING TIPS

In addition to critical thinking, a variety of testing strategies can be utilized in standardized testing. For example, in a timed multiple-choice test, students should answer the questions of which they are **certain**, skipping over questions that require more time to think. This will allow the student to devote the appropriate amount of time to harder questions, without running the risk of earning a lower score for running out of time. Test-takers should read questions carefully, looking out for words such as *first* or *usually*. These words can be very important when selecting the best response. When faced with a tough question, students should avoid selecting answers that use the terms *always* and *never*. Correct answers are most often worded with **less absolute** language, such as the phrases *in most cases* or *usually*. Students should also be cautious when answering questions that imply a cause-and-effect relationship. When selecting an answer for this type of question, avoid options that state one thing is causing another. Instead, select a more conservative option that states the two things are somehow connected.

PROCESS OF ELIMINATION

Standardized tests are most commonly organized into questions with four possible answer choices. For each question, there is a 1 in 4 chance (25%) that the student will select the correct answer. This also means there is a 3 in 4 chance (75%) that the student will select the wrong answer. The odds seem to favor the student answering incorrectly. By simply **eliminating** the obviously incorrect answers, students can increase the odds of selecting the correct answer. If there are four possible answer choices, eliminating two of those answers will give the student a 50% chance of answering the question correctly. By the simple process of elimination, a student can increase his chances of answering a question correctly even if he knows very little about the subject.

MULTIPLE-CHOICE QUESTIONS

In standardized multiple-choice tests, there are three levels of test questions: recall, application, and analysis.

RECALL QUESTIONS

In standardized multiple-choice tests, there are three levels of test questions: recall, application, and analysis. **Recall questions** require the test-taker simply to remember a piece of information. An example of a recall question is a definition. The question may ask the student to select the best definition of a word that is either contained within a sentence or provided in a more straightforward form. Recall questions will not require the student to analyze or apply knowledge. Once a student identifies a recall question, she can answer it directly (if she knows the correct answer) or she can begin to eliminate incorrect answers to increase her odds of answering correctly.

When answering a recall-level question, students often either know the answer or do not. When a student does not immediately know the correct answer, he can try a memory trick. Namely, he should move on to another question or think of something else entirely. By giving his mind a distraction, and then returning to the troublesome question, the answer will often become clear. Students may also use **visual association** when learning material. For example, in order to remember that arteries carry blood away from the heart, a student might picture the heart as a museum filled with art, which is stolen by a thief. By picturing a thief stealing art, the student associates the word *art* with the word *arteries*, thus remembering that arteries carry blood away from the heart. Another method is the **comparison strategy**. By finding similarities between pieces of information, students can more readily retain knowledge. For example, arteries carry blood away from the heart. Both *artery* and *away* begin with the letter *a*.

Application Questions

Application questions require that students use the knowledge they have learned. Students may be asked to **apply** the knowledge they have acquired from textbooks and apply it to a real-life situation. For example, a question may provide a brief scenario described in paragraph form. A question will ask the student to use the information presented in the paragraph. In general, the questions will be asked in the form of "if you know this about X, what can be assumed about Y?" These questions will present all of the information students need within the question. By carefully reading the questions and examining the answer choices, students should be able to locate the correct answer.

Analysis Questions

Analysis-level questions are the most complex of the three levels. For this type of problem, students must carefully read the question, dissect it, and then study the **interaction** between its various parts. Students may find that analysis-level questions require them to identify what piece of information is missing. Students should read each answer choice provided and examine how well that piece fits into the puzzle. The student should consider whether the answer choice actually provides a solution, or whether it simply produces more questions. As with all test questions, students improve their chances of success by eliminating the obviously incorrect choices.

Preparing for Standardized Exams

Standardized testing can be a stressful situation for students. It is crucial that students begin studying material **early** so that they have plenty of time to prepare. By studying early, students can avoid all-night cram sessions that deprive them of sleep, nutrition, and mental health. Students should avoid overly emotional interactions prior to a test, because this can cause increased anxiety, which could lead to decreased performance. At least ten days prior to the test, the student should begin taking multivitamins, eating properly, getting plenty of rest, and exercising. All of these things will give the body what it needs to perform at its highest level on test day.

Personality Profile

The Admission Assessment test will include 15 items designed to gauge your **personality type**. Although there are no wrong answers to these questions, it is a good idea to learn the conceptual framework underlying the personality profile. The primary distinction made by these questions is between the extroverted and introverted personality types.

Extroverted Personality Type

The extroverted personality type is characterized by a desire to be **around other people**. Extroverted individuals draw energy from their interaction with others. Extroverts are likely to enjoy social gatherings, and are most successful when working in **collaboration** with other people. Extroverts are more talkative, gregarious, and assertive of their own desires than are introverts.

Introverted Personality Type

The introverted personality type is characterized by a desire to be alone and **away from other people**. Introversion should not be confused with antisocial personality disorder; there is no pathology associated with normal introversion. Introverts tend to be imaginative and thoughtful, and often enjoy activities like reading, distance running, and writing. Introverts tend to be more successful when they are allowed to work **independently**. For introverts, social interaction can be depleting and exhausting. Introverts often report a need to "recharge" by spending time alone. Introverts prefer to observe activities before participating, and tend to be more analytical than extroverts.

Learning Styles

The Admission Assessment will include 14 items designed to gauge your **learning style**. As with the personality profile, there are no incorrect answers to these questions. However, it is a good idea to be acquainted with the seven common learning styles: spatial, auditory-musical, linguistic, kinesthetic, mathematical, interpersonal, and intrapersonal.

Spatial Learning Style

Students with the spatial learning style (also known as the visual learning style) learn best by using pictures and **images**. They find it is easier to retain information that is presented in a table or chart. They prefer to use a map to orient themselves rather than relying on a set of written directions. Color-coding information is a helpful method of teaching for student with this learning style.

Auditory-Musical Learning Style

Students with the auditory-musical learning style (also known as the aural learning style) learn best by using **sound**, and especially music. These students have a natural sense of rhythm and harmony, and find it easy to remember the words to songs. Often, these students unconsciously drum out a beat on their desk or keep up a constant rhythm of toe taps under their chair. They can improve their retention of new information by placing it into a rhyme or setting it to a familiar tune. These students often have success using **mnemonics** based on popular songs.

Linguistic Learning Style

Students with the linguistic learning style (also known as the verbal learning style) learn best by using **words**, whether spoken or written. These students like to express themselves with words, and are very receptive to the language used in texts and by teachers. They will also have a natural facility for wordplay, and will enjoy word-based puzzles and games. Students with a linguistic learning style will find it easy to retain the information they read, and should be able to express themselves clearly in writing. They enjoy reading texts aloud, and benefit from mnemonics based on wordplay and common expressions.

Kinesthetic Learning Style

Students with the kinesthetic learning style (also known as the physical learning style) learn best by using **physical movement** and gesture. These students retain information that they receive through their sense of touch. Often, students with a kinesthetic style of learning will be able to retain spoken information better when their **hands** are kept occupied. For instance, studies have shown that kinesthetic learners pick up their multiplication tables faster when they are allowed to bounce a ball while practicing. These students also love to make models and three-dimensional representations of the things they have learned.

Mathematical Learning Style

Students with the mathematical learning style (also known as the logical learning style) learn best by using systems of **logic** and analytical reasoning. These students are great at recognizing patterns, and are quick to discern the logical system underlying a set of information. These students prefer to work through problems in a **systematic manner**, and thrive in highly structured learning environments. A student with a mathematical learning style will appreciate being given a list of the tasks to be accomplished over a certain interval. These students excel in the sciences and any other area that calls for rigorous, systematic thinking.

Interpersonal Learning Style

Students with the interpersonal learning style (also known as the social learning style) learn best when working in **collaboration** with other people. These students are good communicators, and have no problem making their meaning plain to other people. They are also sensitive to the concerns of other people, and have a genuine interest in preserving harmony within the work group. Interpersonal learners work best in **groups**, and often exhibit strong **leadership** skills. These students enjoy role-playing exercises and peer-review assignments. They may become frustrated or bored when asked to work alone for a long time.

Intrapersonal Learning Style

Students with the intrapersonal learning style (also known as the solitary learning style) learn best by **themselves**. These students become frustrated when working in a group, and prefer to act independently. They often need a period of **reflection** before initiating an activity. They often excel at reading and writing. Student with an intrapersonal learning style will thrive in structured learning environments, and will prefer consistency to chaos. These students may become over-stimulated by contact with other people, and require frequent opportunities to recharge with solitude and contemplation. Intrapersonal learners tend to be reserved and thoughtful, but capable of developing strong relationships with a few select peers.

HESI Practice Test #1

Want to take this practice test in an online interactive format?
Check out the bonus page, which includes interactive practice questions and much more: **mometrix.com/bonus948/hesia2**

Mathematics (Video Explanations Available)

We now have video explanations for every math question in this practice test. Visit **mometrix.com/academy/hesi-a2-math-explanations/** or scan this QR code to access these videos.

1. Solve for x: $2x + 4 = x - 6$.

a. $x = -12$
b. $x = 10$
c. $x = -16$
d. $x = -10$

2. Evaluate the expression $\frac{2a}{3b} + 5a - 7b$ when $a = 21$ and $b = 7$.

____

3. A car lot has an inventory of 476 cars. If 36 people bought cars in the week after the inventory was taken, how many cars will remain in inventory at the end of that week?

________ cars

4. Is 45,064 divisible by 8? Explain why.

a. Yes, because it is even.
b. Yes, because the number formed by the last three digits is divisible by 8.
c. Yes, because it begins with an even digit.
d. No, because the last two digits form an even number.

5. If a chef can make 25 pastries in a day, how many can he make in a week?

________ pastries

6. What is the least common multiple of 6 and 10?

____

7. Four nurse midwives open a joint practice together. They use a portion of the income to pay for various expenses for the practice. Each nurse midwife contributes $2,000 per month. One of them allocates $\frac{1}{2}$ of her funds to pay an office administrator and another $\frac{1}{10}$ for office supplies. What is the total fraction of her budget that is spent on the office administrator and office supplies?

a. $\frac{3}{5}$
b. $\frac{2}{12}$
c. $\frac{2}{20}$
d. $\frac{1}{20}$

8. Billy rides his bicycle 5 miles for each morning that he works his paper route. One morning this week, he rode an extra mile to visit with his grandparents. At the end of the week, he had ridden 21 miles. How many mornings did he deliver papers? Support your answer with an equation.

a. 3 mornings; $6x + 3 = 21$
b. 4 mornings; $21x - 5 = 22$
c. 4 mornings; $5x + 1 = 21$
d. 4 mornings; $6x + 3 = 21$

9. A woman must earn $250 in the next four days to pay a traffic ticket. How much will she have to earn each day?

a. $45.50
b. $62.50
c. $75.50
d. $100.50

10. Report all decimal places: 3.7 + 7.289 + 4 =

____

11. A man earns $15.23 per hour and gets a raise of $2.34 per hour. What is his new hourly rate of pay?

a. $12.89
b. $15.46
c. $17.57
d. $23.40

12. Erma has her eye on two sweaters at her favorite clothing store, but she has been waiting for the store to offer a sale. This week, the store advertises that all clothing purchases, including sweaters, come with an incentive: 25% off a second item of equal or lesser value. One sweater is $50 and the other is $44. If Erma purchases the sweaters during the sale, what will she spend?

$________

13. Nora earns $4 per hour at her waitressing job and today received $29 in tips. From her shift today, she earned a total of $53 from both tips and hourly wages. Write an equation from the information given and determine how many hours Nora worked today.

a. $4x + 29 = 53$; Nora worked 6 hours.
b. $29x + 4 = 53$; Nora worked 2 hours.
c. $53x - 29 = 4$; Nora worked 2 hours.
d. $4x - 29 = 53$; Nora worked 9 hours.

14. Simplify the following expression: $\frac{2}{3} \div \frac{4}{15} \times \frac{5}{8}$.

a. $\frac{25}{16}$
b. $\frac{5}{4}$
c. $\frac{17}{8}$
d. 2

15. Karen goes to the grocery store with $40. She buys a carton of milk for $1.85, a loaf of bread for $3.20, and a bunch of bananas for $3.05. How much money does she have left?

a. $30.95
b. $31.90
c. $32.10
d. $34.95

16. Four friends go shopping. They purchase items that cost $6.65 and $159.23. If they split the cost evenly, how much will each friend have to pay?

a. $26.64
b. $39.81
c. $41.47
d. $55.30

17. Simplify the following expression:

$$7 + 16 - (5 + 6 \times 3) - 10 \times 2$$

____

18. Roger's car gets an average of 25 miles per gallon. If his gas tank holds 16 gallons, about how far can he drive on a full tank?

a. 41 miles
b. 100 miles
c. 320 miles
d. 400 miles

19. The gas tank in a lawn mower holds up to one liter of gasoline. The gas can used to fill the gas tank of the mower is measured in gallons. Given that there are approximately 3,785 milliliters in a gallon of water, how much of a gallon of gas is needed to fill an empty gas tank of the lawn mower?

a. 0.26 gal
b. 0.20 gal
c. 3.79 gal
d. 1.90 gal

20. Express the answer in simplest form: $\frac{2}{3} + \frac{2}{7} =$

a. $\frac{20}{21}$
b. $\frac{4}{10}$
c. $\frac{4}{21}$
d. $\frac{2}{5}$

21. Zachary starts his first work shift at 1615. He wants to set an alarm on his phone for 45 minutes before so he knows when to leave for his shift. If his phone uses a 12-hour clock, what time should he set his alarm for?

a. 3:30 PM
b. 4:15 PM
c. 3:30 AM
d. 5:00 AM

22. Aaron worked $2\frac{1}{2}$ hours on Monday, $3\frac{3}{4}$ hours on Tuesday, and $7\frac{2}{3}$ hours on Thursday. How many hours did he work in all?

a. $10\frac{5}{6}$
b. $12\frac{1}{2}$
c. $13\frac{1}{4}$
d. $13\frac{11}{12}$

23. A woman wants to stack two small bookcases beneath a window that is $26\frac{1}{2}$ inches from the floor. The larger bookcase is $14\frac{1}{2}$ inches tall. The other bookcase is $8\frac{3}{4}$ inches tall. How tall will the two bookcases be when they are stacked together?

a. 12 inches tall
b. $23\frac{1}{4}$ inches tall
c. $35\frac{1}{4}$ inches tall
d. 41 inches tall

24. Express the answer in simplest form: $\frac{23}{24} - \frac{11}{24} =$

a. $\frac{11}{23}$
b. $\frac{1}{2}$
c. $\frac{2}{3}$
d. $\frac{12}{24}$

25. Express the answer in simplest form: $3\frac{4}{7} - 2\frac{3}{14} =$

a. $2\frac{3}{14}$
b. $1\frac{1}{14}$
c. $1\frac{5}{14}$
d. $2\frac{3}{7}$

26. Express the answer in simplest form: Dean has brown, white, and black socks. One-third of his socks are white; one-sixth of his socks are black. What fraction of his socks are brown?

a. $\frac{1}{3}$
b. $\frac{2}{6}$
c. $\frac{1}{2}$
d. $\frac{3}{4}$

27. Express the answer in simplest form: A recipe calls for $1\frac{1}{2}$ cups of sugar, $3\frac{2}{3}$ cups of flour, and $\frac{2}{3}$ of a cup of milk. If you want to double the recipe, what will be the total amount of cups of ingredients required?

a. $11\frac{2}{3}$
b. 8
c. $12\frac{1}{6}$
d. $6\frac{2}{3}$

28. Express your answer as a mixed number in simplest form: $4\frac{1}{3} \times \frac{2}{7} =$

a. $6\frac{1}{3}$
b. $3\frac{7}{10}$
c. $\frac{8}{21}$
d. $1\frac{5}{21}$

29. Evaluate the expression $8x + 3y - z + 14$ when $x = 2$, $y = 4$, and $z = 11$.

____

30. Express the answer as a mixed number or fraction in simplest form: $\frac{5}{8} \div \frac{1}{5} =$

a. $\frac{1}{8}$
b. $2\frac{3}{4}$
c. $3\frac{1}{3}$
d. $3\frac{1}{8}$

31. What is 6:30 AM in military time?

a. 0630
b. 0930
c. 1230
d. 1830

32. Round to the nearest whole number: Bill got $\frac{7}{9}$ of the answers right on his chemistry test. On a scale of 1 to 100, what numerical grade would he receive if the score is rounded to the nearest whole number?

____

33. Convert $15\frac{2}{3}$ to an improper fraction.

a. $\frac{22}{3}$
b. $\frac{17}{3}$
c. $\frac{47}{3}$
d. $\frac{43}{3}$

34. Margery is planning a vacation, and she has added up the total potential cost. Her round-trip airfare will cost $572. Her hotel cost is $89 per night, and she will be staying at the hotel for five nights. She has allotted a total of $150 for sightseeing during her trip, and she expects to spend about $250 on meals. As she books the hotel, she is told that she will receive a discount of 10% off the price of $89 for each additional night after the first night she stays there. Taking this discount into consideration, what is the amount that Margery expects to spend on her vacation?

$_________

35. Change the fraction to a decimal and round to the hundredths place: $4\frac{3}{7} =$

____

36. Change the decimal to the simplest equivalent proper fraction: 3.78 =

a. $3\frac{3}{4}$
b. $3\frac{7}{8}$
c. $3\frac{39}{50}$
d. $3\frac{78}{100}$

37. Change the decimal to the simplest equivalent proper fraction: $0.07 =$

a. $\frac{7}{10}$
b. $\frac{0.07}{10}$
c. $\frac{7}{100}$
d. $\frac{70}{100}$

38. Solve for x: $2x - 7 = 3$.

a. $x = 4$
b. $x = 3$
c. $x = -2$
d. $x = 5$

39. Sarah and Elizabeth take a test in their calculus class at school. They are competing for valedictorian, so they want to compare how they did on their tests. Sarah got $\frac{4}{9}$ questions correct, and Elizabeth, who chose to answer 2 bonus questions, got $\frac{5}{11}$ questions correct. Who did better on the calculus test and how did the girls figure it out?

a. Elizabeth because $\frac{4}{9} > \frac{5}{11}$.
b. Sarah because $\frac{5}{11} < \frac{4}{9}$.
c. Elizabeth because $\frac{4}{9} < \frac{5}{11}$.
d. Sarah because $\frac{4}{9} < \frac{5}{11}$.

40. Two-thirds of the students in Mr. Garcia's class are boys. If there are 27 students in the class, how many of them are girls?

_________ girls

41. A bag holds 17 green marbles, 10 blue marbles, and 9 red marbles. Express the ratio of red marbles to total marbles in simplest form.

a. 4: 36
b. 3: 12
c. 9: 36
d. 1: 4

42. Solve for x:

$7{:}\,42 :: 4{:}\,x$

a. 12
b. 48
c. 24
d. 16

43. Change the decimal to a percent: $0.64 =$

a. 0.64%
b. 64%
c. 6.4%
d. 0.064%

44. Solve the following equation: $x + 16 = 3x + 32$.

a. $-16 = 2x$
b. $x = -8$
c. $x = -16$
d. $x = -32$

45. Susan decided to celebrate getting her first nursing job by purchasing a new outfit. She bought a dress for $69.99 and a pair of shoes for $39.99. She also bought accessories for $34.67. What was the total cost of Susan's outfit, including accessories?

$________

46. The expression $m^3 \times m^8$ is given. Simplify.

a. m^{-5}
b. m^5
c. m^{11}
d. m^{24}

47. Change the percent to a decimal: $17.6\% =$

a. 17.6
b. 1.76
c. 0.176
d. 0.0176

48. Change the percent to a decimal: $126\% =$

____

49. Change the fraction to a percent and round to the nearest whole number: $\frac{2}{9} =$

a. 20%
b. 21%
c. 22%
d. 23%

50. In a town of 24,821 people, about one fifth of the population is under the age of 20. Of those, approximately three fourths attend local K–12 schools. If the number of students in each grade is about the same, how many first graders likely reside in the town?

a. Fewer than 150
b. Between 150 and 200
c. Between 200 and 250
d. More than 250

51. A woman has $450 in a bank account. She earns 0.5% interest on her end-of-month balance. How much interest will she earn for the month?

$________

52. Round to the nearest percentage point: Gerald made 13 out of the 22 shots he took in the basketball game. What was his shooting percentage?

a. 13%
b. 22%
c. 59%
d. 67%

53. Round to the nearest whole number: What is 18% of 600?

a. 108
b. 76
c. 254
d. 176

54. Round to the tenths place: What is 6.4% of 32?

a. 1.8
b. 2.1
c. 2.6
d. 2.0

55. Danny is doing a workout program that requires 300 push-ups. Danny wants to divide the push-ups over the span of 5 days. This means that Danny will be completing 20% of the push-ups each day. How many push-ups will Danny do each day?

a. 61 push-ups per day
b. 68 push-ups per day
c. 60 push-ups per day
d. 64 push-ups per day

Reading Comprehension

Questions 1 to 4 pertain to the following passage:

It is most likely that you have never had diphtheria. You probably don't even know anyone who has suffered from this disease. In fact, you may not even know what diphtheria is. Similarly, diseases like whooping cough, measles, mumps, and rubella may all be unfamiliar to you. In the nineteenth and early twentieth centuries, these illnesses struck hundreds of thousands of people in the United States each year, mostly children, and tens of thousands of people died. The names of these diseases were frightening household words. Today, they are all but forgotten. That change happened largely because of vaccines.

You probably have been vaccinated against diphtheria. You may even have been exposed to the bacterium that causes it, but the vaccine prepared your body to fight off the disease so quickly that you were unaware of the infection. Vaccines take advantage of your body's natural ability to learn how to combat many disease-causing germs, or microbes. What's more, your body remembers how to protect itself from the microbes it has encountered before. Collectively, the parts of your body that remember and repel microbes are called the immune system. Without the proper functioning of the immune system, the simplest illness—even the common cold—could quickly turn deadly.

On average, your immune system needs more than a week to learn how to fight off an unfamiliar microbe. Sometimes, that isn't enough time. Strong microbes can spread through your body faster than the immune system can fend them off. Your body often gains the upper hand after a few weeks, but in the meantime you are sick. Certain microbes are so virulent that they can overwhelm or escape your natural defenses. In those situations, vaccines can make all the difference.

Traditional vaccines contain either parts of microbes or whole microbes that have been altered so that they don't cause disease. When your immune system confronts these harmless versions of the germs, it quickly clears them from your body. In other words, vaccines trick your immune system in order to teach your body important lessons about how to defeat its opponents.

1. What is the main idea of the passage?

a. The nineteenth and early twentieth centuries were a dark period for medicine.
b. You have probably never had diphtheria.
c. Traditional vaccines contain altered microbes.
d. Vaccines help the immune system function properly.

2. Which statement is NOT a detail from the passage?

a. Vaccines contain microbe parts or altered microbes.
b. The immune system typically needs a week to learn how to fight a new disease.
c. The symptoms of disease do not emerge until the body has learned how to fight the microbe.
d. A hundred years ago, children were at the greatest risk of dying from now-treatable diseases.

3. What is the meaning of the word *virulent* as it is used in the third paragraph?

a. Tiny
b. Malicious
c. Contagious
d. Annoying

4. What is the author's primary purpose in writing the essay?

a. To entertain
b. To persuade
c. To inform
d. To analyze

Questions 5 to 8 pertain to the following passage:

Foodborne illnesses are contracted by eating food or drinking beverages contaminated with bacteria, parasites, or viruses. Harmful chemicals can also cause foodborne illnesses if they have contaminated food during harvesting or processing. Foodborne illnesses can cause symptoms ranging from upset stomach to diarrhea, fever, vomiting, abdominal cramps, and dehydration. Most foodborne infections are undiagnosed and unreported, though the Centers for Disease Control and Prevention estimates that every year about 76 million people in the United States become ill from pathogens in food. About 5,000 of these people die.

Harmful bacteria are the most common cause of foodborne illness. Some bacteria may be present at the point of purchase. Raw foods are the most common source of foodborne illnesses because they are not sterile; examples include raw meat and poultry contaminated during slaughter. Seafood may become contaminated during harvest or processing. One in 10,000 eggs may be contaminated with Salmonella inside the shell. Produce, such as spinach, lettuce, tomatoes, sprouts, and melons, can become contaminated with Salmonella, Shigella, or Escherichia coli (E. coli). Contamination can occur during growing, harvesting, processing, storing, shipping, or final preparation. Sources of produce contamination vary, as these foods are grown in soil and can become contaminated during growth, processing, or distribution. Contamination may also occur during food preparation in a restaurant or a home kitchen. The most common form of contamination from handled foods is the calicivirus, also called the Norwalk-like virus.

When food is cooked and left out for more than two hours at room temperature, bacteria can multiply quickly. Most bacteria don't produce an odor or change in color or texture, so they can be impossible to detect. Freezing food slows or stops bacteria's growth, but does not destroy the bacteria. The microbes can become reactivated when the food is thawed. Refrigeration also can slow the growth of some bacteria. Thorough cooking is required to destroy the bacteria.

5. What is the subject of the passage?

a. Foodborne illnesses
b. The dangers of uncooked food
c. Bacteria
d. Proper food preparation

6. Which statement is NOT a detail from the passage?

a. Every year, more than 70 million Americans contract some form of foodborne illness.
b. Once food is cooked, it cannot cause illness.
c. Refrigeration can slow the growth of some bacteria.
d. The most common form of contamination in handled foods is calicivirus.

7. What is the meaning of the word *pathogens* as it is used in the first paragraph?

a. Diseases
b. Vaccines
c. Disease-causing substances
d. Foods

8. What is the meaning of the word *sterile* as it is used in the second paragraph?

a. Free of bacteria
b. Healthy
c. Delicious
d. Impotent

Questions 9 to 12 pertain to the following passage:

There are a number of health problems related to bleeding in the esophagus and stomach. Stomach acid can cause inflammation and bleeding at the lower end of the esophagus. This condition, usually associated with the symptom of heartburn, is called esophagitis, or inflammation of the esophagus. Sometimes a muscle between the esophagus and stomach fails to close properly and allows the return of food and stomach juices into the esophagus, which can lead to esophagitis. In another unrelated condition, enlarged veins (varices) at the lower end of the esophagus rupture and bleed massively. Cirrhosis of the liver is the most common cause of esophageal varices. Esophageal bleeding can be caused by a tear in the lining of the esophagus (Mallory-Weiss syndrome). Mallory-Weiss syndrome usually results from vomiting, but may also be caused by increased pressure in the abdomen from coughing, hiatal hernia, or childbirth. Esophageal cancer can cause bleeding.

The stomach is a frequent site of bleeding. Infections with Helicobacter pylori (H. pylori), alcohol, aspirin, aspirin-containing medicines, and various other medicines (such as nonsteroidal anti-inflammatory drugs [NSAIDs]—particularly those used for arthritis) can cause stomach ulcers or inflammation (gastritis). The stomach is often the site of ulcer disease. Acute or chronic ulcers may enlarge and erode through a blood vessel, causing bleeding. Also, patients suffering from burns, shock, head injuries, cancer, or those who have undergone extensive surgery may develop stress ulcers. Bleeding can also occur from benign tumors or cancer of the stomach, although these disorders usually do not cause massive bleeding.

9. What is the main idea of the passage?

a. The digestive system is complex.
b. Of all the digestive organs, the stomach is the most prone to bleeding.
c. Both the esophagus and the stomach are subject to bleeding problems.
d. Esophagitis afflicts the young and old alike.

10. Which statement is NOT a detail from the passage?

a. Alcohol can cause stomach bleeding.
b. Ulcer disease rarely occurs in the stomach.
c. Benign tumors rarely result in massive bleeding.
d. Childbirth is one cause of Mallory-Weiss syndrome.

11. What is the meaning of the word *rupture* as it is used in the first paragraph?

a. Tear
b. Collapse
c. Implode
d. Detach

12. What is the meaning of the word *erode* as it is used in the second paragraph?

a. Avoid
b. Divorce
c. Contain
d. Wear away

Questions 13 to 16 pertain to the following passage:

We met Kathy Blake while she was taking a stroll in the park . . . by herself. What's so striking about this is that Kathy is completely blind, and she has been for more than 30 years.

The diagnosis from her doctor was retinitis pigmentosa, or RP. It's an incurable genetic disease that leads to progressive visual loss. Photoreceptive cells in the retina slowly start to die, leaving the patient visually impaired.

"Life was great the year before I was diagnosed," Kathy said. "I had just started a new job; I just bought my first new car. I had just started dating my now-husband. Life was good. The doctor had told me that there was some good news and some bad news. 'The bad news is you are going to lose your vision; the good news is we don't think you are going to go totally blind.' Unfortunately, I did lose all my vision within about 15 years."

Two years ago, Kathy got a glimmer of hope. She heard about an artificial retina being developed in Los Angeles. It was experimental, but Kathy was the perfect candidate.

Dr. Mark Humayun is a retinal surgeon and biomedical engineer. "A good candidate for the artificial retina device is a person who is blind because of retinal blindness," he said. "They've lost the rods and cones, the light-sensing cells of the eye, but the rest of the circuitry is relatively intact. In the simplest rendition, this device basically takes a blind person and hooks them up to a camera."

It may sound like the stuff of science fiction . . . and just a few years ago it was. A camera is built into a pair of glasses, sending radio signals to a tiny chip in the back of the retina. The chip, small enough to fit on a fingertip, is implanted surgically and stimulates the nerves that lead to the vision center of the brain. Kathy is one of twenty patients who have undergone surgery and use the device.

It has been about two years since the surgery, and Kathy still comes in for weekly testing at the University of Southern California's medical campus. She scans back and forth with specially made, camera-equipped glasses until she senses objects on a screen and then touches the objects. The low-resolution image from the camera is still enough to make out the black stripes on the screen. Impulses are sent from the camera to the 60 receptors that are on the chip in her retina. So, what is Kathy seeing?

"I see flashes of light that indicate a contrast from light to dark—very similar to a camera flash, probably not quite as bright because it's not hurting my eye at all," she replied.

Humayun underscored what a breakthrough this is and how a patient adjusts. "If you've been blind for 30 or 50 years, (and) all of a sudden you get this device, there is a period of learning," he said. "Your brain needs to learn. And it's literally like seeing a baby crawl—to a child walk—to an adult run."

While hardly perfect, the device works best in bright light or where there is a lot of contrast. Kathy takes the device home. The software that runs the device can be upgraded. So, as the software is upgraded, her vision improves. Recently, she was outside with her husband on a moonlit night and saw something she hadn't seen for a long time.

"I scanned up in the sky (and) I got a big flash, right where the moon was, and pointed it out. I can't even remember how many years ago it's been that I would have ever been able to do that."

This technology has a bright future. The current chip has a resolution of 60 pixels. Humayun says that number could be increased to more than a thousand in the next version.

"I think it will be extremely exciting if they can recognize their loved ones' faces and be able to see what their wife or husband or their grandchildren look like, which they haven't seen," said Humayun.

Kathy dreams of a day when blindness like hers will be a distant memory. "My eye disease is hereditary," she said. "My three daughters happen to be fine, but I want to know that if my grandchildren ever have a problem, they will have something to give them some vision."

13. What is the primary subject of the passage?

a. A new artificial retina
b. Kathy Blake
c. Hereditary disease
d. Dr. Mark Humayun

14. What is the meaning of the word *progressive* as it is used in the second paragraph?

a. Selective
b. Gradually increasing
c. Diminishing
d. Disabling

15. Which statement is NOT a detail from the passage?

a. The use of an artificial retina requires a special pair of glasses.
b. Retinal blindness is the inability to perceive light.
c. Retinitis pigmentosa is curable.
d. The artificial retina performs best in bright light.

16. What is the author's intention in writing the essay?

a. To persuade
b. To entertain
c. To analyze
d. To inform

Questions 17 to 21 pertain to the following passage:

Usher syndrome is the most common condition that affects both hearing and vision. The major signs of Usher syndrome are hearing loss and an eye disorder called retinitis pigmentosa, or RP. Retinitis pigmentosa causes night blindness and a loss of peripheral vision (side vision) through the progressive degeneration of the retina. The retina, which is crucial for vision, is a light-sensitive tissue at the back of the eye. As RP progresses, the field of vision narrows, until only central vision (the ability to see straight ahead) remains. Many people with Usher syndrome also have severe balance problems.

There are three clinical types of Usher syndrome. In the United States, types 1 and 2 are the most common. Together, they account for approximately 90 to 95 percent of all cases of juvenile Usher syndrome. Approximately three to six percent of all deaf and hearing-disabled children have Usher syndrome. In developed countries, such as the United States, about four in every 100,000 newborns have Usher syndrome.

Usher syndrome is inherited as an autosomal recessive trait. The term autosomal means that the mutated gene is not located on either of the chromosomes that determine sex; in other words, both males and females can have the disorder and can pass it along to a child. The word recessive means that in order to have Usher syndrome, an individual must receive a mutated form of the Usher syndrome gene from each parent. If a child has a mutation in one Usher syndrome gene but the other gene is normal, he or she should have normal vision and hearing. Individuals with a mutation in a gene that can cause an autosomal recessive disorder are called carriers, because they carry the mutated gene but show no symptoms of the disorder. If both parents are carriers of a mutated gene for Usher syndrome, they will have a one-in-four chance of producing a child with Usher syndrome.

Usually, parents who have normal hearing and vision do not know if they are carriers of an Usher syndrome gene mutation. Currently, it is not possible to determine whether an individual without a family history of Usher syndrome is a carrier. Scientists at the National Institute on Deafness and Other Communication Disorders (NIDCD) are hoping to change this, however, as they learn more about the genes responsible for Usher syndrome.

17. What is the main idea of the passage?

a. Usher syndrome is an inherited condition that affects hearing and vision.
b. Some people are carriers of Usher syndrome.
c. Usher syndrome typically skips a generation.
d. Scientists hope to develop a test for detecting the carriers of Usher syndrome.

18. What is the meaning of the word *signs* as it is used in the first paragraph?

a. Qualifications
b. Conditions/diseases
c. Subjective markers
d. Measurable indicators

19. Which statement is NOT a detail from the passage?

a. Types 1 and 2 Usher syndrome are the most common in the United States.
b. Usher syndrome affects both hearing and smell.
c. Right now, there is no way to identify a carrier of Usher syndrome.
d. Central vision is the ability to see straight ahead.

20. What is the meaning of the word *juvenile* as it is used in the second paragraph?

a. Bratty
b. Serious
c. Occurring in children
d. Improper

21. What is the meaning of the word *mutated* as it is used in the third paragraph?

a. Selected
b. Altered
c. Composed
d. Destroyed

Questions 22 to 27 pertain to the following passage:

The immune system is a network of cells, tissues, and organs that defends the body against attacks by foreign invaders. These invaders are primarily microbes—tiny organisms such as bacteria, parasites, and fungi—that can cause infections. Viruses also cause infections, but are too primitive to be classified as living organisms. The human body provides an ideal environment for many microbes. It is the immune system's job to keep the microbes out or destroy them.

The immune system is amazingly complex. It can recognize and remember millions of different enemies, and it can secrete fluids and cells to wipe out nearly all of them. The secret to its success is an elaborate and dynamic communications network. Millions of cells, organized into sets and subsets, gather and transfer information in response to an infection. Once immune cells receive the alarm, they produce powerful chemicals that help to regulate their own growth and behavior, enlist other immune cells, and direct the new recruits to trouble spots.

Although scientists have learned much about the immune system, they continue to puzzle over how the body destroys invading microbes, infected cells, and tumors without harming healthy tissues. New technologies for identifying individual immune cells are now allowing scientists to determine quickly which targets are triggering an immune response. Improvements in microscopy are permitting the first-ever observations of living B cells, T cells, and other cells as they interact within lymph nodes and other body tissues.

In addition, scientists are rapidly unraveling the genetic blueprints that direct the human immune response, as well as those that dictate the biology of bacteria, viruses, and parasites. The combination of new technology with expanded genetic information will no doubt reveal even more about how the body protects itself from disease.

22. What is the main idea of the passage?

a. Scientists fully understand the immune system.
b. The immune system triggers the production of fluids.
c. The body is under constant invasion by malicious microbes.
d. The immune system protects the body from infection.

23. Which statement is NOT a detail from the passage?

a. Most invaders of the body are microbes.
b. The immune system relies on excellent communication.
c. Viruses are extremely sophisticated.
d. The cells of the immune system are organized.

24. What is the meaning of the word *ideal* as it is used in the first paragraph?

a. Thoughtful
b. Confined
c. Hostile
d. Perfect

25. Which statement is NOT a detail from the passage?

a. Scientists can now see T cells.
b. The immune system ignores tumors.
c. The ability of the immune system to fight disease without harming the body remains mysterious.
d. The immune system remembers millions of different invaders.

26. What is the meaning of the word *enlist* as it is used in the second paragraph?

a. Call into service
b. Write down
c. Send away
d. Put across

27. What is the author's primary purpose in writing the essay?

a. To persuade
b. To analyze
c. To inform
d. To entertain

Questions 28 to 31 pertain to the following passage:

The federal government regulates dietary supplements through the United States Food and Drug Administration (FDA). The regulations for dietary supplements are not the same as those for prescription or over-the-counter drugs. In general, the regulations for dietary supplements are less strict.

To begin with, a manufacturer does not have to prove the safety and effectiveness of a dietary supplement before it is marketed. A manufacturer is permitted to say that a dietary supplement addresses a nutrient deficiency, supports health, or is linked to a particular body function (such as immunity), if there is research to support the claim. Such a claim must be followed by the words "This statement has not been evaluated by the Food and Drug Administration. This product is not intended to diagnose, treat, cure, or prevent any disease."

Also, manufacturers are expected to follow certain good manufacturing practices (GMPs) to ensure that dietary supplements are processed consistently and meet quality standards. Requirements for GMPs went into effect in 2008 for large manufacturers and are being phased in for small manufacturers through 2010.

Once a dietary supplement is on the market, the FDA monitors safety and product information, such as label claims and package inserts. If it finds a product to be unsafe, it can take action against the manufacturer and/or distributor and may issue a warning or require that the product be removed from the marketplace. The Federal Trade Commission (FTC) is responsible for regulating product advertising; it requires that all information be truthful and not misleading.

The federal government has taken legal action against a number of dietary supplement promoters or websites that promote or sell dietary supplements because they have made false or deceptive statements about their products or because marketed products have proven to be unsafe.

28. What is the main idea of the passage?

a. Manufacturers of dietary supplements have to follow good manufacturing practices.
b. The FDA has a special program for regulating dietary supplements.
c. The federal government prosecutes those who mislead the general public.
d. The FDA is part of the federal government.

29. Which statement is NOT a detail from the passage?

a. Promoters of dietary supplements can make any claims that are supported by research.
b. GMP requirements for large manufacturers went into effect in 2008.
c. Product advertising is regulated by the FTC.
d. The FDA does not monitor products after they enter the market.

30. What is the meaning of the phrase *phased in* as it is used in the third paragraph?

a. Stunned into silence
b. Confused
c. Implemented in stages
d. Legalized

31. What is the meaning of the word *deceptive* as it is used in the fifth paragraph?

a. Misleading
b. Malicious
c. Illegal
d. Irritating

Questions 32 to 35 pertain to the following passage:

Anemia is a condition in which there is an abnormally low number of red blood cells (RBCs). This condition also can occur if the RBCs don't contain enough hemoglobin, the iron-rich protein that makes the blood red. Hemoglobin helps RBCs carry oxygen from the lungs to the rest of the body.

Anemia can be accompanied by low numbers of RBCs, white blood cells (WBCs), and platelets. Red blood cells are disc-shaped and look like doughnuts without holes in the center. They carry oxygen and remove carbon dioxide (a waste product) from your body. These cells are made in the bone marrow and live for about 120 days in the bloodstream. Platelets and WBCs also are made in the bone marrow. White blood cells help fight infection. Platelets stick together to seal small cuts or breaks on the blood vessel walls and to stop bleeding.

If you are anemic, your body doesn't get enough oxygenated blood. As a result, you may feel tired or have other symptoms. Severe or long-lasting anemia can damage the heart, brain, and other organs of the body. Very severe anemia may even cause death.

Anemia has three main causes: blood loss, lack of RBC production, or high rates of RBC destruction. Many types of anemia are mild, brief, and easily treated. Some types can be prevented with a healthy diet or treated with dietary supplements. However, certain types of anemia may be severe, long lasting, and life threatening if not diagnosed and treated.

If you have the signs or symptoms of anemia, you should see your doctor to find out whether you have the condition. Treatment will depend on the cause and severity of the anemia.

32. What is the main idea of the passage?

a. Anemia presents in a number of forms.
b. Anemia is a potentially dangerous condition characterized by low numbers of RBCs.
c. Anemia is a deficiency of WBCs and platelets.
d. Anemia is a treatable condition.

33. Which statement is NOT a detail from the passage?

a. There are different methods for treating anemia.
b. Red blood cells remove carbon dioxide from the body.
c. Platelets are made in the bone marrow.
d. Anemia is rarely caused by blood loss.

34. What is the meaning of the word *oxygenated* as it is used in the third paragraph?

a. Containing low amounts of oxygen
b. Containing no oxygen
c. Consisting entirely of oxygen
d. Containing high amounts of oxygen

35. What is the meaning of the word *severity* as it is used in the fifth paragraph?

a. Seriousness
b. Disconnectedness
c. Truth
d. Swiftness

Questions 36 to 39 pertain to the following passage:

Contrary to previous reports, drinking four or more cups of coffee a day does not put women at risk of rheumatoid arthritis (RA), according to a new study partially funded by the National Institute of Arthritis and Musculoskeletal and Skin Diseases (NIAMS). The study concluded that there is little evidence to support a connection between consuming coffee or tea and the risk of RA among women.

Rheumatoid arthritis is an inflammatory autoimmune disease that affects the joints. It results in pain, stiffness, swelling, joint damage, and loss of function. Inflammation most often affects the hands and feet and tends to be symmetrical. About one percent of the U.S. population has rheumatoid arthritis.

Elizabeth W. Karlson, M.D., and her colleagues at Harvard Medical School and Brigham and Women's Hospital in Boston, Massachusetts, used the Nurses' Health Study, a long-term investigation of nurses' diseases, lifestyles, and health practices, to examine possible links between caffeinated beverages and RA risk. The researchers were able to follow up with more than 90 percent of the original pool of 83,124 participants who answered a 1980 food frequency questionnaire, and no links were found. They also considered changes in diet and habits over a prolonged period of time, and when the results were adjusted for other factors, such as cigarette smoking, alcohol consumption, and oral contraceptive use, the outcome still showed no relationship between caffeine consumption and risk of RA.

Previous research had suggested an association between consuming coffee or tea and RA risk. According to Dr. Karlson, the data supporting that conclusion were inconsistent. Because the information in the older studies was collected at only one time, she says, consideration was not given to the other factors associated with RA, such as cigarette smoking and changes in diet and lifestyle over a follow-up period. The new study presents a more accurate picture of caffeine and RA risk.

36. What is the main idea of the passage?

a. In the past, doctors have cautioned older women to avoid caffeinated beverages.
b. Rheumatoid arthritis affects the joints of older women.
c. A recent study found no link between caffeine consumption and RA among women.
d. Cigarette smoking increases the incidence of RA.

37. Which statement is NOT a detail from the passage?

a. Alcohol consumption is linked with RA.
b. The original data for the study came from a 1980 questionnaire.
c. Rheumatoid arthritis most often affects the hands and feet.
d. This study included tens of thousands of participants.

38. What is the meaning of the word *symmetrical* as it is used in the second paragraph?

a. Affecting both sides of the body in corresponding fashion
b. Impossible to treat
c. Sensitive to the touch
d. Asymptomatic

39. What is the author's primary purpose in writing the essay?

a. To entertain
b. To inform
c. To analyze
d. To persuade

Questions 40 to 43 refer to the following passage:

Exercise is vital at every age for healthy bones. Not only does exercise improve bone health, but it also increases muscle strength, coordination, and balance, and it leads to better overall health. Exercise is especially important for preventing and treating osteoporosis.

Like muscle, bone is living tissue that responds to exercise by becoming stronger. Young women and men who exercise regularly generally achieve greater peak bone mass (maximum bone density and strength) than those who do not. For most people, bone mass peaks during the third decade of life. After that time, we can begin to lose bone. Women and men older than age 20 can help prevent bone loss with regular exercise. Exercise maintains muscle strength, coordination, and balance, which in turn prevent falls and related fractures. This is especially important for older adults and people with osteoporosis.

Weight-bearing exercise is the best kind of exercise for bones, which forces the muscle to work against gravity. Some examples of weight-bearing exercises are weight training, walking, hiking, jogging, climbing stairs, tennis, and dancing. Swimming and bicycling, on the other hand, are not weight-bearing exercises. Although these activities help build and maintain strong muscles and have excellent cardiovascular benefits, they are not the best exercise for bones.

40. What is the main idea of the passage?

a. Weight-bearing exercise is the best for bones.
b. Exercise increases balance.
c. Exercise improves bone health.
d. Women benefit from regular exercise more than men.

41. What is the meaning of the word *vital* as it is used in the first paragraph?

a. Deadly
b. Important
c. Rejected
d. Nourishing

42. Which statement is NOT a detail from the passage?

a. Tennis is a form of weight-bearing exercise.
b. Most people reach peak bone mass in their twenties.
c. Swimming is not good for the bones.
d. Bone is a living tissue.

43. What is the meaning of the word *fractures* as it is used in the second paragraph?

a. Breaks
b. Agreements
c. Tiffs
d. Fevers

Questions 44 to 47 pertain to the following passage:

Searching for medical information can be confusing, especially for first-timers. However, if you are patient and stick to it, you can find a wealth of information. Your community library is a good place to start your search for medical information. Before going to the library, you may find it helpful to make a list of topics you want information about and questions you have. Your list of topics and questions will make it easier for the librarian to direct you to the best resources.

Many community libraries have a collection of basic medical references. These references may include medical dictionaries or encyclopedias, drug information handbooks, basic medical and nursing textbooks, and directories of physicians and medical specialists (listings of doctors). You may also find magazine articles on a certain topic. Look in the Reader's Guide to Periodical Literature for articles on health and medicine from consumer magazines.

Infotrac, a CD-ROM computer database available at libraries or on the Web, indexes hundreds of popular magazines and newspapers, as well as medical journals such as the Journal of the American Medical Association and New England Journal of Medicine.

Your library may also carry searchable computer databases of medical journal articles, including MEDLINE/PubMed or the Cumulative Index to Nursing and Allied Health Literature. Many of the databases or indexes have abstracts that provide a summary of each journal article. Although most community libraries don't have a large collection of medical and nursing journals, your librarian may be able to get copies of the articles you want. Interlibrary loans allow your librarian to request a copy of an article from a library that carries that particular medical journal. Your library may charge a fee for this service. Articles published in medical journals can be technical, but they may be the most current source of information on medical topics.

44. What is the main idea of the passage?

a. Infotrac is a useful source of information.
b. The community library offers numerous resources for medical information.
c. Searching for medical information can be confusing.
d. There is no reason to prepare a list of topics before visiting the library.

45. What is the meaning of the word *popular* as it is used in the third paragraph?

a. Complicated
b. Old-fashioned
c. Beloved
d. For the general public

46. Which statement is NOT a detail from the passage?

a. Abstracts summarize the information in an article.
b. Having a prepared list of questions enables the librarian to serve you better.
c. Infotrac is a database on CD-ROM.
d. The articles in popular magazines can be hard to understand.

47. What is the meaning of the word *technical* as it is used in the fourth paragraph?

a. Requiring expert knowledge
b. Incomplete
c. Foreign
d. Plagiarized

Refer to the following for questions 48 - 51:

But all this—the mysterious, far-reaching hair-line trail, the absence of sun from the sky, the tremendous cold, and the strangeness and weirdness of it all—made no impression on the man. It was not because he was long used to it. He was a newcomer in the land, a chechaquo, and this was his first winter. The trouble with him was that he was without imagination. He was quick and alert in the things of life, but only in the things, and not in the significances. Fifty degrees below zero meant eighty-odd degrees of frost. Such fact impressed him as being cold and uncomfortable, and that was all. It did not lead him to meditate upon his frailty as a creature of temperature, and upon man's frailty in general, able only to live within certain narrow limits of heat and cold; and from there on it did not lead him to the conjectural field of immortality and man's place in the universe. Fifty degrees below zero stood for a bite of frost that hurt and that must be guarded against by the use of mittens, ear-flaps, warm moccasins, and thick socks. Fifty degrees below zero was to him just precisely fifty degrees below zero. That there should be anything more to it than that was a thought that never entered his head.

. . . .

At the man's heels trotted a dog, a big native husky, the proper wolf-dog, gray-coated and without any visible or temperamental difference from its brother, the wild wolf. The animal was depressed by the tremendous cold. It knew that it was no time for travelling. Its instinct told it a truer tale than was told to the man by the man's judgment. In reality, it was not merely colder than fifty below zero; it was colder than sixty below, than seventy below. It was seventy-five below zero. Since the freezing-point is thirty-two above zero, it meant that one hundred and seven degrees of frost obtained. The dog did not know anything about thermometers. Possibly in its brain there was no sharp consciousness of a condition of very cold such as was in the man's brain. But the brute had its instinct. It experienced a vague but menacing apprehension that subdued it and made it slink along at the man's heels, and that made it question eagerly every unwonted movement of the man as if expecting him to go into camp or to seek shelter somewhere and build a fire. The dog had learned fire, and it wanted fire, or else to burrow under the snow and cuddle its warmth away from the air.

[Adapted from Jack London, "To Build a Fire" (1902)]

48. What is the point of view used in this passage?

a. First person
b. First person plural
c. Third person limited
d. Third person omniscient

49. What message does the passage reflect when it mentions immortality and man's place in the universe?

a. Humans are frail
b. Humans are stronger than nature
c. Humans will one day attain immortality
d. Humans are smarter than animals

50. In what way does the narrator say the dog is better off than the man?

a. The dog is better equipped for the cold because of its fur
b. The dog has a better conscious idea of what the cold means
c. The dog's instinct guides it, while the man's intellect fails him
d. The dog understands mankind's place in the universe

51. Which statement best captures the author's meaning in the statement, "The trouble with him was that he was without imagination"?

I. The man was not smart
II. The man did not need imagination because he was rational
III. The man did not have the foresight to realize that he was putting himself in danger

a. I only
b. II only
c. III only
d. I and II

Refer to the following for questions 52 - 55:

Forest Manager: Salvage logging is removing dead or dying forest stands that are left behind by a fire or disease. This practice has been used for several decades. These dead or dying trees become fuel that feeds future fires. The best way to lower the risk of forest fires is to remove the dead timber from the forest floor. Salvage logging followed by replanting ensures the reestablishment of desirable tree species.

For example, planting conifers accelerates the return of fire-resistant forests. Harvesting timber helps forests by reducing fuel load, thinning the forest stands, and relieving competition between trees. Burned landscapes leave black surfaces and ash layers that have very high soil temperatures. These high soil temperatures can kill many plant species. Logging mixes the soil. So, this lowers surface temperatures to more normal levels. The shade from material that is left behind by logging also helps to lower surface temperatures. After an area has been salvage logged, seedlings in the area start to grow almost immediately. However, this regrowth can take several years in areas that are not managed well.

Ecology professor: Salvage logging moves material like small, broken branches to the forest floor. These pieces can become fuel for more fires. The removal of larger, less flammable trees leaves behind small limbs and increases the risk of forest fires. In unmanaged areas, these pieces are found more commonly on the tops of trees where they are unavailable to fires. Logging destroys old forests that are more resistant to wildfires. So, this creates younger forests that are more open to fires. In old forests, branches of bigger trees are higher above the floor where fires may not reach.

Replanting after wildfires creates monoculture plantations where only a single crop is planted. This monoculture allows less biological diversity. Also, it allows plants to be less resistant to disease. So, this increases the chance of fire. Salvage logging also upsets natural forest regrowth by killing most of the seedlings that grow after a wildfire. It breaks up the soil and increases erosion. Also, it removes most of the shade that is needed for young seedlings to grow.

52. Which of the following is NOT a supporting detail for the forest manager's argument?

a. "This practice has been used for decades."
b. "Logging mixes the soil. So, this lowers surface temperatures to more normal levels."
c. "After an area has been salvage logged, seedlings in the area start to grow almost immediately."
d. "Salvage logging is removing dead or dying forest stands that are left behind by a fire or disease."

53. A study compared two plots of land that were managed differently after a fire. Plot A was salvage logged. Plot B was left unmanaged. After a second fire, they compared two plant groups between Plots A and B. They found that both plant groups burned worse in Plot A than in Plot B. Whose viewpoint do these results support?

a. only the manager
b. only the professor
c. both the manager and professor
d. neither the manager nor the professor

54. What is the main idea of the forest manager's argument?

a. Salvage logging is helpful because it removes dead or dying timber from the forest floor. So, this lowers the risk of future fires.
b. Salvage logging is helpful because it has been practiced for many decades.
c. Salvage logging is harmful because it raises soil temperatures above normal levels. So, this threatens the health of plant species.
d. Salvage logging is helpful because it gives shade for seedlings to grow after a wildfire.

55. Whose viewpoints would potentially be confirmed by a future study looking at the spreading out and regrowth of seedlings for many years after a wildfire in managed and unmanaged forests?

a. only the manager
b. only the professor
c. both the manager and professor
d. neither the manager nor professor

Vocabulary

1. *Generous* most nearly means

a. giving
b. truthful
c. selfish
d. harsh

2. What is the meaning of the word *prognosis*?

a. Forecast
b. Description
c. Outline
d. Schedule

3. What is the name for any substance that stimulates the production of antibodies?

a. Collagen
b. Hemoglobin
c. Lymph
d. Antigen

4. What is the best definition for the word *abstain*?

a. Offend
b. Retrain
c. To refrain from
d. Defenestrate

5. Select the meaning of the underlined word in this sentence:

Jerry held out hope for recovery, in spite of the <u>ominous</u> results from the lab.

a. Threatening
b. Emboldening
c. Destructive
d. Insightful

6. What is the meaning of the word *incidence*?

a. Random events
b. Sterility
c. Autonomy
d. Rate of occurrence

7. Select the word that means "water loving."

a. Homologous
b. Hydrophilia
c. Dipsomaniac
d. Hydrated

8. Select the meaning of the underlined word in this sentence:

The occluded artery posed a significant threat to the long-term health of the patient.

a. Closed
b. Deformed
c. Enlarged
d. Engorged

9. What is the best description for the word *potent*?

a. Frantic
b. Determined
c. Feverish
d. Powerful

10. Select the meaning of the underlined word in this sentence:

The doctors were less concerned with Bill's respiration than with the precipitous rise in his blood pressure.

a. Detached
b. Sordid
c. Encompassed
d. Steep

11. Select the meaning of the underlined word in this sentence:

It is vital for the victim of a serious accident to receive medical attention immediately.

a. Recommended
b. Discouraged
c. Essential
d. Sufficient

12. Select the meaning of the underlined word in this sentence:

The math test was quite challenging.

a. reasonable
b. lengthy
c. difficult
d. simple

13. What is the best description for the word *insidious*?

a. Stealthy
b. Deadly
c. Collapsed
d. New

14. Select the word that means "take into the body."

a. Congest
b. Ingest
c. Collect
d. Suppress

15. What is the meaning of the word *proscribe*?

a. Anticipate
b. Prevent
c. Defeat
d. Forbid

16. Select the meaning of the underlined word in this sentence.

Wracked by abdominal pain, the victim of food poisoning moaned and rubbed his distended belly.

a. Concave
b. Sore
c. Swollen
d. Empty

17. Select the meaning of the underlined word in this sentence:

Despite the absence of overt signs, Dr. Harris suspected that Alicia might be suffering from the flu.

a. Concealed
b. Apparent
c. Expert
d. Delectable

18. Select the word that means "something added to resolve a deficiency or obtain completion."

a. Supplement
b. Complement
c. Detriment
d. Acumen

19. Select the word that means "a violent seizure."

a. Revelation
b. Nutrient
c. Contraption
d. Paroxysm

20. What is the meaning of *carnivore*?

a. Hungry
b. Meat-eating
c. Infected
d. Demented

21. What is the meaning of *belligerent*?

a. Retired
b. Sardonic
c. Pugnacious
d. Acclimated

22. Select the word that means "on both sides."

a. Bilateral
b. Insufficient
c. Bicuspid
d. Congruent

23. *Instructor* most nearly means

a. pupil
b. teacher
c. survivor
d. dictator

24. Select the meaning of the underlined word in this sentence:

The medication should only be taken if the old symptoms <u>recur</u>.

a. Occur again
b. Survive
c. Collect
d. Desist

25. Select the word that means "likely to change."

a. Venereal
b. Motile
c. Labile
d. Entrail

26. What is the best description for the word *flaccid*?

a. Defended
b. Limp
c. Slender
d. Outdated

27. Select the word that means "both male and female."

a. Monozygotic
b. Heterogeneous
c. Homologous
d. Androgynous

28. What is the meaning of *terrestrial*?

a. Alien
b. Earthly
c. Foreign
d. Domestic

29. Select the word that means "improper or unfortunate."

a. Allocated
b. Untoward
c. Flaccid
d. Dilated

30. Select the meaning of the underlined word in this sentence:

At first, Gerald suspected that he had caught the disease at the office; later, though, he concluded that it was endogenous.

a. Contagious
b. Painful to the touch
c. Continuous
d. Growing from within

31. What is the meaning of *symptom*?

a. Result
b. Subjective indication
c. Side effect
d. Precondition

32. Select the word that means "intrusive."

a. Convulsive
b. Destructive
c. Invasive
d. Connective

33. What is the meaning of *parameter*?

a. Guideline
b. Standard
c. Manual
d. Variable

34. Select the meaning of the underlined word in this sentence:

The audience applauded after the woman concluded her presentation.

a. delivered
b. prepared
c. attended
d. finished

35. Select the word that means "empty."

a. Holistic
b. Void
c. Concrete
d. Maladjusted

36. Select the meaning of the underlined word in this sentence:

Though chemotherapy had sent her cancer into remission, Glenda remained lethargic and depressed.

a. Nauseous
b. Sluggish
c. Contagious
d. Elated

37. Select the word that means "offsetting."

a. Compensatory
b. Defensive
c. Untoward
d. Confused

38. Select the word that means "degeneration or wasting away."

a. Dystrophy
b. Entropy
c. Atrophy
d. Apathy

39. What is the best description for the word *discrete*?

a. Calm
b. Subtle
c. Hidden
d. Separate

40. Select the meaning of the underlined word in this sentence:

In order to minimize scarring, the nurse reused the <u>site</u> of the previous injection.

a. Syringe
b. Location
c. Artery
d. Hole

41. Select the meaning of the underlined word in this sentence:

As a veteran of many flu seasons, the nurse knew how to minimize her <u>exposure</u> to the disease.

a. Laying open
b. Prohibition
c. Connection
d. Dislike

42. What is the meaning of *exacerbate*?

a. Implicate
b. Aggravate
c. Heal
d. Decondition

43. Select the word that means "nerve cell."

a. Neutron
b. Nucleus
c. Neuron
d. Neutral

44. Select the word that means "unfavorable."

a. Liberated
b. Adverse
c. Convenient
d. Occluded

45. *Residence* most nearly means

a. home
b. area
c. plan
d. resist

46. Select the meaning of the underlined word in this sentence:

Dr. Grant ignored Mary's particular symptoms, instead administering a holistic treatment for her condition.

a. Insensitive
b. Ignorant
c. Specialized
d. Concerned with the whole rather than the parts

47. What is the best description for the word *suppress*?

a. Stop
b. Push up
c. Release
d. Strain

48. Select the word that means "about to happen."

a. Depending
b. Offending
c. Suspending
d. Impending

49. Select the meaning of the underlined word in this sentence:

The dermatologist was struck by the symmetric patterns of scarring on the patient's back.

a. Scabbed
b. Painful to the touch
c. Occurring in corresponding parts at the same time
d. Geometric

50. Select the word that means "open."

a. Inverted
b. Patent
c. Convent
d. Converted

51. Select the meaning of the underlined word in this sentence:

Despite an increase in the <u>volume</u> of his urine, the patient still reported bloating.

a. Quality
b. Length
c. Quantity
d. Loudness

52. What is the meaning of *repugnant*?

a. Destructive
b. Selective
c. Collective
d. Offensive

53. Select the word that means "enlarge."

a. Dilate
b. Protrude
c. Confuse
d. Occlude

54. What is the best description for the word *intact*?

a. Collapsed
b. Disconnected
c. Unbroken
d. Free

55. Select the word that means "the ability to enter, contact, or approach."

a. Ingress
b. Excess
c. Access
d. Success

Grammar

1. Choose the verb that correctly completes the sentence.

Claude Monet is a famous painter whose well-known painting ____ Water Lilly Pond.

a. include
b. includes
c. included
d. including

2. Which word is NOT spelled correctly in the context of the following sentence?

Dr. Vargas was surprised that the prescription had effected Ron's fatigue so dramatically.

a. Surprised
b. Prescription
c. Effected
d. Fatigue

3. Select the word that makes this sentence grammatically correct:

Is the new student coming out to lunch with ____?

a. we
b. our
c. us
d. they

4. Select the word or phrase that makes this sentence grammatically correct:

___ picking up groceries one of the things you are supposed to do?

a. Is
b. Am
c. Is it
d. Are

5. Select the word that makes the following sentence grammatically correct.

These days, you can't ___ learning how to use a computer.

a. not
b. evading
c. despite
d. avoid

6. Which word is NOT spelled correctly in the context of the following sentence?

The climate hear is inappropriate for snow sports such as skiing.

a. Climate
b. Hear
c. Inappropriate
d. Skiing

7. Select the word or phrase that makes the following sentence grammatically correct.

____ screaming took the shopkeeper by surprise.

a. We
b. They
c. Them
d. Our

8. Select the word or phrase that makes the following sentence grammatically correct.

Why did we ____ try so hard?

a. has to
b. haven't
c. had to
d. have to

9. Select the word that makes the following sentence grammatically correct.

Tracey wore her hair in a French braid, ____ was the style at the time.

a. among
b. it
c. that
d. which

10. Select the phrase that makes the following sentence grammatically correct.

Working ________ the mission of the entire committee.

a. to peace is
b. toward peace was
c. to peace was
d. toward peace am

11. Select the phrase that makes the following sentence grammatically correct.

Janet called her ________ run after a squirrel.

a. dog, who had
b. dog that had
c. dog, that had
d. dog who had

12. Choose the word that best completes the sentence.

The teacher _____ her students when they gave the wrong answer.

a. applauded
b. belittled
c. commended
d. praised

13. Select the correct word for the blank in the following sentence.

After completing the intense surgery, Dr. Capra needed a long ____.

a. brake
b. break
c. brink
d. broke

14. Select the correct word for the blank in the following sentence.

The other day, Stan ____ reviewing his class notes in preparation for the final exam.

a. begins
b. begun
c. begin
d. began

15. Select the word or phrase that makes the following sentence grammatically correct.

It makes sense to maintain your current prescriptions, ____ they have worked so well in the past.

a. although
b. despite that
c. since
d. but

16. Select the word or phrase that makes the following sentence grammatically correct.

It seems like his blood pressure ___ every week.

a. rises
b. raises
c. raise
d. rise

17. Select the word or phrase that makes the following sentence correct.

____ their similar training, the two professionals drew radically different conclusions.

a. Because of
b. Among
c. Despite
d. Now that

18. Select the word or phrase that makes the following sentence grammatically correct.

Each of the two European capitals ____ named after a famous leader.

a. are
b. am
c. as
d. is

19. Which word is NOT used correctly in the context of the following sentence?

Before you walk any further, beware of the approaching traffic.

a. Before
b. Further
c. Beware
d. Approaching

20. What word is used incorrectly in the following sentence?

The little boy sat the red block atop the stack.

a. Little
b. Sat
c. Atop
d. Stack

21. Select the word or phrase that makes the following sentence grammatically correct.

Even though she was new, Lauren knew that ___ the patient's name would be an ethical violation.

a. divulge
b. to divulge
c. to divulging
d. divulged

22. Select the word or phrase that makes the following sentence grammatically correct.

The attendant looked ____ at everything related to the problem.

a. close
b. closet
c. closely
d. closedly

23. Choose the word that best completes the sentence.

James exclaimed dramatically, "I'm so ______ that I could eat an immense meal!"

a. congested
b. nauseated
c. satisfied
d. starved

24. What word or phrase is used incorrectly in the following sentence?

Henry intuitively understood the doctor's illusion to his long-term depression.

a. Intuitively
b. Illusion
c. Long-term
d. Depression

25. Select the correct word for the blank in the following sentence.

If you want to join the club, you ____ contact the coach by Thursday.

a. would
b. should
c. did
d. have

26. Select the word that makes the following sentence grammatically correct.

Andy has ____ up a law practice of his own.

a. seat
b. set
c. sit
d. sat

27. Select the word or phrase that makes the following sentence grammatically correct.

He decided to buy a large coal furnace because he felt it would be _______ than a woodstove.

a. more efficient
b. efficienter
c. more efficienter
d. efficiency

28. What word is used incorrectly in the following sentence?

It is amazing how many soccer players has developed knee problems over the years.

a. Many
b. Players
c. Has
d. Developed

29. Select the word that makes the following sentence grammatically correct.

She asked ___ to take her around the corner to the drugstore.

a. him
b. his
c. he
d. his'

30. Select the word or phrase that makes the following sentence grammatically correct.

Felix was pleased ____ the progress he had made in his program.

a. among
b. with
c. regards
d. besides

31. Select the word or phrase that makes the following sentence grammatically correct.

After waking up, Dean eyed the cheesecake _________.

a. hungry
b. hungriest
c. hungrily
d. more hungry

32. Which word is NOT used correctly in the context of the following sentence?

After ringing up the nails, the cashier handed Nedra her recipe and change.

a. Ringing
b. Cashier
c. Recipe
d. Change

33. Select the correct word for the blank in the following sentence.

Sharon felt ____ about how her speech had gone.

a. well
b. good
c. finely
d. happily

34. Choose the word that best completes the sentence.

Yesterday's rainfall was a mere shower, but today's storm ______ hailstones down on us.

a. dripped
b. drizzled
c. hurled
d. trickle

35. What word is used incorrectly in the following sentence?

Brendan spent the day lying a brick foundation on the site.

a. Site
b. On
c. Spent
d. Lying

36. Select the word or phrase that makes this sentence grammatically correct:

Children _____ obey their parents tend to do better in school.

a. who
b. which
c. should
d. to

37. Select the word or phrase that makes this sentence grammatically correct:

The development committee ____ a bargain with the city planners.

a. striked
b. stroke
c. struck
d. strike

38. Select the word or phrase that makes this sentence grammatically correct:

A child is not yet old enough to know what is healthy for _______.

a. him or her
b. them
c. it
d. she or he

39. Select the word or phrase that makes this sentence grammatically correct:

Theo was in great shape; he ______ all the way back to the pier.

a. swam
b. swimmed
c. swum
d. swim

40. Select the phrase that makes this sentence grammatically correct:

_________ went to the movies after having dinner at Lenny's.

a. Her and I
b. Her and me
c. She and I
d. She and me

41. Select the word or phrase that makes this sentence grammatically correct:

Before turning in, Brian made sure to ____ the alarm clock.

a. sat
b. sit
c. set
d. setted

42. What word is used incorrectly in the following sentence?

The dashboard shaked as he revved the engine.

a. Dashboard
b. Shaked
c. As
d. Revved

43. Select the word or phrase that makes this sentence grammatically correct:

_____ way he looked, Ted saw people milling about.

a. Moreover
b. Whichever
c. Whomever
d. Whether

44. Select the correct word for the blank in the following sentence.

The buried treasure had ____ there for centuries.

a. laid
b. layed
c. lain
d. laint

45. Choose the verb that correctly completes the sentence.

Since she moved into her own place, Janet ____ her own cooking.

a. has been doing
b. does
c. did
d. is doing

46. Select the word that makes this sentence grammatically correct:

In order to serve each patient better, the clinic decided to see ____ patients overall.

a. less
b. fewer
c. lesser
d. few

47. Select the word or phrase that makes this sentence grammatically correct:

It wasn't until ____ the interview that Kim realized she had forgotten her list of questions.

a. despite
b. after
c. among
d. between

48. Which word is used incorrectly in the following sentence?

The video store is on the way, so we should stop by and rent one.

a. Video
b. Way
c. By
d. One

49. Select the word that makes the following sentence grammatically correct.

____ are the best eye doctors in this county?

a. Who
b. Which
c. Whom
d. What

50. Select the word that makes this sentence grammatically correct:

While he was an apprentice, Steve ____ a great deal of time in the studio.

a. spends
b. spent
c. spended
d. spend

51. Select the word that correctly completes the following sentence.

The intern was surprised by the _______ of pain he was in after his first day of work.

a. amount
b. frequency
c. number
d. amplitude

52. What word is used incorrectly in the following sentence?

Whoever wrote the letter forgot to sign their name.

a. Whoever
b. Wrote
c. Their
d. Name

53. Select the word or phrase that makes this sentence grammatically correct:

The child's fever was ___ high for him to lie comfortably in bed.

a. to
b. much
c. too
d. more

54. Select the word or phrase that makes the following sentence grammatically correct.

Sometimes, the condition _________ with an unusual symptom—vertigo.

a. presence
b. presents
c. present
d. prescience

55. Which word is NOT used correctly in the context of the following sentence?

There is no real distinction among the two treatment protocols recommended online.

a. Real
b. Among
c. Protocols
d. Online

Biology

1. Chromosomes are located within the:

a. Cell body
b. Dendrites
c. Axon
d. Synapse

1. If an organism is AaBb, which of the following combinations in the gametes is impossible?

a. AB
b. aa
c. aB
d. Ab

3. What is the typical result of mitosis in humans?

a. Two diploid cells
b. Two haploid cells
c. Four diploid cells
d. Four haploid cells

4. How does water affect the temperature of a living thing?

a. Water increases temperature.
b. Water keeps temperature stable.
c. Water decreases temperature.
d. Water does not affect temperature.

5. Which of the following is *not* a product of the Krebs cycle?

a. Carbon dioxide
b. Oxygen
c. Adenosine triphosphate (ATP)
d. Energy carriers

6. What kind of bond connects sugar and phosphate in DNA?

a. Hydrogen
b. Ionic
c. Covalent
d. Overt

7. Pollination involves which plant parts?

a. Xylem and petiole
b. Apical meristem and floral meristem
c. Anther and stigma
d. Root hairs and stroma

8. What is the second part of an organism's scientific name?

a. Species
b. Phylum
c. Population
d. Kingdom

9. How are lipids different than other organic molecules?

a. They are indivisible.
b. They are not water soluble.
c. They contain zinc.
d. They form long proteins.

10. Which of the following is NOT a steroid?

a. Cholesterol
b. Estrogen
c. Testosterone
d. Hemoglobin

11. Which of the following properties is responsible for the passage of water through a plant?

a. Cohesion
b. Adhesion
c. Osmosis
d. Evaporation

12. Which hormone is produced by the pineal gland?

a. Insulin
b. Testosterone
c. Melatonin
d. Epinephrine

13. Which part of the cell serves as the control center for all cell activity?

a. Nucleus
b. Cell membrane
c. Cytoplasm
d. Mitochondria

14. What is the name of the organelle that organizes protein synthesis?

a. Mitochondrion
b. Nucleus
c. Ribosome
d. Vacuole

15. During which phase is the chromosome number reduced from diploid to haploid?

a. S phase
b. Interphase
c. Mitosis
d. Meiosis I

16. What is the name for a cell that does NOT contain a nucleus?

a. Eukaryote
b. Bacteria
c. Prokaryote
d. Cancer

17. What is the name for the physical presentation of an organism's genes?

a. Phenotype
b. Species
c. Phylum
d. Genotype

18. Which of the following forms of water is the densest?

a. Liquid
b. Steam
c. Ice
d. All forms of water have the same density.

19. What part of a plant system responds to stimuli by releasing water via transpiration, except during adverse conditions like a drought when it closes up to prevent the plant from dehydration?

a. Pith
b. Stomata
c. Guard cells
d. Sepals

20. What is the longest phase in the life of a cell?

a. Prophase
b. Interphase
c. Anaphase
d. Metaphase

21. Which of the following is NOT found within a bacterial cell?

a. Mitochondria
b. DNA
c. Vesicles
d. Ribosome

22. Which of the following is a protein?

a. Cellulose
b. Hemoglobin
c. Estrogen
d. ATP

23. Which of the following structures is NOT involved in translation?

a. tRNA
b. mRNA
c. Ribosome
d. DNA

24. Which of the following is necessary for cell diffusion?

a. Water
b. Membrane
c. ATP
d. Gradient

25. How are organisms, such as snakes, cacti, and coyotes, able to survive in harsh desert conditions?

a. Over thousands of years, these organisms have developed adaptations to survive in arid climates.
b. These organisms migrate out of the desert during the summer months, only living in the desert for a portion of the year.
c. Snakes, cacti, and coyotes work together to find sources of food and water.
d. Snakes, cacti, and coyotes are all aquatic species that live in ponds and rivers during the hot day.

26. How many different types of nucleotides are there in DNA?

a. One
b. Two
c. Four
d. Eight

27. Which of the following cell types has no nucleus?

a. Platelet
b. Red blood cell
c. White blood cell
d. Phagocyte

28. Which part of aerobic respiration uses oxygen?

a. Osmosis
b. Krebs cycle
c. Glycolysis
d. Electron transport system

29. Which of the following is the most general taxonomic category?

a. Kingdom
b. Phylum
c. Genus
d. Order

30. What is the name of the process by which a bacterial cell splits into two new cells?

a. Mitosis
b. Meiosis
c. Replication
d. Fission

Chemistry

1. In a single replacement reaction, what products could result from these reactants in the following chemical equation?

$$2Al + Fe_2O_3 \rightarrow$$

a. $AlO_3 + Fe_2$
b. $2Fe_2 + 2AlO_3$
c. $Al_2O_3 + 2Fe$
d. $2AlFeO_3$

2. Which of the following substances allows for the fastest diffusion?

a. Gas
b. Solid
c. Liquid
d. Plasma

3. What is the oxidation number of hydrogen in CaH_2?

a. +1
b. −1
c. 0
d. +2

4. Which of the following does NOT exist as a diatomic molecule?

a. Boron
b. Fluorine
c. Oxygen
d. Nitrogen

5. What is another name for aqueous HI?

a. Hydroiodate acid
b. Hydrogen monoiodide
c. Hydrogen iodide
d. Hydriodic acid

6. Which of the following could be an empirical formula?

a. C_4H_8
b. C_2H_6
c. CH
d. C_3H_6

7. Which of the following statements describes a chemical property of water?

a. Water has a pH of 1.
b. A water molecule contains 2 hydrogen atoms and 1 oxygen atom.
c. A water molecule contains 2 oxygen atoms and 1 hydrogen atom.
d. The chemical formula for water is HO_2.

8. What is the name for the reactant that is entirely consumed by the reaction?

a. Limiting reactant
b. Reducing agent
c. Reaction intermediate
d. Reagent

9. What is the name for the horizontal rows of the periodic table?

a. Groups
b. Periods
c. Families
d. Sets

10. What is the mass (in grams) of 7.35 mol water?

a. 10.7 g
b. 18 g
c. 132 g
d. 180.6 g

11. Which of the following orbitals is the last to fill?

a. 1*s*
b. 3*s*
c. 4*p*
d. 6*s*

12. What is the name of the binary molecular compound NO_5?

a. Nitro pentoxide
b. Ammonium pentoxide
c. Nitrogen pentoxide
d. Pentnitrogen oxide

13. An atom has 5 protons, 5 neutrons, and 6 electrons. What is the electric charge of this atom?

a. Neutral
b. Positive
c. Negative
d. Undetermined

14. What is the mass (in grams) of 1.0 mol oxygen gas?

a. 12 g
b. 16 g
c. 28 g
d. 32 g

15. Which kind of radiation has no charge?

a. Beta
b. Alpha
c. Delta
d. Gamma

16. What is the name of the state in which forward and reverse chemical reactions are occurring at the same rate?

a. Equilibrium
b. Constancy
c. Stability
d. Toxicity

17. What is 119 K in degrees Celsius?

a. 32 °C
b. −154 °C
c. 154 °C
d. −32 °C

18. What is the SI unit of energy?

a. Ohm
b. Joule
c. Henry
d. Newton

19. What is oxidation?

a. The exchange of carbon dioxide for oxygen
b. The reduction of the number of chromosomes per cell
c. Cave formations resulting from the dripping of mineralized water
d. A change in the chemical composition of iron

20. What is the name of the device that separates gaseous ions by their mass-to-charge ratio?

a. Mass spectrometer
b. Interferometer
c. Magnetometer
d. Capacitance meter

21. Which material has the lowest specific heat?

a. Water
b. Wood
c. Aluminum
d. Glass

22. What is the name for a reaction in which electrons are transferred from one atom to another?

a. Combustion reaction
b. Synthesis reaction
c. Redox reaction
d. Double-displacement reaction

23. What are van der Waals forces?

a. The weak forces of attraction between two molecules
b. The strong forces of attraction between two molecules
c. Hydrogen bonds
d. Conjugal bonds

24. Which of the following gases effuses the fastest?

a. Cl_2
b. O_2
c. N_2
d. H_2

25. Which of the following quantities do *catalysts* alter to control the rate of a chemical reaction?

a. Substrate energy
b. Activation energy
c. Inhibitor energy
d. Promoter energy

26. Which of the following elements is NOT involved in many hydrogen bonds?

a. Fluorine
b. Carbon
c. Oxygen
d. Nitrogen

27. What is the mass (in grams) of 0.350 mol copper?

a. 12.5 g
b. 14.6 g
c. 18.5 g
d. 22.2 g

28. How many *d* orbitals are there in a *d* subshell?

a. 5
b. 7
c. 9
d. 11

29. What is the name for the number of protons in an atom?

a. Atomic identity
b. Atomic mass
c. Atomic weight
d. Atomic number

30. Which of the following elements is an alkali metal?

a. Magnesium
b. Rubidium
c. Hydrogen
d. Chlorine

Anatomy and Physiology

1. During the *anaphase* of mitosis, the ______________, originally in pairs, separate from their daughters and move to the opposite ends (or poles) of the cell.

a. Chromosomes
b. Spindle fibers
c. Centrioles
d. Nuclear membranes

2. What is the name of the structure that prevents food from entering the airway?

a. Trachea
b. Esophagus
c. Diaphragm
d. Epiglottis

3. Which substance makes up the pads that provide support between the vertebrae?

a. Bone
b. Cartilage
c. Tendon
d. Fat

4. How many different types of tissue are there in the human body?

a. Four
b. Six
c. Eight
d. Ten

5. What is the name of the outermost layer of skin?

a. Dermis
b. Epidermis
c. Subcutaneous tissue
d. Hypodermis

6. Which hormone stimulates milk production in the breasts during lactation?

a. Norepinephrine
b. Antidiuretic hormone
c. Prolactin
d. Oxytocin

7. How does meiosis differ from mitosis?

a. Meiosis is used to repair the body. Mitosis is used to break down the body.
b. Meiosis is used for asexual reproduction of single-celled organisms. Mitosis is used for sexual reproduction of multicellular organisms.
c. Meiosis only occurs in humans. Mitosis only occurs in plants.
d. Meiosis produces cells that are genetically different. Mitosis produces cells that are genetically identical.

8. Which of the following structures has the lowest blood pressure?

a. Arteries
b. Arteriole
c. Venule
d. Vein

9. Which of the heart chambers is the most muscular?

a. Left atrium
b. Right atrium
c. Left ventricle
d. Right ventricle

10. Within which part of the brain is sensory information interpreted?

a. Cerebrum
b. Hindbrain
c. Cerebellum
d. Medulla oblongata

11. Which of the following proteins is produced by cartilage?

a. Actin
b. Estrogen
c. Collagen
d. Myosin

12. Which component of the nervous system is responsible for lowering the heart rate?

a. Central nervous system
b. Sympathetic nervous system
c. Parasympathetic nervous system
d. Distal nervous system

13. A normal human sperm must contain:

a. An X chromosome
b. A Y chromosome
c. 23 chromosomes
d. Both an X and a Y chromosome

14. Which type of substance breaks down to form urea?

a. Lipid
b. Protein
c. Carbohydrate
d. Iron

15. What is the name for a joint that can only move in two directions?

a. Hinge
b. Insertion
c. Ball and socket
d. Flange

16. In which of the following muscle types are the filaments arranged in a disorderly manner?

a. Cardiac
b. Smooth
c. Skeletal
d. Rough

17. How much air does an adult inhale in an average breath?

a. 500 mL
b. 750 mL
c. 1000 mL
d. 1250 mL

18. Which type of cell secretes antibodies?

a. Bacterial cell
b. Viral cell
c. Lymph cell
d. Plasma cells

19. Which of the following describes one responsibility of the integumentary system?

a. Distributing vital substances (such as nutrients) throughout the body
b. Blocking pathogens that cause disease
c. Sending leaked fluids from the cardiovascular system back to the blood vessels
d. Storing bodily hormones that influence gender traits

20. Which force motivates filtration in the kidneys?

a. Osmosis
b. Smooth muscle contraction
c. Peristalsis
d. Blood pressure

21. Which of the following hormones decreases the concentration of blood glucose?

a. Insulin
b. Glucagon
c. Growth hormone
d. Glucocorticoids

22. Which structure controls the hormones secreted by the pituitary gland?

a. Hypothalamus
b. Adrenal gland
c. Testes
d. Pancreas

23. How much of a female's blood volume is composed of red blood cells?

a. 10%
b. 25%
c. 40%
d. 70%

24. Which type of cholesterol is considered to be the best for health?

a. LDL
b. HDL
c. VLDL
d. VHDL

25. The digestion of starch begins:

a. In the mouth
b. In the stomach
c. In the pylorus
d. In the duodenum

26. Where are the vocal cords located?

a. Bronchi
b. Trachea
c. Larynx
d. Epiglottis

27. Where does gas exchange occur in the human body?

a. Alveoli
b. Bronchi
c. Larynx
d. Pharynx

28. Which structure of the nervous system carries action potential in the direction of a synapse?

a. Cell body
b. Axon
c. Neuron
d. Myelin

29. Where is the parathyroid gland located?

a. Neck
b. Back
c. Side
d. Brain

30. What is the name of the process in the lungs by which oxygen is transported from the air to the blood?

a. Osmosis
b. Diffusion
c. Dissipation
d. Reverse osmosis

Physics

1. A motorcycle weighs twice as much as a bicycle and is moving twice as fast. Which of the following statements is true?

a. The motorcycle has four times as much kinetic energy as the bicycle.
b. The motorcycle has eight times as much kinetic energy as the bicycle.
c. The bicycle and the motorcycle have the same kinetic energy.
d. The bicycle has four times as much kinetic energy as the motorcycle.

2. Starting from rest, a bicyclist accelerates in one direction at a constant 2 m/s^2. What is his instantaneous speed after 10 seconds?

a. 2 m/s
b. 5 m/s
c. 20 m/s
d. 40 m/s

3. A merry-go-round three meters in diameter takes 20 seconds to make a full rotation with no external forces acting on it. What is the linear speed of a horse at the edge of the merry-go-round?

a. 0.15 m/s
b. 0.47 m/s
c. 0.24 m/s
d. 0.94 m/s

4. If the average speed of the molecules in a gas increases, which of the following must be true?

a. The temperature of the gas increases.
b. The pressure of the gas increases.
c. The volume of the gas increases.
d. The volume of the gas decreases.

Question 5 pertains to the following graph of displacement from equilibrium versus time for a point on a vibrating string:

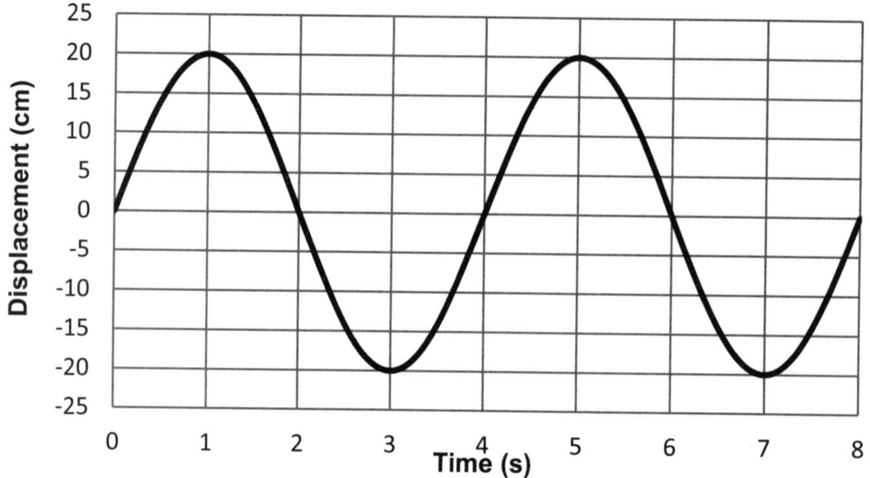

5. Which of the following characteristics of the wave can NOT be determined from the graph?

a. Amplitude
b. Frequency
c. Period
d. Wavelength

6. A roller coaster car travels on a frictionless track along a flat section before entering a loop, the top of which is ten meters higher than the flat section. What is the minimum speed at which the car must be traveling along the flat section in order to reach the top of the loop?

a. 5 m/s
b. 7 m/s
c. 10 m/s
d. 14 m/s

7. If a glass rod is rubbed with a cloth made of polyester, what will the resulting charge be on each material?

a. The charge on the glass rod is positive and the charge on the cloth is negative.
b. The charge on the glass rod is negative and the charge on the cloth is positive.
c. The charge on the glass rod is neutral and the charge on the cloth is positive.
d. The charge on the glass rod and the cloth both become neutral.

8. A crane lifts a crate 10 meters off the ground and then lowers it onto a platform 6 meters above the ground. If the crate has a weight of 1,000 N, what is the net work done by the crane?

a. 14,000 J
b. 10,000 J
c. 6,000 J
d. 4,000 J

9. A soccer ball with a mass of 0.4 kg rolls toward a soccer player at a speed of 1 m/s. He kicks the ball, giving it a speed of 8 m/s in the opposite direction. What impulse did his kick produce on the soccer ball?

a. 0.4 (kg · m)/s
b. 2.8 (kg · m)/s
c. 3.2 (kg · m)/s
d. 3.6 (kg · m)/s

10. Three students pull ropes attached to a ring as shown in the diagram. One student pulls due south with a force of 100 N, another pulls due east with an unknown force, and the third pulls in some direction north-northwest with a force of 115 N. The ring does not move. What is the magnitude of the unknown force, rounded to the nearest whole number?

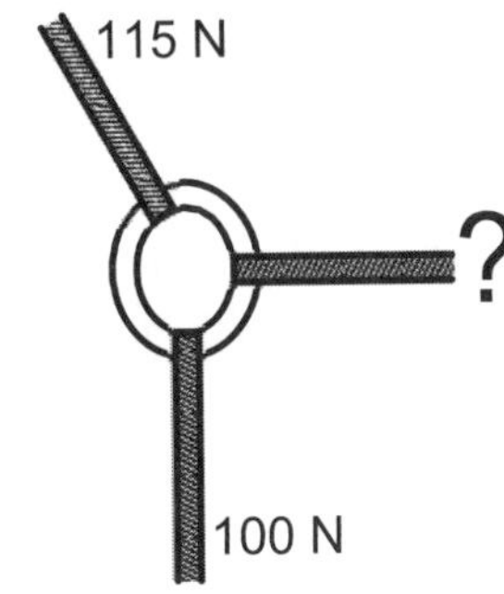

a. 15 N
b. 57 N
c. 81 N
d. 108 N

11. When you walk barefoot on a hot sidewalk, what process is primarily responsible for heat transfer from the sidewalk to your foot?

a. Conduction
b. Convection
c. Radiation
d. None of the above

12. Which of the following observations provides the best evidence that sound can travel through solid objects?

a. Sound waves cannot travel through a vacuum.
b. The atoms of a solid are packed tightly together.
c. If you knock on a solid object, it makes a sound.
d. You can hear a sound on the other side of a solid wall.

13. The pilot of an eastbound plane determines wind speed relative to his aircraft. He measures a wind velocity of 320 km/h, with the wind coming from the east. An observer on the ground sees the plane pass overhead, and measures its velocity as 290 km/h. What is the wind velocity relative to the observer?

a. 30 km/h east-to-west
b. 30 km/h west-to-east
c. 320 km/h east-to-west
d. 290 km/h east-to-west

14. In the circuit pictured, what is the current at point A?

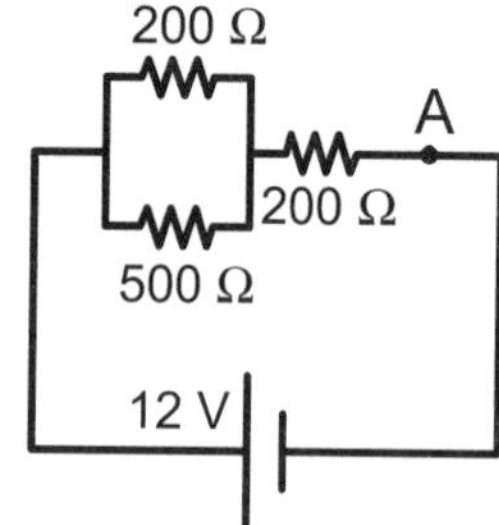

a. 13.3 mA
b. 35 mA
c. 60 mA
d. 154 mA

15. Jim exerts a force of 320 N to push a heavy barrel along a floor surface with significant friction. He manages to impart to the barrel an acceleration of $0.13\ \text{m/s}^2$. If the barrel has a mass of 200 kg, what is the magnitude of the force of friction acting on the barrel?

a. 26 N
b. 147 N
c. 294 N
d. 320 N

16. A light ray passes from air into a block of amber, as shown in this diagram. What is the index of refraction of amber?

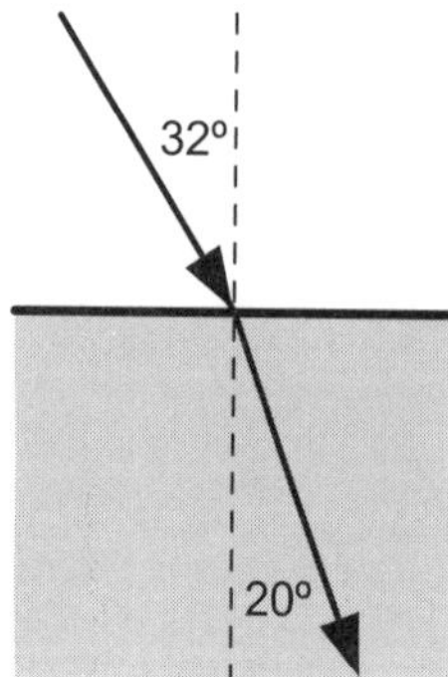

a. 1.11
b. 1.55
c. 1.60
d. 1.66

17. Which of the following best explains why medical imaging machines use x-rays instead of visible light?

a. X-rays have shorter wavelengths than visible light, which lets them penetrate matter more easily.
b. X-rays have longer wavelengths than visible light, which lets them penetrate matter more easily.
c. X-rays have shorter wavelengths than visible light, which means they are more energetic.
d. X-rays have longer wavelengths than visible light, which means they are less energetic.

18. A scientist mixes two chemicals together, and they produce a violent reaction, generating considerable heat. Where did the thermal energy come from to heat up the chemicals?

a. The kinetic energy of the molecules in the chemicals
b. Potential energy inherent in the atomic bonds in the molecules of the chemicals
c. Absorbed from the surrounding air
d. Nowhere; the energy was completely created by the reaction

19. According to Ohm's Law, how are voltage and current related in an electrical circuit?

a. Voltage and current are inversely proportional to one another.
b. Voltage and current are directly proportional to one another.
c. Voltage acts to oppose the current along an electrical circuit.
d. Voltage acts to decrease the current along an electrical circuit.

20. A sled with a mass of 100 kg slides on an icy lake. It collides with another sled with a mass of 80 kg. Before the collision, the first sled was traveling at a speed of 4.0 m/s, and the second sled was stationary. After the collision, the first sled was traveling at a speed of 1.0 m/s. How fast was the second sled traveling after the collision?

a. 3.0 m/s
b. 3.8 m/s
c. 4.3 m/s
d. 5.0 m/s

21. In which of the following materials would you expect sound waves to travel most rapidly?

a. Air
b. Aluminum
c. Rubber
d. Water

22. The graph below shows the velocity of a go-cart over time. At which of the labeled points on the graph is the go-cart's acceleration greatest?

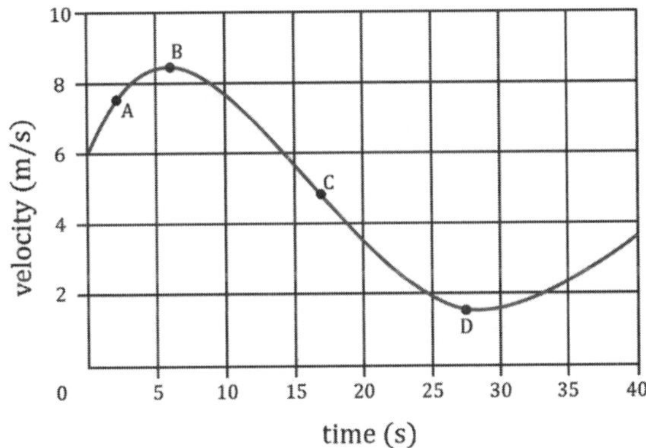

a. Point A
b. Point B
c. Point C
d. Point D

23. Which of the following best explains why radiation therapy is used to treat cancer?

a. The strong electromagnetic forces in the radiation pull cancer cells apart.
b. The waves of the radiation have just the right frequency to destructively interfere with the cancer cells.
c. The high frequency of the radiation causes cancer cells to vibrate so fast they shake themselves apart.
d. The high-energy photons, or charged particles, of the radiation impact and damage vital molecules in the cancer cells, killing them.

24. In the circuit diagrammed, what is the current through the 100 Ω resistor?

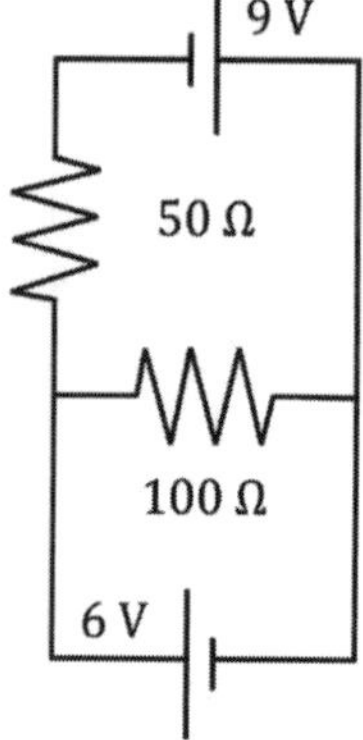

a. 60 mA
b. 300 mA
c. 3.30 A
d. 16.7 A

25. In which of the following scenarios is work NOT applied to the object?

a. Mario moves a book from the floor to the top shelf.
b. A book drops off the shelf and falls to the floor.
c. Mario pushes a box of books across the room.
d. Mario balances a book on his head.

26. Which of the following is an example of heat transfer through convection?

a. A microwave cooking food
b. A pancake cooking on an electric burner
c. A planet heated by the sun
d. A coastline heated by a warm ocean current

27. A boy whirls a ball on a string, spinning it in a circle 1.5 meters in diameter. The ball completes two revolutions every second. If the mass of the ball is 80 grams, what is the tension in the string?

a. 0.59 N
b. 1.2 N
c. 9.5 N
d. 19 N

28. A 100-gram weight hangs motionless from a massless spring. If the weight is pulled down 40 centimeters from this equilibrium position, stretching the spring, what other information is needed to calculate the amount of work done on the spring?

a. The length of the spring when no mass is hung from it
b. The elastic potential energy of the stretched spring
c. The time it took to pull the weight down
d. None, there is already enough information to conclude no work was done on the spring

29. A boy swings on a rope over a lake. When he steps off of the ledge to start his swing, he is 2.0 meters above the lake surface. At the bottom of the swing, just as he lets go of the rope, he is 0.5 meters above the surface. What is the boy's horizontal speed at the bottom of the swing?

a. 5.4 m/s
b. 6.3 m/s
c. 7.7 m/s
d. 8.9 m/s

30. The graph below displays the displacement from equilibrium over time of a point on a vibrating string. What is the amplitude of the vibration?

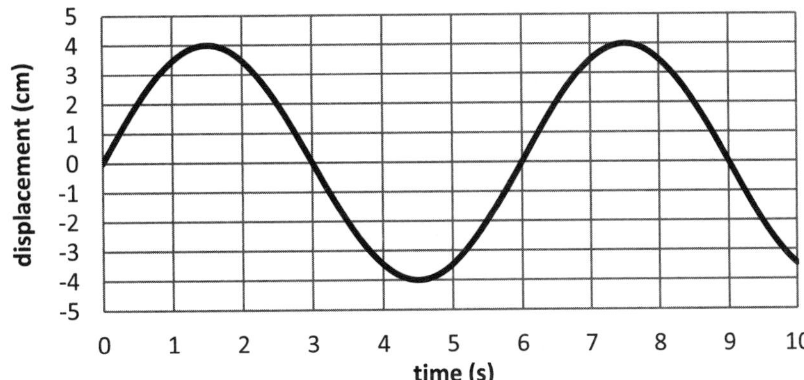

a. 3 s
b. 4 cm
c. 6 s
d. 8 cm

Answer Key and Explanations for Test #1

Mathematics (Video Explanations Available)

We now have video explanations for every math question in this practice test. Visit mometrix.com/academy/hesi-a2-math-explanations/ or scan this QR code to access these videos.

1. D: Begin by subtracting 4 from both sides, then subtract x from both sides:

$$2x + 4 - 4 = x - 6 - 4$$
$$2x = x - 10$$
$$2x - x = x - 10 - x$$
$$x = -10$$

2. 58: To evaluate the expression, first substitute the given values into the expression.

$$\frac{2(21)}{3(7)} + 5(21) - 7(7)$$

From here, simplify using the order of operations.

$$\frac{42}{21} + 5(21) - 7(7)$$

$$2 + 105 - 49$$

$$107 - 49$$

$$58$$

3. 440: To find the number of cars remaining, subtract the number of cars that were sold from the original number:

$$476 - 36 = 440$$

4. B: A number is divisible by 8 if the number formed by the last three digits is divisible by 8. In this case, the number formed by the last three digits (064) is 64, which is divisible by 8. This means that 45,064 is also divisible by 8.

5. 175: There are 7 days in a week. Knowing that the chef can make 25 pastries in a day, the weekly number can be calculated:

$$25 \times 7 = 175$$

6. 30: For small numbers like 6 and 10, the LCM can be determined by simply listing the multiples of each number and then looking for the lowest multiple that appears in both lists.

Multiples of 6: 6, 12, 18, 24, **30**, ...

Multiples of 10: 10, 20, **30**, ...

Lowest multiple in common: 30

7. A: The second midwife allocates $\frac{1}{2}$ of her funds for an office administrator plus another $\frac{1}{10}$ for office supplies. We need to add $\frac{1}{2}$ and $\frac{1}{10}$ by first finding a common denominator.

$$\frac{1}{2}+\frac{1}{10}=\frac{5}{10}+\frac{1}{10}=\frac{6}{10}$$

Now, simplify $\frac{6}{10}$ by dividing the numerator and denominator by their greatest common factor, which is 2.

$$\frac{6 \div 2}{10 \div 2}=\frac{3}{5}$$

8. C: To write the equation for this problem, first decide what x represents. We want to know how many days Billy worked his paper route this week, so x (the unknown) will represent the number of days he worked. Now, notice that Billy rides 5 miles each time he works the paper route. This number describes the *rate* at which he rides daily, so the equation will have 5 multiplied by x.

$$5x$$

We are told that one day during the week, Billy rides an extra mile. Because of this, the equation will include the term $+1$.

$$5x+1$$

We also are told that Billy rides a total of 21 miles over the week. This will be the number on the other side of the equation.

$$5x+1=21$$

Now, solve for x. Start by subtracting 1 from both sides.

$$5x+1-1=21-1$$
$$5x=20$$

Then, divide both sides by 5.

$$\frac{5x}{5}=\frac{20}{5}$$

$$x=4$$

Billy worked his paper route four mornings this week.

9. B: The woman has four days to earn \$250. To find the amount she must earn each day, divide the amount she must earn (\$250) by 4:

$$\frac{\$250}{4} = \$62.50$$

10. 14.989: To solve this problem, you must know how to add a series of numbers when some of the numbers include decimals. As with addition problems 1 and 2, the most important first step is to set up the proper vertical alignment. This step is even more important when working with decimals. Be sure that all of the decimal points are in alignment; in other words, the 7 in 3.7 should be above the 2 in 7.289. Since the final term, 4, is a whole number, we assume a 0 in the tenths place. Similarly, you may assume zeros in the hundredths and thousandths places, if you prefer to have a digit in every relevant place. Then beginning at the rightmost place value (in this case, the thousandths), add the terms together as you would with whole numbers. The decimal point of the sum should be aligned with the decimal points of the terms.

11. C: To calculate his new salary, add his raise to his original salary:

$$\$15.23 + \$2.34 = \$17.57$$

12. 83: Erma's sale discount will be applied to the less expensive sweater, so she will receive the \$44 sweater for 25% off. This amounts to a discount of \$11, so the cost of the sweater will be \$33. Added to the cost of the \$50 sweater, which is not discounted, Erma's total is \$83.

13. A: To write an equation from the information given, first determine "what is the unknown?" In this case, the unknown is how many hours Nora worked. So x will represent the number of hours.

Since Nora is paid \$4 per hour in wages, part of her pay is calculated by multiplying 4 by x. The rest of her pay comes from tips, which are added on top of her hourly pay. Her total pay per shift can be written as $4x + \text{tips} = \text{total}$.

For today's shift, Nora received \$29 in tips and her total pay was \$53. The equation is then $4x + 29 = 53$.

To solve for x, first subtract 29 from both sides.

$$4x + 29 - 29 = 53 - 29$$
$$4x = 24$$

Now, divide both sides by 4.

$$\frac{4x}{4} = \frac{24}{4}$$

$$x = 6$$

So, Nora worked six hours today.

14. A: To simplify, proceed using the order of the operations: $\frac{2}{3} \div \frac{4}{15} = \frac{2}{3} \times \frac{15}{4} = \frac{30}{12}$, which simplifies to $\frac{5}{2}$. Next, multiply $\frac{5}{2}$ by $\frac{5}{8}$. The result is $\frac{25}{16}$.

15. B: To solve this problem, you must know how to solve word problems involving decimal subtraction. In this scenario, Karen starts out with a certain amount of money and spends some of it on groceries. To calculate how much money she has left, simply subtract the money spent from the original figure: 40– 1.85– 3.20– 3.05. There is no reason to include the dollar sign in your calculations, so long as you remember that it exists. You cannot subtract the costs of these items at the same time, so you must either subtract them one by one or add them up and subtract the sum from 40. Either way will generate the right answer.

16. C: Find the total cost of the items:

$$\$6.65 + \$159.23 = \$165.88$$

Then, calculate how much each individual will owe:

$$\frac{\$165.88}{4} = \$41.47$$

17. -20: Simplify this expression by using the order of operations (PEMDAS). First, simplify the parentheses. Remember, the order of operations has to be followed within parentheses, so multiply before you add.

$$7 + 16 - (5 + 6 \times 3) - 10 \times 2$$

$$7 + 16 - (5 + 18) - 10 \times 2$$

$$7 + 16 - 23 - 10 \times 2$$

Then, simplify the multiplication.

$$7 + 16 - 23 - 20$$

Finally, add and subtract from left to right.

$$7 + 16 - 23 - 20 = -20$$

18. D: This problem requires you to understand word problems involving mileage rates and multiplication. The problem states that the car gets an average 25 miles per gallon; in other words, every gallon of fuel powers the car for approximately 25 miles. If the car holds 16 gallons of gas, then, and each of these gallons provides 25 miles of travel, you can set up the following equation: 25 miles/gallon × 16 gallons = 400 miles. Since the first term has gallons in the denominator and the second term has gallons in what would be the numerator (if it were expressed as 16 gallons/1), these units cancel each other out and leave only miles.

19. A: To convert liters to gallons, first convert milliliters to liters. Converting from one metric unit to another requires moving the decimal point in the given measurement to the left or right to determine the value for the required metric unit. The table below shows the prefixes of some of the more common metric units involving volume.

Prefix	kilo-	hecto-	deka-		deci-	centi-	milli-
Symbol	k	h	da		d	c	m
Unit Measure	10^3	10^2	10^1	$10^0 = 1$	10^{-1}	10^{-2}	10^{-3}

When converting a given metric unit that has a smaller unit of measure than the required metric unit, we can move the decimal point for the number having the smaller metric unit the same number of places to the left that it takes to get to the larger metric unit in the table. Since the milliliter metric unit is three places from the liter metric unit, we can move the decimal point that is at the end of 3,785 mL three places to the left to convert it to liters.

$$3.\underset{\smile}{7}\underset{\smile}{8}\underset{\smile}{5}. = 3.785$$

So, 3,785 mL = 3.785 L.

Alternatively, we could multiply 3,785 mL by a power of ten to the negative third power to get:

$$3{,}785 \times 10^{-3} = 3{,}785 \times \frac{1}{1{,}000} = \frac{3{,}785}{1{,}000} = 3.785$$

Thus, there are approximately 3.785 liters in one gallon of water so, 3.785 L = 1 gal.

Then, to see how much of a gallon of water is in one liter, divide both sides of the equality above by 3.785.

$$\frac{3.785 \text{ L}}{3.785} = \frac{1 \text{ gal}}{3.785}$$
$$1 \text{ L} = 0.264 \text{ gal}$$

To the nearest hundredth of a gallon, a liter of water is 0.26 gallons.

20. A: This problem requires you to understand addition of fractions with unlike denominators. The denominator is the bottom term in a fraction; the top term is called the numerator. In order to perform addition with fractions, all of the terms must have the same denominator. In order to derive the lowest common denominator in this problem, you must list the multiples for 3 and 7 until you find one that both have in common. In increasing order, multiples of 3 are 3, 6, 9, 12, 15, 18, and 21; multiples of 7 are 7, 14, and 21. The least common multiple is 21. This is also the lowest common denominator for the two fractions. To convert each term into a fraction with this common denominator, you must multiply both numerator and denominator by the same number. To make the denominator of $\frac{2}{3}$ into 21, you must multiply by 7; therefore, you must also multiply the numerator, 2, by 7. The new fraction is $\frac{14}{21}$. For the second term, you must multiply numerator and denominator by 3: $\frac{2}{7} \times \frac{3}{3} = \frac{6}{21}$. The new addition problem is $\frac{14}{21} + \frac{6}{21} = \frac{20}{21}$. Remember that when adding fractions, only the numerators are combined.

21. A: To convert a 24-hour time to 12-hour time, start by subtracting 1200, if the number is greater than 1200.

$$1615 - 1200 = 0415$$

This number corresponds to the 12-hour time in the afternoon, so Zachary's shift starts at 4:15 PM. Since he wants to set an alarm for 45 minutes before, subtract 45 minutes from 4:15 PM, which is 3:30 PM. Therefore, Zachary should set his alarm for 3:30 PM so he knows when to leave for his shift.

22. D: This problem requires you to understand addition involving mixed numbers. The calculation required by this problem is straightforward: In order to find the number of hours Aaron worked, add up the three mixed numbers. To make this possible, you will need to find the least common multiple of 2, 4, and 3 so that you can establish a common denominator. The lowest common denominator for this problem is 12. You can either add up the whole numbers separately from the fractions or convert the mixed numbers into improper fractions and add them in that form. Either way will yield the correct answer.

23. B: Add to solve. The height of the window from the floor is not needed in this equation. It is extra information. You only need to add the heights of the two bookcases. Convert the fractions so that they have a common denominator. After you add, simplify the fraction.

$$\begin{aligned} 14\frac{1}{2} + 8\frac{3}{4} &= 14\frac{2}{4} + 8\frac{3}{4} \\ &= 22\frac{5}{4} \\ &= 23\frac{1}{4} \end{aligned}$$

24. B: To solve this problem, you must understand subtraction involving fractions with like denominators. As with addition involving fractions with like denominators, you should only subtract the numerators. So, this problem is solved $\frac{23}{24} - \frac{11}{24} = \frac{12}{24}$. This answer can be simplified by dividing by the greatest common factor (a factor is any number that can be divided into the given number equally). The factors of 12 are 1, 2, 3, 4, 6, and 12. The factors of 24 are 1, 2, 3, 4, 6, 8, 12, and 24. The greatest common factor of 12 and 24 is 12, so divide both numerator and denominator by 12 to reduce the answer to its simplest form: $\frac{12 \div 12}{24 \div 12} = \frac{1}{2}$.

25. C: This problem requires you to understand subtraction with mixed numbers. In order to perform this problem, you must look at the fractions separately from the whole numbers. To subtract $\frac{4}{7} - \frac{3}{14}$, the two fractions must have the same denominator. Since 14 is a multiple of 7, you only have to alter the first term. Multiply both numerator and denominator by 2: $\frac{4}{7} \times \frac{2}{2} = \frac{8}{14}$. Then subtract: $\frac{8}{14} - \frac{3}{14} = \frac{5}{14}$. Now subtract the whole numbers: $3 - 2 = 1$. Putting the whole number and fraction together yields $1\frac{5}{14}$.

26. C: To solve this problem, you must know how to solve word problems requiring fraction addition and subtraction. You are given the proportions of Dean's socks that are white and black. The best approach to this problem is adding together the two known quantities and subtracting the sum from 1. First you need to find a common denominator for $\frac{1}{3}$ and $\frac{1}{6}$. The lowest common multiple of these two numbers is 6, so convert $\frac{1}{3}$ by multiplying the numerator and denominator by 2. The new equation will be $\frac{2}{6} + \frac{1}{6} = \frac{3}{6}$. This sum is equivalent to $\frac{1}{2}$, meaning that half of Dean's socks are either white or black. The other half, then, are brown, meaning the calculation will look like this: $\frac{2}{2} - \frac{1}{2} = \frac{1}{2}$.

27. A: This problem requires you to understand word problems involving the addition and multiplication of mixed numbers and improper fractions. To begin with, convert the three mixed numbers to improper fractions by multiplying the whole number by the denominator and adding the product to the numerator. The resulting fractions will be $\frac{3}{2}$ (sugar), $\frac{11}{3}$ (flour), and $\frac{2}{3}$ (milk). Then find the least common multiple of 2 and 3, which is 6, and convert the three fractions so that they have this denominator: $\frac{9}{6}$ (sugar), $\frac{22}{6}$ (flour), and $\frac{4}{6}$ (milk). Add these fractions together and multiply the sum by two to double the recipe: $\frac{9}{6}+\frac{22}{6}+\frac{4}{6}=\frac{35}{6}$. $\frac{35}{6}\times 2=\frac{70}{6}=\frac{35}{3}$. Finally, convert this improper fraction to a simple mixed number by dividing numerator by denominator and simplifying the leftover fraction: $\frac{35}{3}=11\frac{2}{3}$.

28. D: To solve this problem, you must know how to multiply mixed numbers and fractions. Unlike fraction addition and subtraction, fraction multiplication does not require a common denominator. However, it is necessary to convert mixed numbers into improper fractions. This is done by multiplying the whole number by the denominator and adding the product to the numerator: in this case, $4\times 3+1=13$. So the problem is now $\frac{13}{3}\times\frac{2}{7}$. Fraction multiplication is performed by multiplying numerator by numerator and denominator by denominator: $\frac{13\times 2}{3\times 7}=\frac{26}{21}$. This improper fraction can be converted into a mixed number by dividing numerator by denominator, which gives $1\frac{5}{21}$.

29. 31: To evaluate this expression, first substitute all the given values into the expression.

$$8(2)+3(4)-(11)+14$$

From here, simplify using the order of operations.

$$16+12-11+14$$

$$28-11+14$$

$$17+14$$

$$31$$

30. D: To solve this problem, you must know how to divide fractions. The process of dividing fractions is similar to that of multiplying fractions, except that the second term must first be inverted, or replaced with its reciprocal. Once this is done, the numerator is multiplied by the numerator, and the denominator is multiplied by the denominator. This problem can be solved by multiplying $\frac{5}{8}$ by the reciprocal of $\frac{1}{5}$, which is $\frac{5}{1}$ or 5: $\frac{5\times 5}{8\times 1}=\frac{25}{8}$. Finally, convert this improper fraction into a mixed number according to the usual procedure.

31. A: Military time is based off a 24-hour clock, so if the 12-hour time is AM, the first two digits of the military time will be 00-11, and if it is PM, the first two digits of the military time will be 12-23. Since we are working with 6:00 AM, the first two digits of military time will be 06. The last two digits of military time comes from the minutes, so 6:30 AM in military time is 0630.

32. 78: To solve this problem, you must know how to convert a fraction into a ratio. In this problem, you are being asked to convert the fraction into a value on a scale from 1 to 100, which is basically like being asked to convert it into a percentage. To do so, divide the numerator by the denominator. The answer will be a repeating seven: 0.777.... Calculate to the thousandths place and move the decimal two places to the right in order to determine the value. Because the digit in the thousandths place is a 7, you will round up the digit to the left to establish the final answer, 78.

33. C: Multiply 15 by 3 and add 2 to get the numerator, 47, over the original denominator, 3.

34. 1381.40: Start by adding up the costs of the trip, excluding the hotel cost: $\$572+\$150+\$250=\$972$. Then, calculate what Margery will spend on the hotel. The first of her five nights at the hotel will cost her \$89. For each of the other four nights, she will get a discount of 10% per night, or \$8.90. This discount of \$8.90 multiplied by the four nights is \$35.60. The total she would have spent on the five nights without the discount is \$445. With the discount, the amount goes down to \$409.40. Add this amount to the \$972 for a grand total of \$1,381.40.

35. 4.43: To solve this problem, you must know how to convert mixed numbers into decimals. Perhaps the easiest way to perform this operation is to convert the mixed number into an improper fraction and then divide the numerator by the denominator. Convert the mixed number into an improper fraction by multiplying the whole number by the denominator and adding the product to the numerator: $4 \times 7 + 3 = 31$, so the improper fraction is $\frac{31}{7}$. Next divide 31 by 7, according to the same procedure used in problems 7 and 8. Remember that when you have to add 0 to 31 in order to continue your calculations, you must put a decimal point directly above in the quotient. Also, since the problem asks you to round to the hundredths place, you must solve the problem to the nearest thousandth.

36. C: This problem requires you to understand the conversion of decimals into mixed numbers. 3.78 has value into the hundredths place, so your fraction will have a denominator of 100. There are three whole units and seventy-eight hundredths, a mixed number that can be written as $3\frac{78}{100}$. Next, you must simplify this fraction. The only common factor of 78 and 100 is 2, so divide both numerator and denominator by 2: $\frac{78 \div 2}{100 \div 2} = \frac{39}{50}$. This fraction cannot be simplified any further, so the answer is $3\frac{39}{50}$.

37. C: To solve this problem, you must know how to convert decimals into fractions. Remember that all of the numbers to the right of a decimal point represent values less than one. So, a decimal number such as this will not include any whole numbers when it is converted into a fraction. The 7 is in the hundredths place, so the number is properly expressed as $\frac{7}{100}$. The fraction cannot be simplified because 7 and 100 do not share any factors besides one.

38. D: Use inverse operations to solve the two-step equation for x.

$$2x - 7 = 3$$
$$2x - 7 + 7 = 3 + 7$$
$$2x = 10$$
$$\frac{2x}{2} = \frac{10}{2}$$
$$x = 5$$

39. C: To determine who did better on the test, compare the two fractions: $\frac{4}{9}$ and $\frac{5}{11}$. The two fractions can be compared by using cross multiplication. When cross multiplying, multiply the numerator of the first fraction by the denominator of the second fraction: $4 \times 11 = 44$. This number corresponds to the first fraction. Then, multiply the denominator of the first fraction by the numerator of the second fraction: $9 \times 5 = 45$. This number corresponds to the second fraction. From here, compare the two numbers: $44 < 45$. This means that the first fraction $\left(\frac{4}{9}\right)$ is less than the second fraction $\left(\frac{5}{11}\right)$: $\frac{4}{9} < \frac{5}{11}$. Since Elizabeth got $\frac{5}{11}$ questions correct on her test, she did better than Sarah.

40. 9: This problem requires you to understand how to approach word problems involving fractions and ratios. You are given the total number of students in the class and the fraction of students who are boys. With this information, you can determine the number of boys by multiplying $\frac{2}{3}$ by 27. You will find that there are 18 boys in the class. You can then find the number of girls by subtracting the number of boys from the total number of students: $27 - 18 = 9$. There are nine girls in the class.

41. D: There are 9 red marbles and 36 total marbles. This can be expressed as the ratio $9 : 36$. This can be simplified by dividing both 9 and 36 by their greatest common factor (9). The ratio $9 : 36$ becomes $1 : 4$.

42. C: Set up the proportion as a pair of equivalent fractions: $\frac{7}{42} = \frac{4}{x}$. Then solve for x. To do this, you must cross-multiply (producing $7x = 168$), and then divide both sides by 7. Your calculations should determine that $x = 24$.

43. B: To solve this problem, you must know how to convert a decimal into a percent. A percentage is a number expressed in terms of hundredths. When we say, for instance, that a candidate received 55% of the vote, we mean that she received 55 out of every 100 votes cast. When we say that the sales tax is 6%, we mean that for every 100 cents in the price another 6 cents are added to the final cost. To convert a decimal into a percentage, multiply it by 100 or just shift the decimal point two places to the right. In this case, by moving the decimal point two places to the right you can calculate the correct answer, 64%.

44. B: To solve the equation, isolate the variable on one side.

Subtract x from each side:

$$16 = 2x + 32$$

Subtract 32 from each side.

$$-16 = 2x$$

Divide both sides by 2:

$$x = -8$$

45. 144.65: To determine the total cost of Susan's outfit, add the costs of all her purchases.

$$\$69.99 + \$39.99 + \$34.67 = \$144.65$$

46. C: To simplify the expression using the laws of exponents, we use the multiplication rule which states that when two terms with exponents that have the same base are being multiplied, we can keep the base and add the exponents. In this case, we keep the base m and add the exponents, $3 + 8$, which equals 11. Therefore, the simplified form of the expression $m^3 \times m^8$ is equal to m^{11}.

47. C: This problem requires you to understand the conversion of percentages into decimals. A percentage is an amount out of 100; 17.6%, then, is equivalent to 17.6 out of 100, or $\frac{17.6}{100}$. A percentage can be converted into decimal form by dividing it by 100, or, more simply, by shifting the decimal point two places to the left. Therefore, 17.6% is equivalent to 0.176.

48. 1.26: To solve this problem, you must know how to convert percentages into decimals. Remember that a percentage is really just an expression of a value in terms of hundredths. That is, 25% is the same as 25 out of 100. To convert a percentage into a decimal, shift the decimal point two places to the left. In this case, the decimal point is assumed to be after the six in 126%. By shifting the decimal point two places to the left, you find that the equivalent decimal is 1.26.

49. C: This problem requires you to understand how to convert fractions into percentages. To do so, divide the numerator by the denominator. Remember that the instructions ask you to round your quotient to the nearest whole number. The quotient will be an endlessly repeating 0.2, which means that you will round down to 22%. You only need to solve this equation to the thousandths place in order to obtain sufficient information to answer the question.

50. D: The population is approximately 25,000, so one fifth of the population consists of about 5,000 individuals under age 20. Three fourths of 5,000 is 3,750, the approximate number of students in grades K-12. Since there are thirteen grades, there are about 288 students in each grade. So, the number of first graders is likely more than 250.

51. 2.25: Calculate 0.5% of $450:

$$\$450 \times 0.005 = \$2.25$$

This is the amount of interest she will earn.

52. C: To solve this problem, you must know how to convert a fraction into a percentage. Gerald made 13 out of 22 shots, a performance that can also be expressed by the fraction $\frac{13}{22}$. To convert this fraction into a percentage, divide the numerator by the denominator. Once you derive the initial 5 in the quotient, you can be fairly certain that answer choice C is correct. Whenever possible, try to take these kinds of shortcuts to save yourself some time.

53. 108: This problem requires you to understand how to find equivalencies involving percentages. One way to solve this problem is to set up the equation $\frac{18}{100} = \frac{x}{600}$. In words, this equation states that 18 out of 100 is equal to some unknown value out of 600. The first step in solving such an equation is to cross-multiply; in other words, $18 \times 600 = 100x$. This produces $10{,}800 = 100x$, a problem that can be solved for x by dividing both sides by 100. This calculation shows that $x = 108$, meaning that 108 is 18% of 600. A simpler way is to remember that the word "of" in mathematics means to multiply. To multiply 18% by 600, convert the percentage to a decimal by moving the decimal point two places to the left: 0.18. Then multiply 0.18 and 600 to get 108.

54. D: To solve this problem, you must know how to find equivalencies involving percentages. To begin, set up the following equation: $\frac{6.4}{100} = \frac{x}{32}$. Next cross-multiply: $6.4 \times 32 = 100x$. This produces $204.8 = 100x$, which is solved for x by dividing both sides of the equation by 100. The value of x is 2.048, which is rounded to 2.0. Or change the percent to a decimal, 0.064, and multiply by 32 to obtain 2.048 and round to 2.0.

55. C: First, figure out what the question is asking. Since we are given the total number of push-ups he wants to do and the percent he will do each day, the question is asking: what is 20 percent of 300?

Next, turn the question into an algebraic equation.

$$x = 0.2(300)$$

Finally, multiply to solve for x.

$$x = 60$$

Reading Comprehension

1. D: The main idea of this passage is that vaccines help the immune system function properly. Identifying main ideas is one of the key skills tested by the HESI exam. One of the common traps that many test-takers fall into is assuming that the first sentence of the passage will express the main idea. Although this will be true for some passages, often the author will use the first sentence to attract interest or to make an introductory, but not central, point. On this question, if you assume that the first sentence contains the main idea, you will mistakenly choose answer B. Finding the main idea of a passage requires patience and thoroughness; you cannot expect to know the main idea until you have read the entire passage. In this case, a diligent reading will show you that answer choices A, B, and C express details from the passage, but only answer choice D is a comprehensive summary of the author's message.

2. C: This passage does not state that the symptoms of disease will not emerge until the body has learned to fight the disease. The reading comprehension section of the HESI exam will include several questions that require you to identify details from a passage. The typical structure of these questions is to ask you to identify the answer choice that contains a detail not included in the passage. This question structure makes your work a little more difficult, because it requires you to confirm that the other three details are in the passage. In this question, the details expressed in answer choices A, B, and D are all explicit in the passage. The passage never states, however, that the symptoms of disease do not emerge until the body has learned how to fight the disease-causing microbe. On the contrary, the passage implies that a person may become quite sick and even die before the body learns to effectively fight the disease.

3. B: In the third paragraph, the word *virulent* means "malicious." The reading comprehension section of the HESI exam will include several questions that require you to define a word as it is used in the passage. Sometimes the word will be one of those used in the vocabulary section of the exam; other times, the word in question will be a slightly difficult word used regularly in academic and professional circles. In some cases, you may already know the basic definition of the word. Nevertheless, you should always go back and look at the way the word is used in the passage. The HESI exam will often include answer choices that are legitimate definitions for the given word, but which do not express how the word is used in the passage. For instance, the word *virulent* could in some circumstances mean contagious or annoying. However, since the passage is not talking about transfer of the disease and is referring to a serious illness, malicious is the more appropriate answer.

4. C: The author's primary purpose in writing this essay is to inform. The reading comprehension section of the HESI exam will include a few questions that ask you to determine the purpose of the author. The answer choices are always the same: The author's purpose is to entertain, to persuade, to inform, or to analyze. When an author is *writing to entertain*, he or she is not including a great deal of factual information; instead, the focus is on vivid language and interesting stories. *Writing to persuade* means "trying to convince the reader of something." When a writer is just trying to provide the reader with information, without any particular bias, he or she is *writing to inform*. Finally, *writing to analyze* means to consider a subject already well known to the reader. For instance, if the above passage took an objective look at the pros and cons of various approaches to fighting disease, we would say that the passage was a piece of analysis. Because the purpose of this passage is to present new information to the reader in an objective manner, however, it is clear that the author's intention is to inform.

5. A: The subject of this passage is foodborne illnesses. Identifying the subject of a passage is similar to identifying the main idea. Do not assume that the first sentence of the passage will declare the subject. Oftentimes, an author will approach his or her subject by first describing some related, familiar subject. In this passage, the author does introduce the subject of the passage in the first sentence. However, it is only by reading the rest of the passage that you can determine the subject. One way to figure out the subject of a passage is to identify the main idea of each paragraph, and then identify the common thread in each.

6. B: This passage never states that cooked food cannot cause illness. Indeed, the first sentence of the third paragraph states that harmful bacteria can be present on cooked food that is left out for two or more hours. This is a direct contradiction of answer choice B. If you can identify an answer choice that is clearly contradicted by the text, you can be sure that it is not one of the ideas advanced by the passage. Sometimes the correct answer to this type of question will be something that is contradicted in the text; on other occasions, the correct answer will be a detail that is not included in the passage at all.

7. C: In the first paragraph, the word *pathogens* means "disease-causing substances." The vocabulary you are asked to identify in the reading comprehension section of the HESI exam will tend to be health related. The makers of the HESI are especially interested in your knowledge of the terminology used by doctors and nurses. Some of these words, however, are rarely used in normal conversation, so they may be unfamiliar to you. The best way to determine the meaning of an unfamiliar word is to examine how it is used in context. In the last sentence of the first paragraph, it is clear that pathogens are some substances that cause disease. Note that the pathogens are not diseases themselves; we would not say that an uncooked piece of meat "has a disease," but rather that consuming it "can cause a disease." For this reason, answer choice C is better than answer choice A.

8. A: In the second paragraph, the word *sterile* means "free of bacteria." This question provides a good example of why you should always refer to the word as it is used in the text. The word *sterile* is often used to describe "a person who cannot reproduce." If this definition immediately came to mind when you read the question, you might have mistakenly chosen answer D. However, in this passage the author describes raw foods as *not sterile*, meaning that they contain bacteria. For this reason, answer choice A is the correct response.

9. C: The main idea of the passage is that both the esophagus and the stomach are subject to bleeding problems. The structure of this passage is simple: The first paragraph discusses bleeding disorders of the esophagus, and the second paragraph discusses bleeding disorders of the stomach. Remember that statements can be true, and can even be explicitly stated in the passage, and can yet not be the main idea of the passage. The main idea given in answer choice A is perhaps true, but is too general to be classified as the main idea of the passage.

10. B: The passage never states that ulcer disease rarely occurs in the stomach. On the contrary, in the second paragraph the author states that ulcer disease *can* affect the blood vessels in the stomach. The three other answer choices can be found within the passage. The surest way to answer a question like this is to comb through the passage, looking for each detail in turn. This is a time-consuming process, however, so you may want to follow any initial intuition you have. In other words, if you are suspicious of one of the answer choices, see if you can find it in the passage. Often you will find that the detail is expressly contradicted by the author, in which case you can be sure that this is the right answer.

11. A: In the first paragraph, the word *rupture* means "tear." All of the answer choices are action verbs that suggest destruction. In order to determine the precise meaning of rupture, then, you must examine its usage in the passage. The author is describing a condition in which damage to a vein causes internal bleeding. Therefore, it does not make sense to say that the vein has *collapsed* or *imploded*, as neither of these verbs suggests a ripping or opening in the side of the vein. Similarly, the word *detach* suggests an action that seems inappropriate for a vein. It seems quite possible, however, for a vein to *tear*: Answer choice A is correct.

12. D: In the second paragraph, the word *erode* means "wear away." Your approach to this question should be the same as for question 11. Take a look at how the word is used in the passage. The author is describing a condition in which ulcers degrade a vein to the point of bleeding. Obviously, it is not appropriate to say that the ulcer has *avoided*, *divorced*, or *contained* the vein. It *is* sensible, however, to say that the ulcer has *worn away* the vein.

13. A: The primary subject of the passage is a new artificial retina. This question is a little tricky, because the author spends so much time talking about the experience of Kathy Blake. As a reader, however, you have to ask yourself whether Mrs. Blake or the new artificial retina is more essential to the story. Would the author still be interested in the story if a different person had the artificial retina? Probably. Would the author have written about Mrs. Blake if she hadn't gotten the artificial retina? Almost certainly not. Really, the story of Kathy Blake is just a way for the author to make the artificial retina more interesting to the reader. Therefore, the artificial retina is the primary subject of the passage.

14. B: In the second paragraph, the word *progressive* means "gradually increasing." The root of the word is *progress*, which you may know means "advancement toward a goal." With this in mind, you may be reasonably certain that answer choice B is correct. It is never a bad idea to examine the context, however. The author is describing *progressive visual loss*, so you might be tempted to select answer choice C or D, since they both suggest loss or diminution. Remember, however, that the adjective *progressive* is modifying the noun *loss*. Since the *loss* is increasing, the correct answer is B.

15. C: The passage never states that retinitis pigmentosa (RP) is curable. This question may be somewhat confusing, since the passage discusses a new treatment for RP. However, the passage never declares that researchers have come up with a cure for the condition; rather, they have developed a new technology that allows people who suffer from RP to regain some of their vision. This is not the same thing as curing RP. Kathy Blake and others like her still have RP, though they have been assisted by this new technology.

16. D: The author's intention in writing this essay is to inform. You may be tempted to answer that the author's intention is to entertain. Indeed, the author expresses his message through the story of Kathy Blake. This story, however, is not important by itself. It is clearly included as a way of explaining the new camera glasses. If the only thing the reader learned from the passage was the story of Kathy Blake, the author would probably be disappointed. At the same time, the author is not really trying to persuade the reader of anything. There is nothing controversial about these new glasses: Everyone is in favor of them. The mission of the author, then, is simply to inform the reader.

17. A: The main idea of the passage is that Usher syndrome is an inherited condition that affects hearing and vision. Always be aware that some answers may be included in the passage but not the main idea. In this question, answer choices B and D are both true details from the passage, but neither of them would be a good summary of the article. One way to approach this kind of question is to consider what you would be likely to say if someone asked you to describe the article in a single sentence. Often, the sentence you come up with will closely mimic one of the answer choices. If so, that answer choice is probably correct.

18. D: In the first paragraph, the word signs means "measurable indicators." The word sign is used frequently in medical contexts, though many people do not entirely understand its meaning. Signs are those objective (measurable) indicators of illness that can be observed by someone besides the person with the illness. A stomachache, for instance, is not technically considered a sign, since it cannot be observed by anyone other than the person who has it, and therefore must be expressed by the individual experiencing it. This would be known as a symptom. Change in vital signs, a failed hearing test, or a low Snellen (vision) chart score, however, would all be considered signs because practitioners can measure or observe them. The best definition for signs, then, is "measurable indicators," that is, objective markers of a disease or condition.

19. B: The passage does not state that Usher syndrome affects both hearing and smell. On the contrary, the passage only states that Usher syndrome affects hearing and vision. You should not be content merely to note that sentence in the passage and select answer choice B. In order to be sure, you need to quickly scan the passage to determine whether there is any mention of problems with the sense of smell. This is because the mention of impaired hearing and vision does not make it impossible for smell to be damaged as well. It is a good idea to practice scanning short articles for specific words. In this case, you would want to scan the article looking for words like *smell* and *nose*.

20. C: In the second paragraph, the word *juvenile* means "occurring in children." Examine the context in which the word is used. Remember that the context extends beyond just the immediate sentence in which the word is found. It can also include adjacent sentences and paragraphs. In this case, the word *juvenile* is immediately followed by a further explanation of Usher syndrome as it appears in children. You can be reasonably certain, then, that juvenile Usher syndrome is the condition as it presents in children. Although the word *juvenile* is occasionally used in English to describe immature or annoying behavior, it is clear that the author is not here referring to a *bratty* form of Usher syndrome.

21. B: In the third paragraph, the word *mutated* means "altered." This word comes from the same root as mutant; a *mutant* is an organism in which the chromosomes have been changed somehow. The context in which the word is used makes it clear that the author is referring to a scenario in which one of the parent's chromosomes has been altered. One way to approach this kind of problem is to substitute the answer choice into the passage to see if it still makes sense. Clearly, it would not make sense for a chromosome to be *selected*, since chromosomes are passed on and inherited without conscious choice. Neither does it make sense for a chromosome to be destroyed, because a basic fact of biology is that all living organisms have chromosomes.

22. D: The main idea of the passage is that the immune system protects the body from infection. The author repeatedly alludes to the complexity and mystery of the immune system, so it cannot be true that scientists fully understand this part of the body. It is true that the immune system triggers the production of fluids, but this description misses the point. Similarly, it is true that the body is under constant invasion by malicious microbes; however, the author is much more interested in the body's response to these microbes. For this reason, the best answer choice is D.

23. C: The passage never states that viruses are extremely sophisticated. In fact, the passage explicitly states the opposite. However, in order to know this you need to understand the word *primitive*. The passage says that viruses are too primitive, or early in their development, to be classified as living organisms. A primitive organism is simple and undeveloped—exactly the opposite of sophisticated. If you do not know the word *primitive*, you can still answer the question by finding all three of the other answer choices in the passage.

24. D: In the first paragraph, the word *ideal* means "perfect." Do not be confused by the similarity of the word *ideal* to *idea* and mistakenly select answer choice A. Take a look at the context in which the word is used. The author is describing how many millions of microbes can live inside the human body. It would not make sense, then, for the author to be describing the body as a *hostile* environment for microbes. Moreover, whether or not the body is a confined environment would not seem to have much bearing on whether it is good for microbes. Rather, the paragraph suggests that the human body is a perfect environment for microbes.

25. B: The passage never states that the immune system ignores tumors. Indeed, at the beginning of the third paragraph, the author states that scientists remain puzzled by the body's ability to fight tumors. This question is a little tricky, because it is common knowledge that many tumors prove fatal to the human body. However, you should not take this to mean that the body does not at least try to fight tumors. In general, it is best to seek out direct evidence in the text rather than to rely on what you already know. You will have enough time on the HESI exam to fully examine and research each question.

26. A: In the second paragraph, the word *enlist* means "call into service." The use of this word is an example of figurative language, the use of a known image or idea to elucidate an idea that is perhaps unfamiliar to the reader. In this case, the author is describing the efforts of the immune system as if they were a military campaign. The immune system *enlists* other cells, and then directs these *recruits* to areas where they are needed. You are probably familiar with *enlistment* and *recruitment* as they relate to describe military service. The author is trying to draw a parallel between the enlistment of young men and women and the enlistment of immune cells. For this reason, "call into service" is the best definition for *enlist.*

27. C: The author's primary purpose in writing this essay is to inform. As you may have noticed, the essays included in the reading comprehension section of the HESI exam were most often written to inform. This should not be too surprising; after all, the most common intention of any writing on general medical subjects is to provide information rather than to persuade, entertain, or analyze. This does not mean that you can automatically assume that "to inform" will be the answer for every question of this type. However, if you are in doubt, it is probably best to select this answer. In this case, the passage is written in a clear, declarative style with no obvious prejudice on the part of the author. The primary intention of the passage seems to be providing information about the immune system to a general audience.

28. B: The main idea of the passage is that the Food and Drug Administration (FDA) has a special program for regulating dietary supplements. This passage has a straightforward structure: The author introduces his subject in the first paragraph and uses the four succeeding paragraphs to elaborate. All of the other possible answers are true statements from the passage but cannot be considered the main idea. One way to approach questions about the main idea is to take sentences at random from the passage and see which answer choice they could potentially support. The main idea should be strengthened or supported by most of the details from the passage.

29. D: The passage never states that the Food and Drug Administration (FDA) ignores products after they enter the market. In fact, the entire fourth paragraph describes the steps taken by the FDA to regulate products once they are available for purchase. In some cases, questions of this type will contain answer choices that are directly contradictory. Here, for instance, answer choices A and B cannot be true if answer choice D is true. If there are at least two answer choices that contradict another answer choice, it is a safe bet that the contradicted answer choice cannot be correct. If you are at all uncertain about your logic, however, you should refer to the passage.

30. C: In the third paragraph, the phrase *phased in* means "implemented in stages." Do not be tempted by the similarity of this phrase to the word *fazed*, which can mean "confused or stunned." The author is referring to manufacturing standards that have already been implemented for large manufacturers and are in the process of being implemented for small manufacturers. It would make sense, then, for these standards to be implemented in *phases*: that is, to be *phased in*.

31. A: In the fifth paragraph, the word *deceptive* means "misleading." The root of the word *deceptive* is the same as for the words *deceive* and *deception*. Take a look at the context in which the word is used. The author states that the FDA prevents certain kinds of advertising. It would be somewhat redundant for the author to mean that the FDA prevents *illegal* advertising; this goes without saying. At the same time, it is unlikely that the FDA spends its time trying to prevent merely *irritating* advertising; the persistent presence of such advertising makes this answer choice inappropriate. Left with a choice between *malicious* and *misleading* advertising, it makes better sense to choose the latter, since being mean and nasty would be a bad technique for selling a product. It is common, however, for an advertiser to deliberately mislead the consumer.

32. B: The main idea of the passage is that anemia is a potentially dangerous condition characterized by low numbers of RBCs (red blood cells). All of the other answer choices are true (although answer C leaves out RBCs), but only answer choice C expresses an idea that is supported by the others. When you are considering a question of this type, try to imagine the answer choices as they would appear on an outline. If the passage above were placed into outline form, which answer choice would be the most appropriate title? Which answer choices would be more appropriate as supporting details? Try to get in the habit of imagining a loose outline as you are reading the passages on the HESI exam.

33. D: The passage never states that anemia is rarely caused by blood loss. On the contrary, in the first sentence of the fourth paragraph the author lists three causes of anemia, and blood loss is listed first. Sometimes, answer choices for this type of question will refer to details not explicitly mentioned in the passage. For instance, answer choice A is true without ever being stated in precisely those terms. Since the passage mentions several different treatments for anemia, however, you should consider the detail in answer choice A to be in the passage. In other words, it is not enough to scan the passage looking for an exact version of the detail. Sometimes, you will have to use your best judgment.

34. D: In the third paragraph, the word *oxygenated* means "containing high amounts of oxygen." This word is not in common usage, so it is absolutely essential for you to refer to its context in the passage. The author states in the second paragraph that anemia is in part a deficiency of the red blood cells that carry oxygen throughout the body. Then in the first sentence of the third paragraph, the author states that anemic individuals do not get enough oxygenated blood. Given this information, it is clear that *oxygenated* must mean carrying high amounts of oxygen, because it has already been stated that anemia consists of a lack of oxygen-rich blood.

35. A: In the fifth paragraph, the word *severity* means "seriousness." This word shares a root with the word *severe*, but not with the word *sever*. As always, take a look at the word as it is used in the passage. In the final sentence of the passage, the author states that the treatment for anemia will depend on the *cause and severity* of the condition. In the previous paragraph, the author outlined a treatment for anemia and indicated that the proper response to the condition varies. The author even refers to the worst cases of anemia as being *severe*. With this in mind, it makes the most sense to define *severity* as seriousness.

36. C: The main idea of the passage is that a recent study found no link between caffeine consumption and rheumatoid arthritis (RA) among women. As is often the case, the first sentence of the passage contains the main idea. However, do not assume that this will always be the case. Furthermore, do not assume that the first sentence of the passage will only contain the main idea. In this passage, for instance, the author makes an immediate reference to the previous belief in the correlation between caffeine and RA. It would be incorrect, however, to think that this means answer choice A is correct. Regardless of whether or not the main idea is contained in the first sentence of the passage, you will need to read the entire text before you can be sure.

37. A: The passage never states that alcohol consumption is linked with RA. The passage does state that the new study took into account alcohol consumption when evaluating the long-term data. This is a good example of a question that requires you to spend a little bit of time rereading the passage. A quick glance might lead you to believe that the new study had found a link between alcohol and RA. Tricky questions like this make it even more crucial for you to go back and verify each answer choice in the text. Working through this question by using the process of elimination is the best way to ensure the correct response.

38. A: In the second paragraph, the word *symmetrical* means "affecting both sides of the body in corresponding fashion." This is an example of a question that is hard to answer even after reviewing its context in the passage. If you have no idea what *symmetrical* means, it will be hard for you to select an answer: All of them sound plausible. In such a case, the best thing you can do is make an educated guess. One clue is that the author has been describing a condition that affects the hands and the feet. Since people have both right and left hands and feet, it makes sense that inflammation would be described as *symmetrical* if it affects both the right and left hand or foot.

39. B: The author's primary purpose in writing this essay is to inform. You may be tempted to select answer choice D on the grounds that the author is presenting a particular point of view. However, there is no indication that the author is trying to persuade the reader of anything. One clear sign that an essay is written to persuade is a reference to what the reader already thinks. A persuasive essay assumes a particular viewpoint held by the reader and then argues against that viewpoint. In this passage, the author has no allegiance to any idea; he or she is only reporting the results of the newest research.

40. C: The main idea of the passage is that exercise improves bone health. This short passage has a simple structure: The author presents the thesis (main idea) and then spends the rest of the essay supporting it. When a passage is as clearly organized as this one, there should be little mystery about the main idea. If you look at the first sentences of paragraphs two and three, you will see that both contain the words *exercise* and *bones*. This is a good sign that either answer choice A or C is correct. Once you note that weight-bearing exercise is not discussed until the final paragraph, it seems clear that the correct answer must be C.

41. B: In the first paragraph, the word *vital* means "important." On first looking at this word, you might note its similarity to other words having to do with life and liveliness: *vitality*, *revive*, and *vivacious*, to name just a few. This knowledge can help guide your response, though you shouldn't make any assumptions based on it. Otherwise, you might mistakenly select answer choice D. The author states that exercise is *vital* for healthy bones. It would not make sense to say that exercise is *nourishing* for healthy bones, because it would also be so for unhealthy bones. The author is not describing the condition of healthy bones, but rather how bones can be made healthy. For this reason, it makes the most sense to select answer choice B.

42. C: The passage never states that swimming is not good for the bones. This question is a little bit tricky, because the author does state that non-weight-bearing forms of exercise, including swimming, are not *as* good for the bones as weight-bearing exercises. However, just because swimming is not as good for the bones as running does not mean that it is bad for the bones. In fact, swimming works every major muscle system of the body and contributes to overall health, which includes bone health. Be on guard for questions like this that try to fool you into putting words in the author's mouth.

43. A: In the second paragraph, the word *fractures* means "breaks." In the second paragraph, the author declares that exercise reduces the risk of falls and fractures. To begin with, it makes sense to assume that broken bones would be one of the possible results of a fall. We are all aware that older people are more likely to break their bones by falling in the shower or on the stairs. On occasion, authors will use the word *fracture* to describe a damaged relationship, which may tempt you to select *tiffs*. In this case, however, the context makes clear that the author is describing broken bones.

44. B: The main idea of the passage is that the community library offers numerous resources for medical information. While most of the articles used in the reading comprehension section of the HESI exam will be about scientific or health-related concepts directly, some will touch on health and medicine in a more indirect manner. In this article, the author outlines some of the useful sources of medical information that can be obtained at the local library. Answer choices A and C are true, but do not express the general, overarching message of the article. Answer choice D is not true and is directly contradicted by the article itself.

45. D: In the third paragraph, the word *popular* means "for the general public." This word is more often used to describe someone or something that is well known or liked, so you might be tempted to select answer choice C. Take a look at the word as it is used in the context of the third paragraph, however. The author states that the library contains popular magazines and newspapers and then adds that the library also contains medical journals. Popular magazines and newspapers, then, are not the same thing as professional trade journals. Because the latter are known to be complicated and technical (that is, requiring professional expertise), you can guess that *popular* magazines are for a general reading audience.

46. D: The passage does not state that the articles in popular magazines can be hard to understand. If you are working in order, you can use your knowledge of the word *popular* to figure out the answer to this question. Specifically, you will know that the word describes publications that are written for a general, nonexpert audience. With this in mind, it seems unlikely that the articles would also be hard to understand. The other three details are explicit in the passage, so the answer must be D.

47. A: In the fourth paragraph, the word *technical* means "requiring expert knowledge." Again, some of the details gleaned from your work in the preceding questions can help you. The word *technical* is used to describe medical journals. As has already been shown, the author states that medical journals are written for an expert audience and can be difficult for a nonprofessional to understand. If this is the case, you can infer that the word *technical* must mean "requiring expert knowledge," answer choice A.

48. D: Choice C is close to being the answer, but Choice D is the best answer because the narrator can enter the consciousness of both the man and the dog, making it third person omniscient. Choices A and B can be ruled out because the narrator does not use the pronouns "I" or "we."

49. A: Choice A offers the best interpretation. The passage refers to immortality and man's place in the universe; the man does not have the imagination to contemplate such issues, and he does not seem to realize the frailty of humans on the planet. Choices B and C contradict or misinterpret the meaning of the passage. Choice D is not really implied by the passage; in fact, the dog's instincts make it seem more intelligent than the man in a certain sense.

50. C: It can be supported by the following quotation: "[The dog's] instinct told it a truer tale than was told to the man by the man's judgment." Choice A may sound possible, but it does not really capture the narrator's main point of comparison. Choice B can be contradicted by the following quotation: "In its brain there was no sharp consciousness of a condition of very cold such as was in the man's brain." There is nothing in the passage to support the claim in Choice D.

51. C: Only interpretation III fits with the meaning of the passage. The narrator's statement that the man lacked imagination means that he did not have the foresight to realize that he was risking his life. Interpretation I is incorrect because the passage reads, "He was quick and alert in the things of life." Interpretation II is incorrect because the quote shows lack of imagination as a danger, not something unneeded.

52. D: Choice D is not a supporting detail because it is a definition of salvage logging. The other choices are supporting details of the Forest Manager's argument.

53. B: Plot A was salvage logged and burned worse than the unmanaged plot (Plot B). This study supports the professor's view that salvage logging increases the risk and severity of fire.

54. A: The question asks which option is the chief argument regarding fire prevention. Choices B and D are not helpful for fire prevention. Choice C is incorrect because logging decreases soil temperature. Choice B is a supporting detail from the passage but is not the main idea. Choice C contradicts the passage. Choice D is not mentioned in the passage.

55. C: Both the manager and the professor discuss the importance of seedling growth after a fire. So, a study looking at the regrowth of seedlings in logged and unmanaged forests would potentially provide support for both arguments (as well as possibly showing problems with both arguments).

Vocabulary

1. A: When it is said that someone is generous, it usually means they are giving and unselfish.

2. A: The best definition for the word *prognosis* is "forecast." A prognosis is a probable result or course of a disease. The prognosis usually includes the likelihood of recovery for the patient. A prognosis is distinct from a *diagnosis*, which is just the description of the patient's condition. Likewise, a *description* is not the same thing as a prognosis, because it does not include a suggestion of what will happen in the future. An *outline* is an organized description of a subject, and therefore is not similar to a prognosis. Finally, a *schedule* is a plan for the future, rather than a prediction.

3. D: The name for a substance that stimulates the production of antibodies is an *antigen*. An antigen is any substance perceived by the immune system as dangerous. When the body senses an antigen, it produces an antibody. *Collagen* is one of the components of bone, tendon, and cartilage. It is a spongy protein that can be turned into gelatin by boiling. *Hemoglobin* is the part of red blood cells that carries oxygen. In order for the blood to carry enough oxygen to the cells of the body, there has to be a sufficient amount of hemoglobin. *Lymph* is a near-transparent fluid that performs a number of functions in the body: It removes bacteria from tissues, replaces lymphocytes in the blood, and moves fat away from the small intestine. Lymph contains white blood cells.

4. C: The best definition for the word *abstain* is "to refrain from." Doctors often ask their patients to abstain from certain behaviors that have a negative impact on health. For example, a patient recovering from a viral infection might be asked to abstain from alcohol, so as to prevent weakening of the immune system. To *offend* is "to annoy or irritate." A health-care worker should take care to avoid offending a patient. *Retrain* means "to teach someone how to do a job again." For instance, a nurse might have to be retrained after a long period of not performing a particular task. To *defenestrate* means "to throw out the window." This word is unlikely to be used in a health context.

5. A: The best synonym for *ominous* as it is used in this sentence is "threatening." An ominous symptom, for instance, is one that suggests the presence of serious disease. The word *emboldening* means "making bold." A patient who is regaining strength might be emboldened to try new and more difficult activities. The word *destructive* means "causing damage, chaos, or loss." A destructive condition or behavior has a negative effect on the patient's health. The word *insightful* means "thoughtful or provocative." As a health practitioner, you should try to be insightful so that you can come up with creative solutions to your patients' problems.

6. D: The word *incidence* means "rate of occurrence." A doctor will often refer to the incidence of a particular disease or condition as a measure of its severity or longevity. *Random events* are referred to as "incidents." *Sterility* means "free of living bacteria and microorganisms." It is absolutely necessary for a medical environment to be sterile so that patients will not get infections. *Autonomy* means "self-control and self-determination." A health-care worker should try to promote the autonomy of the patient whenever possible, although autonomy should never be more important than health and well-being.

7. B: *Hydrophilia* means "water loving." One could say that humans have a hydrophilic body, because our bodies crave constant infusions of water. The word *homologous* means "corresponding or having the same relative position or structure." A *dipsomaniac* is a person who cannot resist alcoholic drinks. Dipsomania is a compulsion that must be treated with behavioral therapy or medications such as Antabuse, which causes a violent physical reaction to alcohol. The word *hydrated* means "full of water or sufficiently full of water." Patients need to be hydrated, and medical workers need to be hydrated while they are performing their duties.

8. A: The closest meaning for the word *occluded* as it is used in this sentence is "closed." Occluded means "blocked or obstructed." The word is commonly used to describe arteries that no longer allow the passage of blood. The word *deformed* means "misshapen or out of the normal shape." Any deformed body part is a cause for concern. The word *engorged* means "overfull, especially of blood or food." The organs of the body may become engorged when they are infected or diseased. *Enlarged* means "made larger."

9. D: The best definition for the word *potent* is "powerful." A strong drug may be referred to as potent. The ability of a man to reproduce is sometimes referred to as his potency. The word *frantic* means "frenzied or anxious." A medical worker should never be frantic when dealing with patients and should do his or her best to keep patients from becoming frantic. The word *determined* means "set on a particular path." Whenever possible, a health-care worker should try to ensure that patients are determined to take the necessary steps toward recovery and good health. The word *feverish* can mean either "having a high temperature" or "being worried and anxious." A feverish patient should be comforted and given plenty of fluids.

10. D: The word *precipitous* as it is used this sentence means "steep." Doctors will often refer to a precipitous change in blood pressure. In general, precipitous changes are dangerous to the health. The word *detached* means "unconnected or aloof." A common example is a detached retina, a condition in which part of the eye becomes disconnected, and vision is damaged. The word *sordid* means "dirty" or "vile." The word *encompassed* means "surrounded or entirely contained within." For instance, a doctor might describe a treatment protocol as encompassing all aspects of the patient's life.

11. C: The word *vital* as it is used this sentence means "essential." Medical workers will often refer to a patient's vital signs, meaning blood pressure, heart rate, and temperature. The word *recommended* means "preferred by some authority." The recommended course of treatment is the one outlined and prescribed by a doctor. The word *discouraged* means "disappointed and doubtful of success." Health-care workers should try to prevent patients from becoming discouraged, since this can further diminish quality of life and chances of recovery. The word *sufficient* means "having enough to accomplish the necessary task." As an example, a doctor might inquire to make sure that a patient is receiving sufficient fluids or food.

12. C: When something is described as challenging, it usually means that it is difficult or demanding.

13. A: The best definition of the word *insidious* is "stealthy." An insidious disease takes root and develops in the body slowly, so that by the time the patient is aware of it, the damage can be severe and even fatal. Cancer is the classic example of insidious disease, because it may take root in the body and develop for a long period without any perceptible signs or symptoms. An insidious disease may be *deadly*, but it is not necessarily so. The words *collapsed* and *new* have no innate relationship to the word *insidious*.

14. B: The word *ingest* means "take into the body." The rate at which a patient ingests food and fluids is important when establishing a treatment protocol. To *congest* is "to fill to excess or to overcrowd." Chest congestion is a common complaint, which may be rooted in serious or minor causes. To *collect* is "to gather together." A health-care worker needs to collect information on patients so as to serve them effectively. To *suppress* means "to hold down or hold back." Patients should be encouraged not to suppress any information during a medical examination; keeping important facts from the doctor or nurse can prevent effective treatment.

15. D: The word *proscribe* means "forbid." A doctor often will proscribe certain foods or behaviors if they would negatively impact patient health. To *anticipate* is "to expect ahead of time." A doctor tries to anticipate how a disease will progress or how a patient will respond to treatment, though it is impossible to do this all the time. To *prevent* is "to keep from happening." Health-care workers try to prevent accidents and mistakes from happening on the job. To *defeat* is "to achieve victory over." The primary goal of treatment is to defeat whatever conditions are adversely affecting the patient's health.

16. C: The word *distended* as it is used in this sentence means "swollen." Doctors will often refer to a distended abdomen, which accompanies gassiness or bloating. The word *concave* means "shaped like the inside of a bowl." Many structures of the human body, for instance the inside of the ear and the arch of the foot, are described as concave. A distended body part may be *sore*, but it is not necessarily so. A distended artery, for instance, may have no accompanying pain. Also, though a distended body part may be *empty*, this is not always the case. In cases of starvation, the stomach may become distended; however, other body parts may become distended from being full to excess.

17. B: The word *overt* as it is used in this sentence means "apparent." Overt signs are those that can be seen by someone other than the person who is experiencing them. A rash is an overt sign; a stomachache is not. The word *concealed* means "hidden." Concealed signs cannot be perceived with the senses; a rise in blood pressure, for instance, is a concealed sign of illness. The word *expert*, used as an adjective, means "knowledgeable about a particular subject." When dealing with an unfamiliar situation, for instance, a doctor might call in an expert practitioner. The word *delectable* means "tasty or delicious."

18. A: The word *supplement* means "something added to resolve a deficiency or obtain completion." A doctor might recommend a particular nutritional supplement to address a patient's needs. A *complement* completes something or makes it perfect. Doctors try to put together complementary treatments that will reinforce and support one another. The word *detriment* means "loss, damage, or injury." A patient should be dissuaded from behaviors that will work to their detriment. The word *acumen* means "expertise" or "special knowledge in some area." A health-care worker will develop acumen based on his or her professional experience.

19. D: The word *paroxysm* means "a violent seizure." A patient who is suffering from paroxysms needs to be stabilized and treated immediately. A *revelation* is "a sudden realization or flash of knowledge." Sometimes, a doctor will puzzle over a case until he or she has a revelation and realizes what needs to be done. A *nutrient* is "something that provides nutrition, or sustenance, to the body." Tests may indicate that a patient needs more of a particular nutrient in order to improve his or her health. A *contraption* is "a mechanical device." Health-care workers must learn how to use all sorts of contraptions in order to perform their duties.

20. B: The word *carnivore* means "meat-eating." A patient who is not a carnivore might be in danger of anemia (iron deficiency) or other malnutrition. On the other hand, excessive consumption of red meat can lead to heart disease and obesity. *Hungry* means "feeling hunger." The word *infected* means "contaminated by germs." An infected body part needs to be sterilized and treated immediately. The word *demented* means "crazy or insane," especially when this behavior is the result of the condition known as dementia. A demented individual may not be able to make health-related decisions.

21. C: The word *belligerent* means "pugnacious." *Pugnacious* means "ready to fight." Belligerent patients may be resistant to treatment and disdainful of the doctor's or nurse's authority. The word *retired* means "withdrawn from business." The word *sardonic* means "mocking or sneering." This word is unlikely to come up in a medical context, though a health-care worker should avoid being sardonic. The word *acclimated* means "used to or accustomed to." Often, it takes a while for patients to become acclimated to a course of treatment or to a new lifestyle imposed upon them by diminishing health.

22. A: The word *bilateral* means "on both sides." This word is typically used to describe conditions that afflict both sides of the body. For instance, a patient suffering from bilateral partial paralysis might have numbness in both his right and left arms. The word *insufficient* means "lacking in necessary qualities." A patient might have insufficient blood flow to a certain area, or an insufficient amount of a certain nutrient. A *bicuspid* is anything that ends in two points. Many teeth are referred to as bicuspids because of their shape. The word *congruent* means "agreeing or in complete accord."

23. B: A teacher provides instruction and information to an individual or group of individuals. An instructor functions in the same capacity, that is, in the practice of teaching.

24. A: The word *recur* as it is used in this sentence means "occur again." Doctors often refer to the recurrence of a disease or symptom. In some cases, the recurrence of a disease indicates that the treatment used in the past was ineffective. *Recur* has the same root as *occur*, with the prefix *re-*, meaning "back or again." To *survive* means "to remain alive." To *collect* means "to bring together into one place." To *desist* means "to cease or stop doing something." A doctor might advise a patient to desist from a certain behavior in order to improve his or her health.

25. C: The word *labile* means "likely to change." This word is often used as a synonym for unstable. Blood pressure that fluctuates rapidly may be described as labile. The word *venereal* is used to describe conditions that relate to sexual intercourse. Venereal disease, for instance, is acquired during sexual contact. Chlamydia, gonorrhea, and syphilis are all examples of venereal disease. The word *motile* means "moving or capable of moving." A doctor will often refer to a part of the body as motile when its movements have been compromised in the past. An *entrail* is one of the internal parts of an animal or human body. It most often refers to the intestines.

26. B: The best description for the word *flaccid* is "limp." A flaccid part of the body is lacking in muscle tone. The word *defended* means "driven danger away from." The word *slender* means "thin or skinny, but not to the extent of being unhealthy." In general, patients who are slender recover better from injury and illness than patients who are overweight or obese. The word *outdated* describes "something that has become irrelevant with age." As medical technology becomes increasingly sophisticated, much of the equipment that used to be essential has now become outdated.

27. D: The word *androgynous* means "both male and female." Some children are born with androgynous characteristics, and their sexuality may remain ambiguous (hard to determine) for their entire life. *Monozygotic* means "derived from one fertilized egg." Identical twins are often referred to as monozygotic because they emerge from an individual zygote (fertilized egg). The word *exogenous* is used to describe "conditions that originate outside of the body." It is not to be confused with *heterogeneous*, which means "having different parts." *Homologous* means "corresponding or having the same relative position." A dog's body is said to be homologous to a cat's because their legs are in the same place.

28. B: The word *terrestrial* means "earthly." It can also be used to refer to things that are from the land rather than from the water. The word *alien*, when used as an adjective, describes "things that are unfamiliar or from an outside source." *Alien* does not only refer to creatures from outer space. A patient who has come down with a mystery ailment might try to identify some contact with alien substances. The word *foreign* is used to describe "people or things that are from some other area or country." In an area where medical procedures are being performed, foreign objects are usually forbidden. The word *domestic* is used to describe "things that are of the home or household."

29. B: The word *untoward* means "improper or unfortunate." Health-care workers should avoid untoward actions when dealing with their patients. This means acting according to the professional code of ethics. *Allocated* means "reserved for a particular purpose." For example, a patient may be put on a specific exercise regimen. The patient then needs to allocate a certain part of the day for this activity, so that it is sure to be done. *Flaccid* means "limp or lacking in muscle tone." If a patient is experiencing any degree of paralysis, the affected part of the body may be flaccid. *Dilated* means "expanded or made larger." The pupils of the eyes become dilated in the dark so that more light can enter the lens.

30. D: The word *endogenous* as it is used in this sentence means "growing from within." Doctors occasionally refer to endogenous cholesterol, which comes from inside the body rather than from the diet. *Contagious* means "capable of spreading from person to person." A person with a contagious disease needs to be kept away from other people. Often, diseases are only contagious for a limited time. *Continuous* means "proceeding on without stopping." If a patient is suffering from continuous back pain, for instance, he or she is experiencing the pain at all times.

31. B: The word symptom means "subjective indication." A symptom is any subjective indication of disease that can be perceived only by the patient. Lower back pain, for instance, is a symptom, because it cannot be perceived by anyone else. Symptoms are distinct from signs, which are apparent to the other people. Bleeding and high blood pressure are both signs. In medicine, an indication is "a sign or symptom that suggests a particular treatment." Signs are objective indications, whereas symptoms are subjective indications, and both are important in determining medical interventions. For example, some rashes are an indication for topical ointment.

32. C: The word *invasive* means "intrusive." An invasive disease seeks to penetrate the body and cause damage. Strep throat, a bacterial infection, is an example of an invasive disease. The word *convulsive* means "afflicted by spasms or seizures." A patient who suffers from epilepsy or extreme fever may become convulsive. Convulsive patients need to be stabilized so that they don't hurt themselves. The word *destructive* is used to describe "things that cause damage, injury, or loss." Health-care workers try to steer patients away from destructive behaviors. The word *connective* is used to describe "structures that bring other things into contact." The connective tissues of the body include cartilage, ligaments, and tendons.

33. A: The word *parameter* means "guideline." A doctor will often lay out certain parameters at the beginning of treatment. These are not specific rules, but rather they are the general ideas that will inform the entire course of treatment. Parameters are the boundaries of treatment. A *standard*, on the other hand, is "an established basis of comparison." A *manual* is "a book that explains how to perform a particular task." A *variable* is "something that changes." The amount of food a patient is given might be considered to be a variable, for example.

34. D: When something is concluded, it means that it is finished or completed.

35. B: The word *void* means "empty." Doctors may refer to a patient's bowels as void when they do not contain any digested food matter. *Holistic* means "concerned with the whole of something rather than with the particular parts." Doctors try to put together a holistic treatment plan so that the patient's general level of health will be improved. *Concrete* is a building material, but the word is also used as an adjective to describe "things that are real, sturdy, and well established." Doctors try to establish concrete standards for measuring a patient's condition, rather than relying on general impressions. *Maladjusted* means "poorly accustomed or acclimated." Although it often takes time for a patient to adjust to a new treatment protocol, some patients will remain maladjusted and require a change in treatment.

36. B: The word *lethargic* as it is used in this sentence means "sluggish." Lethargy is a symptom of many forms of illness. It is also a side effect of chemotherapy. *Nauseous* means "sickened, or suffering from an upset stomach." Nausea is a common side effect of chemotherapy as well; it is just not the one described in this sentence. *Contagious* means "capable of spreading from person to person." Many viral and bacterial infections are contagious. *Elated* means "ecstatic" or "wildly happy." It is usually a good thing when a patient is elated, although manic-depressive patients may alternate between excessive elation and near-suicidal sadness.

37. A: The word *compensatory* means "offsetting." A patient may develop compensatory behaviors to make up for a developing health condition. *Defensive* means "protective" or "intending to repel an attack." Sometimes, patients will feel defensive in the presence of a health professional. *Untoward* means "unfavorable, improper, or unfortunate." Untoward events will inevitably occur during the course of treatment; it is the job of the staff to continue their work regardless. *Confused* means "perplexed or bewildered." Some patients, especially the very young or very old, may become confused during treatment. When confusion is identified, health-care workers should slow down and help the patient feel more comfortable.

38. C: The word *atrophy* means "degeneration or wasting away." Doctors often refer to muscle atrophy, which occurs when a patient is immobile for a long period. Physical therapy and massage are two common ways to prevent muscle atrophy when a patient cannot move because of injury or illness. *Dystrophy* is "weakening, degeneration, or abnormal growth of muscle." You may have heard of muscular dystrophy, a hereditary disease in which the muscles gradually lose their strength. *Entropy* is "the tendency toward chaos and disorder." This term is occasionally used in a medical context to describe a patient's tendency toward decline and decrease in function. It is the job of the health-care worker to fight against entropy. *Apathy* is "a lack of caring." Patients who are suffering from serious injury or illness, especially those who have a poor long-term prognosis, may descend into apathy. A health-care worker should try to use his or her influence to improve mood and combat apathy.

39. D: The best description for the word *discrete* is "separate." Discrete symptoms, for example, are those that do not have any connection to one another, though they spring from the same source. The word *subtle* is used to describe things that are "delicate or mysterious in their meaning or intent." Sometimes, the signs of disease will be subtle. Although today's health-care system has amazing technology for spotting the signs of disease, health-care workers still must be on the lookout for the subtle signs of disease. This is similar in meaning to *discreet*, so pay attention to spelling since *discrete* has a completely different meaning.

40. B: The word *site* as it is used in this sentence means "location." Doctors will often refer to the site of an injection or a planned surgery. A *syringe* is "the device used to inject or withdraw fluid from the body." Medical personnel who specialize in withdrawing blood from patients are called phlebotomists. An *artery* is "a blood vessel that carries blood away from the heart to nourish the rest of the body." Although the site to which the author is referring in this sentence is a *hole*, it will not always be so. For this reason, "hole" cannot be the best definition for *site*.

41. A: The word *exposure* as it is used in this sentence means "laying open." The most common usage of this term is in reference to the sun, although exposure to toxic chemicals is also a major health concern. A doctor will often ask a patient to limit his or her exposure to some environmental element. *Prohibition* is "the act of forbidding." Often, a doctor will place a prohibition on certain behaviors or foods if they are believed to adversely affect health. The words *connection* and *dislike* have no relation to exposure.

42. B: The word *exacerbate* means "aggravate." The first commandment of medical care is "do no harm," which essentially means do nothing to exacerbate the patient's illness or injury. Behaviors or foods that exacerbate the symptoms of illness or injury should be stopped immediately. To *implicate* is "to demonstrate involvement or assign blame." Often, during the examination period, a doctor or nurse will implicate seemingly unrelated behaviors in a patient's condition. Once a behavior has been implicated, the doctor and patient will work together to eliminate its negative effects on health. To *decondition* is "to weaken or diminish the conditioned response to a certain stimulus." Part of working in health care is helping people make positive choices. In part, this is accomplished by deconditioning them to stimuli that provoke a negative response.

43. C: The word *neuron* means "nerve cell." The human body has millions of neurons, with billions of connections between them. A *neutron* is "the part of an atom that has neither positive nor negative charge." Neutrons are located in the nucleus of the atom. The *nucleus* is "the central part of a cell or atom, around which the other parts cluster." The HESI exam requires you to know the names and functions of all the cell parts. *Neutral* means "not taking part in or not taking sides in a dispute." A neutral behavior or medication is one that has neither a positive nor a negative effect on health.

44. B: The word *adverse* means "unfavorable." Unhealthy behaviors have an adverse effect on well-being. *Liberated* means "freed." The general goal of health care is to liberate patients from the negative effects of illness or injury. *Convenient* means "easily accessible and available." When health care is convenient, patients are more likely to acquire it. Health-care workers should strive to make their services convenient for patients whenever possible. *Occluded* means "blocked or closed." Patients with a high level of cholesterol are at risk of developing occluded arteries. Another instance in which the term is used is when a patient is choking: In this case, the patient's airway is said to be occluded.

45. A: A residence is a place where a person lives; the term is often used to refer to someone's home.

46. D: The word *holistic* as it is used in this sentence means "concerned with the whole rather than the parts." Doctors try to consider the patient's health from a holistic perspective; that is, they try to improve health in its entirety rather than to eliminate specific symptoms. The word *insensitive* means "not responsive." The word *ignorant* means "lacking knowledge." Health-care workers cannot be ignorant of the latest findings and information in their field. The word *specialized* means "adapted to or trained in a specific discipline or task." Because of the technological complexity of modern medical practice, most careers in health care are specialized.

47. A: The best description for the word *suppress* is "stop." Sometimes, a patient will suppress their symptoms if they are not psychologically ready to face illness. However, the suppression of illness tends to create other problems. Ultimately, it is better not to suppress illness, but to face it directly.

To *strain* is "to work hard or overextend." This word is used in a couple of different ways in health care. A patient may be suffering from a specific muscle strain after excessive exercise or hyperextension. Also, a doctor may prohibit a patient from straining in his or her professional life if it is causing fatigue and making the patient vulnerable to disease.

48. D: The word *impending* means "about to happen." A doctor might refer to impending symptoms, which are the symptoms the patient is likely to start experiencing in the near future. *Depending* means "relying on or placing trust in." Because most patients have no medical expertise, they are depending on doctors and nurses to choose the appropriate course of action. *Offending* means "annoying or irritating." *Suspending* means "stopping for an undetermined period." If a treatment is not working, for instance, or if it is causing unforeseen negative side effects, then a doctor may suspend it until more information can be gathered.

49. C: The word *symmetric* as it is used in this sentence means "occurring in corresponding parts at the same time." Some illnesses will cause symmetric rashes, meaning that both the right and left sides of the body are afflicted with similarly shaped inflammation. The word *scabbed* means "covered with wounds." The word *geometric* is used to describe "things that resemble the classic geometric shapes, such as the circle, square, or triangle." On occasion, a doctor may use this word to describe the pattern of a wound or rash.

50. B: The word *patent* means "open." Doctors will describe an artery as patent when it allows a free flow of blood. Similarly, a patent airway allows for unrestricted breathing. *Inverted* means turned upside down or backwards. Sometimes, a patient will be inverted in order to stimulate blood flow to certain parts of the body. A *convent* is "a home for nuns or monks." This word has no relevance to health care, but it is included because the HESI exam will sometimes try to tempt you with answer choices that sound like the right answer. The word *converted* means "changed or altered." A patient may have his or her diet converted in order to meet the needs of a treatment protocol.

51. C: The word *volume* as it is used in this sentence means "quantity." Doctors will refer to an increase in the volume of urine or some other body product as an indication of health. Volume is calculated as length × width × height (or depth); it is a three-dimensional measure. *Length*, on the other hand, is "a two-dimensional measure of distance." *Quality* means "degree of excellence." Quantity can be measured in any kind of units. *Loudness* might be the right answer if *volume* were being used in a different way, as "the relative power of a sound." In this sentence, however, the word is not being used to describe a sound.

52. D: The word *repugnant* means "offensive, especially to the senses or the morals." For instance, a patient may find a certain kind of medicine repugnant, in which case the doctor must either figure out a way to disguise the taste or consider a different form of treatment. The word *destructive* means "causing damage, injury, or loss." Patients should be steered away from destructive behaviors. *Selective* means "choosy or capable of making a thoughtful choice." In general, it is good to be selective, although a patient who is too selective about his or her diet may develop a nutritional deficiency. *Collective* means "combined or grouped together to form a whole." Health care seeks to treat the collective symptoms of the patient, rather than to focus on specific problems.

53. A: The word *dilate* means "enlarge." Dilation is often expressed as measurement, typically in units of centimeters. For instance, when the body becomes hot, the arteries dilate and blood rushes to the extremities. To *protrude* means "to stick out." Sometimes when a patient breaks a bone severely, part of the bone will protrude from the skin. To *occlude* means "to close up or block."

Airways and arteries are the most common parts of the body to become occluded. Either of these occlusions needs to be dealt with immediately before other treatment can be administered.

54. C: The best description for the word *intact* is "unbroken." The word can be used in a number of different contexts. For instance, if a patient presents with severe pain in his or her side, the doctor might worry about the possibility of a ruptured appendix. After an X-ray reveals no damage to the appendix, however, the doctor might say that the organ is intact.

55. C: The word *access* means the ability "to enter, contact, or approach." It is important for patients to have easy access to health-care services. If patients do not have convenient access to services, they will be less likely to take actions to improve health. *Ingress* is "entering or going in." In some cases, a doctor will have to perform tests to determine a disease's path of ingress to the body. *Excess* is "too much or an overabundance of something." In general, excess of any kind is bad for the health. Even excessive exercise can be detrimental to health. During an initial examination, the doctor will try to identify areas in which the patient needs attention. *Success* is "the attainment of goals, whether personal, emotional, professional, physical, or financial." Obviously, the success of the patient is the top priority for all health-care workers.

Grammar

1. B: The best option is a present tense singular verb, and this option is *includes.*

2. C: The word *effected* is not spelled correctly in the context of this sentence. In order to answer this question, you need to know the difference between *affect* and *effect.* The former is a verb and the latter is a noun. In other words, *affect* is something that you do and *effect* is something that is. In this sentence, the speaker is describing something that the prescription medication *did.* Therefore, the appropriate word is a verb. *Effect,* however, is a noun. For this reason, instead of *effected* the author should have used the word *affected.*

3. C: The word *us* makes the sentence grammatically correct. *Us* is the objective case of *we.* In this case, *us* is being used as an indirect object. An indirect object is the noun to which the action of the verb refers. In the sentence *He gave her a sandwich,* the indirect object is *her* (and the direct object is *sandwich*). All of the answer choices for this question are in the first-person plural, with the exception of answer choice D, which is in the third-person plural. The appropriate third-person plural form to complete this sentence is *them.*

4. A: The word *is* makes the sentence grammatically correct. In order to answer this question, you need to determine what the object of the verb will be. One way to do this is to rearrange the question as if it were a declarative sentence: *Picking up the groceries ____ one of the things you are supposed to do.* Expressed like this, it is easy to see that the subject of the sentence is "picking up the groceries." This is a third-person singular subject (that is, it is an "it"), so it receives the third-person present indicative verb form, *is.*

5. D: The word *avoid* makes the sentence grammatically correct. To *avoid* is to keep from doing something. The sentence states that it is impossible to function in the modern world without learning how to use a computer. The word *evade* has a similar meaning to *avoid,* but the verb form used here does not fit into the sentence correctly. The best way to approach this kind of question on the HESI exam is to read the sentence aloud softly, substituting in the various answer choices. If you used this strategy on question 4, you would immediately notice that answer choice B does not correctly complete the sentence.

6. B: The word *hear* is not spelled correctly in the context of this sentence. The speaker has mixed up the homophones *hear* and *here. Homophones* are words that sound the same but are spelled differently and have a different meaning. Homophones are not to be confused with *homonyms,* which are spelled the same but have a different meaning. In question 5, the author is trying to describe the place where the climate is; that is, he or she is describing the climate *here.* Unfortunately, the author uses the word *hear,* which is a verb meaning "to listen."

7. D: The word *our* makes the sentence grammatically correct. *Our* is the possessive case of *we,* In this case, our is being used as an attributive adjective. An adjective is a word that modifies (or describes) a noun. *Our* is called an attributive adjective because it is attributing (assigning) ownership of the screaming to a particular party, *us.* Answer choices A and D are in the first-person plural; answer choices B and C are in the third-person plural. Neither B nor C, however, is in the possessive case. The sentence could be effectively completed with *their,* but this choice is not available.

8. D: The phrase *have to* makes the sentence grammatically correct. The speaker is trying to express that his group was forced to try hard. For this reason, it is essential for the verb *have* to be used. *Have* is an auxiliary verb indicating obligation. It agrees with the first-person plural pronoun *we.* An auxiliary verb accompanies another verb and makes some alterations in mood or tense. In this case, the addition of the verb *have* indicates that the speaker and others were obliged to try hard. *Can*, *will*, and *have* are all common examples of auxiliary verbs.

9. D: The word *which* makes the sentence grammatically correct. In this sentence, *which* is used as a relative pronoun. A relative pronoun introduces a relative clause, which is so called because it "relates" to the antecedent. The antecedent is the word that the relative pronoun refers to. In this sentence, the antecedent is "French braid," and the subsequent relative clause gives the reader more information about the French braid. Answer choice C is also a relative pronoun, but it is rarely used after a comma.

10. B: The phrase *toward peace was* makes this sentence grammatically correct. The word *toward* is a preposition that can mean "in the direction of" or "with a view to obtaining." It is in this last sense that the word is being used in this sentence. Peace is an abstract concept, not a physical destination that one could actually reach. For this reason, it does not make sense to select answer choices A or C. Answer choice D has an incorrect verb form; since the subject of the sentence is "working toward peace," the third-person singular verb form is correct.

11. A: The phrase *dog, who had* makes the sentence grammatically correct. To begin with, it is necessary for there to be a comma separating these two clauses, because the second clause is nonrestrictive. A clause is considered nonrestrictive if it could not stand by itself and if the rest of the sentence would still make sense were it removed. If the portion of this sentence after the comma were removed, the sentence would be *Janet called her dog*. Obviously, this is still a coherent sentence. Also, *who* is used here instead of *which* because the antecedent, *dog*, has an identity and personality.

12. B: "Wrong answer" is a clue that indicates a negative word. Belittled means to criticize. All the other answer choices have a positive connotation and, therefore, do not fit the intended meaning of the sentence.

13. B: The word *break* correctly completes this sentence. This question hinges on the different meanings that can be assigned to the word *break*. A *break* can be a brief period of rest from work or some tiring activity, or it can be the act of destroying or disconnecting something. The first usage is as a noun, and the second usage is as a verb. In this sentence, the author is expressing that Dr. Capra needed something, which means you should use the noun form. Also, remember that a *brake* is the mechanism for stopping a vehicle.

14. D: The word *began* properly completes the sentence. The sentence begins with the phrase "the other day," which indicates that the action described took place sometime in the recent past. A past tense verb form is appropriate, then. The verb *begun* is the past participle of *begin*. A past participle describes action that took place before but is now complete and is used with "had" or "have." This sentence does not indicate, however, that the action is now complete. For all we know, Stan could still be reviewing his class notes. For this reason, the past tense *began* is the correct answer.

15. C: The word *since* makes the sentence grammatically correct. In this sentence, *since* is being used as a conjunction meaning "because." The word can also be used as an adverb or a preposition indicating an interval from some past time to the present. In this sentence, however, the right answer is indicated by the context. The first part of the sentence states that the current prescription is to be maintained; this suggests that the speaker has a positive attitude toward it. It makes sense, then, that the prescription would have worked well in the past, and that this would be the reason for continuing it.

16. A: The word *rises* makes the sentence grammatically correct. At the heart of this question is the distinction between *rise* and *raise*, which can be summed up in one sentence: To *raise* is to cause to *rise*. This probably requires a little explanation. *Raise* is generally a transitive verb, meaning that it has to be done to something. In other words, it needs an object. One *raises* a window or *raises* a question, but a window or question does not *raise* itself. *Rise*, on the other hand, is typically used as an intransitive verb. This means that it does not take an object. I *rise* from sleep; I do not *rise myself* from sleep. In the sentence for question 14, the blood pressure is doing the action described by the verb, and there is no object. For this reason, *rises* is correct.

17. C: The word *despite* completes the sentence correctly. *Despite* is a preposition meaning "notwithstanding" or "in spite of." A preposition is a word that indicates relationship. *At*, *by*, *with*, and *before* are all prepositions. All of the answer choices for question 15 include prepositions. So in order to answer the question, you need to determine which relationship the author is most likely trying to express. The first clause indicates that the two professionals had similar training, and the second clause that indicates they drew different conclusions. It would not make sense for them to draw different conclusions *because of* their similar training; one would expect both professionals to approach a question in the same way. Answer choices B and D create an incoherent statement when they are substituted into the sentence. The answer must therefore be C.

18. D: The word *is* makes the sentence grammatically correct. In order to answer this question correctly, you need to be able to identify the subject. Although it may seem as if the subject is *the two European capitals*, this is actually a clause related to the subject *each*. *Each* is a singular pronoun, in which two or more things are being considered individually. In this case, each of these things is an "it," so the appropriate verb form will be the third-person singular present indicative *is*.

19. B: The word *further* is not used correctly in the context of this sentence. Here, the word *farther* would be more appropriate. The distinction between *further* and *farther* is likely to appear in at least one question on the HESI exam. For the purposes of the examination, you just need to know that *farther* can be used to describe physical distance, while *further* cannot. In this sentence, the speaker is describing a distance to be walked, which is a physical distance. For this reason, the word *further* is incorrect.

20. B: The word *sat* is used incorrectly in this sentence. The word *set* would be a good substitution for *sat*. The distinction between *sit* and *set* is likely to appear at least once during the HESI exam. *Sit* is an intransitive verb that does not need an object. One does not *sit* something else, one just *sits*. *Set*, meanwhile, is a transitive verb that requires an object. One *sets* an alarm clock or a table, one does not just *set*. In the sentence on question 18, the little boy is placing something, namely the red block. A transitive verb is required, therefore. For this reason, the past tense of *set* (also *set*) is correct, while the past tense of *sit* (*sat*) is not.

21. B: The phrase *to divulge* makes the sentence grammatically correct. *To divulge* is the infinitive form of a verb meaning to "reveal or disclose information." The verb can stay in the present tense because the speaker is describing what Laura knew at a particular time in the past. In other words, the author has already established the past tense with the word *knew*. It would also be appropriate to fill this blank with the word *divulging*. However, this is not one of the answer choices.

22. C: The word *closely* makes the sentence grammatically correct. Remember that an adjective is a word that describes a noun, while an adverb describes an adjective, a verb, or another adverb. In this sentence, you are looking for the right word to describe how the attendant *looked*. This means that you are looking for an adverb. Most of the time, adverbs end in *-ly*. On question 20, answer choices C and D both have this ending. Answer choice D, however, does not really make sense when substituted into the sentence.

23. D: Starved means very hungry. So, if James is famished, he could eat an immense, i.e., very large, meal. Nauseated (B) means sick. So, if James were not well, he could not eat an immense meal. Congested (A) means overly full or stuffed. If James exclaimed that he was congested, he probably would not be interested in any kind of meal. Also, if James were satisfied (C), then he would obviously not be interested in a meal.

24. B: The word *illusion* is used incorrectly in this sentence. Instead, the author should have used the word *allusion*. An illusion is a false or deceptive image. For example, a magician pulling a rabbit out a hat is a famous illusion. The magician does not actually produce the rabbit out of thin air, but is able to create the image of having done so. An *allusion*, on the other hand, is an indirect reference. If the doctor had said something like, "in light of your past issues," and Henry knew that the doctor meant his depression, then the doctor would have made an allusion.

25. B: The word *should* correctly completes the sentence. All of the answer choices are auxiliary verbs, which are verbs that accompany other verbs and add some element of tone or mood. In order to determine the appropriate auxiliary verb for this sentence, you need to take a close look at the context. The *if* that initiates the sentence suggests that the author is making a conditional statement. In other words, in order to join the club, a condition must be met: Namely, the coach must be contacted by Thursday. For this reason, *should* is the appropriate auxiliary verb. When should is placed before a verb, it adds a note of obligation or recommendation. For instance, saying, "You should brush your teeth," is like saying, "Brushing your teeth is a healthful act that you ought to do."

26. B: The word *set* makes the sentence grammatically correct. This questions centers on the distinction between *set* and *sit*. *Set* is transitive and needs to have an object. This means that it has to be done to something (there are a few exceptions, like *the sun sets*). The past tense and past participle of *set* are both *set*. *Sit*, meanwhile, is intransitive and takes no object. You don't sit something; you just sit. The past tense and past participle of *sit* is *sat*. In this case, the blank must be filled by a transitive verb, because the verb is acting on something else: the law practice. For this reason, *set* is the correct answer.

27. A: The phrase *more efficient* makes the sentence grammatically correct. Here, the author is attempting to describe a comparison between two things: the coal furnace and the woodstove. The comparative form of an adjective usually ends with *-er*: *taller*, *wiser*, *cleaner*, for example. In some cases, however, the word *more* is placed in front of the unchanged adjective. As a general rule, multisyllabic words are more likely to use the *more* construction than the *-er* construction. That is the case with *efficient*. Unfortunately, there is no easy rule for memorizing the comparative forms of common English adjectives. Reading is one way to develop a good eye for proper usage.

28. C: The word *has* is used incorrectly in this sentence. The auxiliary verb *have* would be a correct substitution for *has*. *Have* and *has* are auxiliary verbs that, along with *developed*, form a past participle. A past participle is used for action that took place in the past and is now complete. The subject of the sentence is soccer players, which means the verb has to be in the third-person plural. *Has*, however, is the third-person singular. *Have* is in the third-person plural and would therefore be a better choice.

29. A: The word *him* makes the sentence grammatically correct. In this sentence, the blank needs to be filled by a direct object, because you are looking for the person, place, or thing to which the action of the verb is being done. Here, we are looking to identify the person who was asked. For that reason, we need the objective case of *he*, which is *him*. The objective case of *she* is *her*. There will probably be several questions in the grammar section of the HESI exam that require you to differentiate between a pronoun used as a subject and a pronoun used as an object.

30. B: The word *with* makes the sentence grammatically correct. *With* is a preposition that can mean a number of different things. Perhaps the most common meaning of *with* is "in the company of." In this sentence, however, a more accurate meaning is "in regard to." The word *among* is not appropriate here, because progress is not something one could physically be in the middle of. That is, *progress* is not a group of individual things. The word *regards* is not grammatically appropriate for this sentence, although the sentence could be correctly completed with the phrase *with regard to*. Finally, the word *besides* is incorrect because it would not make sense for Felix to not be pleased with his own progress.

31. C: The word *hungrily* makes the sentence grammatically correct. In order to answer this question, you must know the difference between an adjective and an adverb. An adjective modifies a noun. For instance, in the phrase "the delicious meatball," *delicious* is an adjective. An adverb, on the other hand, modifies an adjective, a verb, or another adverb. In the phrase "walking quickly away," *quickly* is an adverb. In the sentence for this question, it seems clear that the answer must modify the verb *eyed*. After all, it would not make much sense for the cheesecake to be hungry. This means that an adverb is required. The adverbial form of *hungry* is *hungrily*.

32. C: The word *recipe* is not used correctly in the context of this sentence. The author of this sentence has apparently confused the word *recipe* and *receipt*. A *recipe* is a list of instructions for making something, usually a food or beverage. You might have a recipe for chocolate chip cookies, for instance. A *receipt*, on the other hand, is a printed acknowledgement of having received a certain amount of money and goods. The slip of paper you are handed after paying for something in a store is a receipt. The HESI exam will most likely contain a few questions that require you to identify mixed-up word choices.

33. B: The word *good* properly completes this sentence. This question centers on the distinction between good and well, and, more generally, between adjectives and adverbs. An adjective is used to describe a noun or a pronoun. In the phrase "the red bicycle," for example, *red* is an adjective describing *bicycle*. An adverb, on the other hand, describes a verb, an adjective, or another adverb. Words that end in *-ly* are usually adverbs, describing the way something is done. As an example, in the phrase "running steadily," *steadily* is an adverb. To succeed on the HESI exam, you need to know that g*ood* is an adjective and *well* is an adverb. In question 30, you are looking for a word that describes how Sharon felt, not one that describes her act of feeling. For this reason, you should select the adjective *good*.

34. C: A shower in terms of weather is a small amount of precipitation. This meaning is reinforced in the sentence by the adjective mere, (i.e., small or minor). The use of *mere* plus the conjunction *but* signals a contrast between the sentence's two clauses: today's storm contrasts with yesterday's mere shower of rainfall. Thus, we know that today's storm must be larger and more powerful than yesterday's. The only word which indicates this is (C), hurled (thrown with great force). A storm would not drip (A) (i.e., leak them slowly and gradually) solid hailstones. A drizzle (B) is a fine rain which is more synonymous with a mere trickle than with a hailstorm. A trickle (D) is a synonym of drizzle and would not be connected with hail.

35. D: The word *lying* is used incorrectly in this sentence. It would be correct to use the verb *laying* instead. The distinction between *laying* and *lying* is tricky. *Laying* is typically used as a transitive verb, meaning that it is done to something. One lays bricks or lays carpet, for instance. Lie, on the other hand, is an intransitive verb: It is not done to something; it is just done. You *lie* on the floor, for instance. The definition of *lay* is to place; to *lie* is to take a horizontal position. In this sentence, the subject (Brendan) is laying something (bricks), so it is incorrect to use the verb *lying*.

36. A: The word *who* makes the sentence grammatically correct. In this sentence, *who* is being used as a relative pronoun: that is, a pronoun introducing a clause that describes a noun already mentioned. The noun being referred to, known as the antecedent, is *children*. Because children are people with a personality and identity, the pronoun *who* is used rather than *which. Which* is used as a relative pronoun when the antecedent is an inanimate object, such as a box or a house.

37. C: The word *struck* makes the sentence grammatically correct. *Struck* is the past tense and past participle of *strike*, meaning "to hit" or "to beat." *Striked* is not a word. In this case, however, the author is using the common expression "struck a bargain." This expression is frequently used to describe deal making or the end of negotiations. These kinds of conversational phrases may be especially difficult for students whose native language is not English. If you are unfamiliar with expressions in English, you may want to pick up a glossary of slang or colloquial expressions.

38. A: The phrase *him or her* makes the sentence grammatically correct. In this case, we are looking for a word or words that can serve as the object of the preposition *for. She* and *he* are nominative forms, meaning that they can only be used as the subject of a sentence or a clause. *Them* can be the object of a preposition, but it is plural and, therefore, cannot correctly refer to the singular subject *a child*. (Incidentally, the use of *they* and *them* to refer to a singular subject is one of the most common grammatical errors, and will almost certainly appear in one or more questions on the HESI exam.) For a similar reason, you cannot use *it* to refer to *a child*. The correct answer, then, is *him or her*.

39. A: The word *swam* makes the sentence grammatically correct. *Swam* is the past tense of the verb *swim*. The context of this sentence makes clear that the action took place in the past; the author uses the past tense verb *was* and describes an action that has already been completed. *Swimmed* is an incorrect verb form. *Swum* is the past participle of *swim*; it would be appropriate if the sentence read *he had swum* or *he has swum*. The absence of these auxiliary verbs means that the simple past tense is appropriate here.

40. C: The phrase *she and I* makes the sentence grammatically correct. The blank needs to be filled by the subject of the sentence. The subject of a sentence or clause is the person, place, or thing that performs the verb. There are a couple of ways to determine that this sentence needs a subject. To begin with, the blank is at the beginning of the sentence, where the subject most often is found. Also, when you read the sentence, you will notice that it is unclear who went to the movies. Because you are looking for the subject, you need the nominative pronouns *she and I*.

41. C: The word *set* makes the sentence grammatically correct. This question requires knowledge of the distinction between *set* and *sit. Set* is a transitive verb meaning "to place in a particular position." Transitive verbs have to be done *to* something. *Sit*, meanwhile, is an intransitive verb meaning "to assume a seated posture." In this case, Brian is performing the action of the verb on something in particular: the alarm clock. For this reason, the verb *set* is appropriate.

42. B: The word *shaked* is incorrect in this sentence. In fact, *shaked* is not a word at all. The past tense of *shake* is *shook*. This is similar to the word *take*, which has as its past tense *took* rather than *taked*. There is no real reason for this, making it yet another usage pattern in English that does not conform to any strict rules. After all, the past tense of *wake* is *waked* rather than *wook*. There is no easy way to know all of these rules and exceptions, but a good way to acquire a sense of standard English usage is to become widely read and use a dictionary.

43. B: The word *whichever* makes the sentence grammatically correct. In this sentence, *whichever* is being used as an adjective modifying *way*. The presence of this adjective indicates that Ted was looking in any number of different ways. *Moreover* is an adverb meaning "in addition" or "besides." *Whomever* is the form of whoever used as a direct object, indirect object, or object of a preposition. *Whether* is a conjunction that suggests alternatives or sets of two choices.

44. C: The word *lain* properly completes the sentence. On this question, the presence of the word *had* is the biggest clue to the right answer. *Had* indicates that the verb phrase is being used as a past participle. A past participle is the verb form used to describe action that took place in the past and has been completed. In other words, the treasure started lying there a long time ago, and its position was fully established in the past. Remember that *lain* is the past participle of *lie*, and *laid* is the past participle of *lay*. The verb here is clearly intransitive (that is, it does not act on something else, it just does something), so the correct form is *lain*.

45. A: The past progressive form indicates that Janet began doing something in the past, and continues to do so today.

46. B: The word *fewer* makes the sentence grammatically correct. The distinction between fewer and less will most likely appear on your HESI exam. In general, *fewer* is used for things that can be counted and *less* is used for things that cannot be counted. So, for instance, one would say "fewer attendees at this year's conference" and "less confidence in the economy." In this sentence, the adjective is modifying *patients*, who of course can be counted quite easily. So, the correct answer is *fewer*.

47. B: The word *after* makes the sentence grammatically correct. *After* is a conjunction meaning "behind in place or position." A conjunction is a part of speech that connects different words, phrase, and ideas. *And*, *but*, and *because* are all conjunctions. In order to find the appropriate word to complete the sentence in question 42, you need to take a close look at the context. The sentence indicates that Kim realized she had forgotten her list of questions at some time relating to the interview. In other words, it seems clear that the blank must be completed with some word relating to time. Kim either made this realization before, during, or after the interview. Since *after* is one of the answer choices, it must be the correct answer.

48. D: The word *one* is used incorrectly in this sentence. Here, *one* is being used as a pronoun: a stand-in for some other noun. The problem is that it is unclear to what it is referring. The only possible reference for *one* is video store, and it does not make sense to say that "we should rent a video store." Most of the time, we would read this sentence and just assume that the author meant that we should rent a video. However, on the HESI exam, you must be alert for unclear wording.

49. A: The word *who* makes this sentence correct. *Who* is an interrogative pronoun that can be either singular or plural. A pronoun is a word that stands in for another noun. In this case, the pronoun is used so that the author can inquire about the noun to which the pronoun is referring. Once the question is answered, the names of the best eye doctors could be substituted for *who* to make a complete sentence. In any case, *who* is appropriate because the pronoun is referring to people who have both personality and identity; if they were objects, it would be appropriate to use *which* or *what*. *Whom* is a pronoun in the objective cases and is therefore not appropriate for this sentence.

50. B: The word *spent* makes this sentence grammatically correct. The sentence is clearly describing action that took place in the past, because the introductory clause begins with the word *while*. It cannot be determined whether this action is ongoing or has been completed. The past tense of the verb *spend* is *spent*. Unfortunately, there is no rule to guide this past tense; as a matter of fact, the past tense of the verb *mend* is *mended*, which might lead you to believe that *spended* is correct. Reading a variety of materials is the best way to develop an ear for proper usage.

51. A: The word *amount* correctly completes this sentence. This question centers on the distinction between *amount* and *number*. An *amount* is a quantity that cannot be counted, while a *number* is a quantity that can be counted. There is no way to count pain, so *amount* is a better word choice than *number*. *Frequency* is rate of occurrence, or how often something happens. If a doctor asks how often a patient gets a migraine, for instance, she is asking about the *frequency* of the headaches. *Amplitude* is the specific breadth or width. Amplitude is mainly used to describe waves; the difference in height between the top of a wave (crest) and the bottom (trough) is the amplitude.

52. C: The word *their* is used incorrectly in this sentence. The problem is that *whoever* as it is used here is a singular subject, while *their* is a plural possessive pronoun. *Whoever* can be either singular or plural, depending on how it is used. In this case, however, because the author is describing a letter writer who forgot to sign the letter, it seems clear that *whoever* is meant as a singular. For this reason, the author should use *his or her* instead of *their*.

53. C: The word *too* makes the sentence grammatically correct. Clearly, the author is trying to express that the child's fever was excessively high. Of the four answer choices, three convey this idea. Only answer choice A (the preposition *to*) can be immediately eliminated. The best way to find the final answer is to substitute each of the answer choices into the sentence and read the result. Answer choice B requires the addition of the word *too* to make any sense and answer choice D does not make sense either. Answer choice C, then, must be the correct answer.

54. B: The word *presents* makes the sentence grammatically correct. The author is referring to the symptoms that will be displayed when a patient has a particular condition: that is, the presentation of the condition. Because the subject of the sentence (*condition*) is singular, it is proper to use the verb form ending in an *s*. For this reason, you should select answer choice B rather than answer choice C. *Presence* is the quality of being there. When a teacher is calling roll and a student responds to his name by saying "present," he is using a form of this word to indicate that he is there. Of course, *present* can also mean a gift. *Prescience*, on the other hand, is foreknowledge, or knowledge ahead of time. You can exercise prescience by learning the content of the HESI exam and practicing with this study guide.

55. B: The preposition *among* is not used correctly in the context of the sentence. In this case, the word *between* would be more appropriate. *Among* and *between* both mean "in the midst of some other things." However, *between* is used when there are only two other things, and *among* is used when there are more than two. For example, it would be correct to say "between first and second base" or "among several friends." In this sentence, the preposition *among* is inappropriate for describing placement amid "two treatment protocols."

Biology

1. A: The cell body contains the nucleus. In all *eukaryotic* cells (cells containing a nucleus), the nucleus is the site where the chromosomes reside. The chromosomes carry the genes, which direct the activities of the neuron.

2. B: It is impossible for an AaBb organism to have the aa combination in the gametes. It is impossible for each letter to be used more than one time, so it would be impossible for the lowercase a to appear twice in the gametes. It would be possible, however, for Aa to appear in the gametes, since there is one uppercase A and one lowercase a. Gametes are the cells involved in sexual reproduction. They are germ cells.

3. A: The typical result of mitosis in humans is two diploid cells. Mitosis is the division of a body cell into two daughter cells. Each of the two produced cells has the same set of chromosomes as the parent. A diploid cell contains both sets of homologous chromosomes. A haploid cell contains only one set of chromosomes, which means that it only has a single set of genes. For the HESI exam, you will need to know about all the different stages of cell division for both human and plant cells.

4. B: Water stabilizes the temperature of living things. The ability of warm-blooded animals, including human beings, to maintain a constant internal temperature is known as homeostasis. Homeostasis depends on the presence of water in the body. Water tends to minimize changes in temperature because it takes a while to heat up or cool down. When the human body gets warm, the blood vessels dilate and blood moves away from the torso and toward the extremities. When the body gets cold, blood concentrates in the torso. This is the reason why hands and feet tend to get especially cold in cold weather. The HESI exam will require you to understand the basic processes of the human body.

5. B: Oxygen is not one of the products of the Krebs cycle. The Krebs cycle is the second stage of cellular respiration. In this stage, a sequence of reactions converts pyruvic acid into carbon dioxide. This stage of cellular respiration produces the phosphate compounds that provide most of the energy for the cell. The Krebs cycle is also known as the citric acid cycle or the tricarboxylic acid cycle. The HESI exam may require you to know all stages of cellular respiration: the process in which a plant cell converts carbon dioxide into oxygen.

6. C: The sugar and phosphate in DNA are connected by covalent bonds. A covalent bond is formed when atoms share electrons. It is very common for atoms to share pairs of electrons. Hydrogen bonds are used in DNA to bind complementary bases together, such as adenine with thymine or guanine with cytosine. An ionic bond is created when one or more electrons are transferred between atoms. Ionic bonds, also known as electrovalent bonds, are formed between ions with opposite charges. There is no such thing as an overt bond in chemistry. The HESI exam will require you to understand and have some examples of these different types of bonds.

7. C: Pollination is the fertilization of plants. It involves the transfer of pollen from the anther to the stigma, either by wind or by insects.

8. A: The second part of an organism's scientific name is its species. The system of naming species is called binomial nomenclature. The first name is the genus, and the second name is the species. In binomial nomenclature, species is the most specific designation. This system enables the same name to be used all around the world, so that scientists can communicate with one another. Genus and species are just two of the categories in biological classification, otherwise known as taxonomy. The levels of classification, from most general to most specific, are domain, kingdom, phylum, class, order, family, genus, and species. As you can see, binomial nomenclature only includes the two most specific categories.

9. B: Unlike other organic molecules, lipids are not water soluble. Lipids are typically composed of carbon and hydrogen. Three common types of lipid are fats, waxes, and oils. Indeed, lipids usually feel oily when you touch them. All living cells are primarily composed of lipids, carbohydrates, and proteins. Some examples of fats are lard, corn oil, and butter. Some examples of waxes are beeswax and carnauba wax. Some examples of steroids are cholesterol and ergosterol.

10. D: Hemoglobin is not a steroid. It is a protein that helps to move oxygen from the lungs to the various body tissues. Steroids can be either synthetic chemicals used to reduce swelling and inflammation or sex hormones produced by the body. Cholesterol is the most abundant steroid in the human body. It is necessary for the creation of bile, though it can be dangerous if the levels in the body become too high. Estrogen is a female steroid produced by the ovaries (in females), testes (in males), placenta, and adrenal cortex. It contributes to adolescent sexual development, menstruation, mood, lactation, and aging. Testosterone is the main hormone produced by the testes; it is responsible for the development of adult male sex characteristics.

11. A: The property of cohesion is responsible for the passage of water through a plant. Cohesion is the attractive force between two molecules of the same substance. The water in the roots of the plant is drawn upward into the stem, leaves, and flowers by the presence of other water molecules. Adhesion is the attractive force between molecules of different substances. Osmosis is a process in which water diffuses through a selectively permeable membrane. Evaporation is the conversion of water from a liquid to a gas.

12. C: Melatonin is produced by the pineal gland. One of the primary functions of melatonin is regulation of the circadian cycle, which is the rhythm of sleep and wakefulness. Insulin helps regulate the amount of glucose in the blood. Without insulin, the body is unable to convert blood sugar into energy. Testosterone is the main hormone produced by the testes; it is responsible for the development of adult male sex characteristics. Epinephrine, also known as adrenaline, performs a number of functions: It quickens and strengthens the heartbeat and dilates the bronchioles. Epinephrine is one of the hormones secreted when the body senses danger.

13. A: The nucleus is the control center for the cell. The cell membrane surrounds the cell and separates the cell from its environment. Cytoplasm is the thick fluid within the cell membrane that surrounds the nucleus and contains organelles. Mitochondria are often called the powerhouse of the cell because they provide energy for the cell to function.

14. C: Ribosomes are the organelles that organize protein synthesis. A ribosome, composed of RNA and protein, is a tiny structure responsible for putting proteins together. The mitochondrion converts chemical energy into a form that is more useful for the functions of the cell. The nucleus is the central structure of the cell. It contains the DNA and administrates the functions of the cell. The vacuole is a cell organelle in which useful materials (for example, carbohydrates, salts, water, and proteins) are stored.

15. D: During meiosis I, the chromosome number is reduced from diploid to haploid. Interphase is the period of the cell cycle that occurs in between divisions of the cell. In meiosis, the homologous chromosomes in a diploid cell separate, reducing the number of chromosomes in each cell by half. Mitosis is the phase of cell division in which the cell nucleus divides. S phase is the part of the mitotic cycle in which DNA is synthesized.

16. C: Prokaryotic cells do not contain a nucleus. A prokaryote is simply a single-celled organism without a nucleus. It is difficult to identify the structures of a prokaryotic cell, even with a microscope. These cells are usually shaped like a rod, a sphere, or a spiral. A eukaryote is an organism containing cells with nuclei. Bacterial cells are prokaryotes, but since there are other kinds of prokaryotes, bacteria cannot be the correct answer to this question. Cancer cells are malignant, atypical cells that reproduce to the detriment of the organism in which they are located.

17. A: Phenotype is the physical presentation of an organism's genes. In other words, the phenotype is the physical characteristics of the organism. Phenotype is often contrasted with genotype, the genetic makeup of an organism. The genotype of the organism is not visible in its presentation, although some of the characteristics encoded in the genes have to do with physical presentation. A phylum is a group of classes that are closely related. A species is a group of like organisms that are capable of breeding together and producing similar offspring.

18. A: Liquid is the densest form of water. Water can exist in three states, depending on temperature. Ranging from coldest to hottest, these states are solid, liquid, and gaseous—or ice, water, and steam. Water freezes at zero degrees Celsius. Although the solidity of ice might lead one to believe that it is the densest form of water, water actually expands about nine percent when it is frozen. This is the reason why ice will float in water. Steam is the least dense form of water.

19. B: A stoma (plural: stomata) is the part of a plant system that responds to stimuli by releasing water via transpiration. It can also close during adverse conditions like a drought to prevent the plant from dehydration. Stomata closure can also be triggered by the presence of bacteria. Pith refers to the central, spongy part of the stem in vascular plants. Guard cells flank stomata and regulate the opening. Sepals are modified leaves that protect the flower bud before it opens.

20. B: Interphase is the longest phase in the life of a cell. Interphase occurs between cell divisions. Prophase is the initial stage of mitosis. It is also the longest stage. During prophase, the chromosomes become visible, and the centrioles divide and position themselves on either side of the nucleus. Anaphase is the third phase of mitosis, in which chromosome pairs divide and take up positions on opposing poles. Metaphase is the second stage of mitosis. In it, the chromosomes align themselves across the center of the cell.

21. A: Bacterial cells do not contain mitochondria. Bacteria are prokaryotes composed of single cells; their cell walls contain peptidoglycans. The functions normally performed in the mitochondria are performed in the cell membrane of the bacterial cell. DNA is the nucleic acid that contains the genetic information of the organism. It is in the shape of a double helix. DNA can reproduce itself and can synthesize RNA. A vesicle is a small cavity containing fluid. A ribosome is a tiny particle composed of RNA and protein, in which polypeptides are constructed.

22. B: Hemoglobin is a protein. Proteins contain carbon, nitrogen, oxygen, and hydrogen. These substances are required for the growth and repair of tissue and the formation of enzymes. Hemoglobin is found in red blood cells and contains iron. It is responsible for carrying oxygen from the lungs to the various body tissues. Adenosine triphosphate (ATP) is a compound used by living organisms to store and use energy. Estrogen is a steroid hormone that stimulates the development of female sex characteristics. Cellulose is a complex carbohydrate that composes the better part of the cell wall.

23. D: Deoxyribonucleic acid (DNA) is not involved in translation. Translation is the process by which messenger RNA (mRNA) messages are decoded into polypeptide chains. Transfer RNA (tRNA) is a molecule that moves amino acids into the ribosomes during the synthesis of protein.

Messenger RNA carries sets of instructions for the conversion of amino acids into proteins from the RNA to the other parts of the cell. Ribosomes are the tiny particles in the cell where proteins are put together. Ribosomes are composed of ribonucleic acid (RNA) and protein.

24. A: Water is required for cell diffusion. Diffusion is the movement of molecules from an area of high concentration to an area of lower concentration. This process takes place in the body in a number of different areas. For instance, nutrients diffuse from partially digested food through the walls of the intestine into the bloodstream. Similarly, oxygen that enters the lungs diffuses into the bloodstream through membranes at the end of the alveoli. In all these cases, the body has evolved special membranes that only allow certain materials through.

25. A: Many organisms, especially organisms that live in harsh conditions such as deserts or frozen icy areas, have developed specific adaptations that allow them to survive. For example, cacti are able to expand to store large amounts of water, coyotes absorb some water from their food, and snakes can escape the heat by hiding within rocks.

26. C: There are four different nucleotides in DNA. Nucleotides are monomers of nucleic acids, composed of five-carbon sugars, a phosphate group, and a nitrogenous base. Nucleotides make up both DNA and RNA. They are essential for the recording of an organism's genetic information, which guides the actions of the various cells of the body. Nucleotides are also a crucial component of adenosine triphosphate (ATP), one of the parts of DNA and a chemical that enables metabolism and muscle contractions.

27. B: Red blood cells do not have a nucleus. These cells are shaped a little like a doughnut, although the hole in the center is not quite open. The other three types of cell have a nucleus. Platelets, which are fragments of cells and are released by the bone marrow, contribute to blood clotting. White blood cells, otherwise known as leukocytes, help the body fight disease. A phagocyte is a cell that can entirely surround bacteria and other microorganisms. The two most common phagocytes are neutrophils and monocytes, both of which are white blood cells.

28. D: The electron transport system enacted during aerobic respiration requires oxygen. This is the last component of biological oxidation. Osmosis is the movement of fluid from an area of high concentration through a partially permeable membrane to an area of lower concentration. This process usually stops when the concentration is the same on either side of the membrane. Glycolysis is the initial step in the release of glucose energy. The Krebs cycle is the last phase of the process in which cells convert food into energy. It is during this stage that carbon dioxide is produced and hydrogen is extracted from molecules of carbon.

29. A: Kingdom is the most general taxonomic category of the choices given. A genus is a group of related species, which are capable of breeding and producing similar offspring. In binomial nomenclature, genus is the first name. An order is any group of similar families. A phylum is any group of closely related classes. The HESI exam requires you to know the name and relative specificity of each taxonomic category. They are listed here in order from most general to most specific: domain, kingdom, phylum, class, order, family, genus, and species.

30. D: Fission is the process of a bacterial cell splitting into two new cells. Fission is a form of asexual reproduction in which an organism divides into two components; each of these two parts will develop into a distinct organism. The two cells, known as daughter cells, are identical. Mitosis, on the other hand, is the part of eukaryotic cell division in which the cell nucleus divides. In meiosis, the homologous chromosomes in a diploid cell separate, reducing the number of chromosomes in each cell by half. In replication, a cell creates duplicate copies of DNA.

Chemistry

1. C: $Al_2O_3 + 2Fe$. In a single replacement reaction equation, $2Al + Fe_2O_3 \rightarrow$ could result in the products $Al_2O_3 + 2Fe$. The reactants of the original equation are aluminum and iron(III) oxide (rust). The products are aluminum oxide and elemental iron. Single replacement reactions occur when one uncombined element replaces another. In this reaction, the aluminum replaces the iron. This reaction is an example of a thermite reaction and generates a large amount of heat and light. It can be used in fireworks or welding.

2. A: Diffusion is fastest through gases. The next fastest medium for diffusion is liquid, followed by plasma, and then solids. In chemistry, diffusion is defined as the movement of matter by the random motions of molecules. In a gas or a liquid, the molecules are in perpetual motion. For instance, in a quantity of seemingly immobile air, molecules of nitrogen and oxygen are constantly bouncing off each other. There is even some miniscule degree of diffusion in solids, which rises in proportion to the temperature of the substance.

3. B: The oxidation number of the hydrogen in CaH_2 is –1. The oxidation number of the hydrogen in CaH_2 is -1. One of the general rules for determining oxidation states applies specifically to hydrogen: When hydrogen is bonded to a nonmetal its oxidation state is +1, but when hydrogen is bonded to a metal its oxidation state is –1. An ion is a charged version of an element. Oxidation number is often referred to as oxidation state. Oxidation number is sometimes used to describe the number of electrons that must be added or removed from an atom in order to convert the atom to its elemental form.

4. A: Boron does not exist as a diatomic molecule. The other possible answer choices, fluorine, oxygen, and nitrogen, all exist as diatomic molecules. A diatomic molecule always appears in nature as a pair: The word diatomic means "having two atoms." With the exception of astatine, all of the halogens are diatomic. Chemistry students often use the mnemonic BrINClHOF (pronounced "brinkelhoff") to remember all of the diatomic elements: bromine, iodine, nitrogen, chlorine, hydrogen, oxygen, and fluorine. Note that not all of these diatomic elements are halogens.

5. D: Hydriodic acid is another name for aqueous HI. In an aqueous solution, the solvent is water. Hydriodic acid is a polyatomic ion, meaning that it is composed of two or more elements. When this solution has an increased amount of oxygen, the *-ate* suffix on the first word is converted to *-ic*. The HESI exam will require you to know the fundamentals of naming chemicals. This process can be quite complex, so you should carefully review this material before your exam.

6. C: CH could be an empirical formula. An empirical formula is the smallest expression of a chemical formula. To be empirical, a formula must be incapable of being reduced. For this reason, answer choices A, B, and D are incorrect, as they could all be reduced to a simpler form. Note that empirical formulas are not the same as compounds, which do not have to be irreducible. Two compounds can have the same empirical formula but different molecular formulas. The molecular formula is the actual number of atoms in the molecule.

7. B: A water molecule contains 2 hydrogen atoms and 1 oxygen atom. Therefore, the chemical formula for water is H_2O. Also, the pH of water is 7.

8. A: A limiting reactant is entirely used up by the chemical reaction. Limiting reactants control the extent of the reaction and determine the quantity of the product. A reducing agent is a substance that reduces the amount of another substance by losing electrons. A reagent is any substance used in a chemical reaction. Some of the most common reagents in the laboratory are sodium hydroxide and hydrochloric acid. The behavior and properties of these substances are known, so they can be effectively used to produce predictable reactions in an experiment.

9. B: The horizontal rows of the periodic table are called periods. The vertical columns of the periodic table are known as groups or families. All of the elements in a group have similar properties. The relationships between the elements in each period are similar as you move from left to right. The periodic table was developed by Dmitri Mendeleev to organize the known elements according to their similarities. New elements can be added to the periodic table without necessitating a redesign.

10. C: The mass of 7.35 mol water is 132 grams. You should be able to find the mass of various chemical compounds when you are given the number of mols. The information required to perform this function is included on the periodic table. To solve this problem, find the molecular mass of water by finding the respective weights of hydrogen and oxygen. Remember that water contains two hydrogen molecules and one oxygen molecule. The molecular mass of hydrogen is roughly 1, and the molecular mass of oxygen is roughly 16. A molecule of water, then, has approximately 18 grams of mass. Multiply this by 7.35 mol, and you will obtain the answer 132.3, which is closest to answer choice C.

11. D: Of these orbitals, the last to fill is $6s$. Orbitals fill in the following order: $1s$, $2s$, $2p$, $3s$, $3p$, $4s$, $3d$, $4p$, $5s$, $4d$, $5p$, $6s$, $4f$, $5d$, $6p$, $7s$, $5f$, $6d$, and $7p$. The number is the orbital number, and the letter is the sublevel identification. Sublevel s has one orbital and can hold a maximum of two electrons. Sublevel p has three orbitals and can hold a maximum of six electrons. Sublevel d has five orbitals and can hold a maximum of 10 electrons. Sublevel f has seven orbitals and can hold a maximum of 14 electrons.

12. C: Nitrogen pentoxide is the name of the binary molecular compound NO_5. The format given in answer choice C is appropriate when dealing with two nonmetals. A prefix is used to denote the number of atoms of each element. Note that when there are seven atoms of a given element, the prefix *hepta-* is used instead of the usual *septa-*. Also, when the first atom in this kind of binary molecular compound is single, it does not need to be given the prefix *mono-*.

13. C: The atom is negatively charged. Neutrons have no charge. Protons have positive charge, and electrons have negative charge that is equal in magnitude. Because the atom has more electrons than protons, the atom has a negative charge.

14. D: The mass of 1.0 mol oxygen gas is 32 grams. The molar mass of oxygen can be obtained from the periodic table. In most versions of the table, the molar mass of the element is directly beneath the full name of the element. There is a little trick to this question. Oxygen is a diatomic molecule, which means that it always appears in pairs. In order to determine the mass in grams of 1.0 mol of oxygen gas, then, you must double the molar mass. The listed mass is 16, so the correct answer to the problem is 32.

15. D: Gamma radiation has no charge. This form of electromagnetic radiation can travel a long distance and can penetrate the human body. Sunlight and radio waves are both examples of gamma radiation. Alpha radiation has a +2 charge. It only travels short distances and cannot penetrate clothing or skin. Radium and uranium both emit alpha radiation. Beta radiation has a –1 charge. It can travel several feet through the air and is capable of penetrating the skin. This kind of radiation can be damaging to health over a long period of exposure. There is no such thing as delta radiation.

16. A: When forward and reverse chemical reactions are taking place at the same rate, a chemical reaction has achieved equilibrium. This means that the respective concentrations of reactants and products do not change over time. In theory, a chemical reaction will remain in equilibrium indefinitely. One of the common tasks in the chemistry lab is to find the equilibrium constant (or set of relative concentrations that result in equilibrium) for a given reaction. In thermal equilibrium, there is no net heat exchange between a body and its surroundings. In dynamic equilibrium, any motion in one direction is offset by an equal motion in the other direction.

17. B: 119 K is equivalent to –154 degrees Celsius. It is likely that you will have to perform at least one temperature conversion on the HESI exam. To convert Kelvin to degrees Celsius, simply subtract 273. To convert degrees Celsius to Kelvin, simply add 273. To convert Kelvin into degrees Fahrenheit, multiply by 9/5 and subtract 460. To convert degrees Fahrenheit to Kelvin, add 460 and then multiply by 5/9. To convert degrees Celsius to degrees Fahrenheit, multiply by 9/5 and then add 32. To convert degrees Fahrenheit to degrees Celsius, subtract 32 and then multiply by 5/9.

18. B: The joule is the SI unit of energy. Energy is the ability to do work or generate heat. In regard to electrical energy, a joule is the amount of electrical energy required to pass a current of one ampere through a resistance of one ohm for one second. In physical or mechanical terms, the joule is the amount of energy required for a force of one newton to act over a distance of one meter. The ohm is a unit of electrical resistance. The henry is a unit of inductance. The newton is a unit of force.

19. D: Oxidation, also known as rusting, is the result of a change in the chemical composition of the iron.

20. A: A mass spectrometer separates gaseous ions according to their mass-to-charge ratio. This machine is used to distinguish the various elements in a piece of matter. An interferometer measures the wavelength of light by comparing the interference phenomena of two waves: an experimental wave and a reference wave. A magnetometer measures the direction and magnitude of a magnetic field. Finally, a capacitance meter measures the capacitance of a capacitor. Some sophisticated capacitance meters may also measure inductance, leakage, and equivalent series resistance.

21. C: Of the given materials, aluminum has the lowest specific heat. The specific heat of a substance is the amount of heat required to raise the temperature of one gram of the substance by one degree Celsius. In some cases, specific heat is expressed as a ratio of the heat required to raise the temperature of one gram of a substance by one degree Celsius to the heat required to raise the temperature of one gram of water by one degree Celsius.

22. C: In a redox reaction, also known as an oxidation-reduction reaction, electrons are transferred from one atom to another. A redox reaction changes the oxidation numbers of the atoms. In a combustion reaction, one material combines with an oxidizer to form a product and generate heat. In a synthesis reaction, multiple chemicals are combined to create a more complex product. In a double-displacement reaction, two chemical compounds trade bonds or ions and create two different compounds. Other common chemical reactions you may need to know for the HESI exam are the acid-base reaction, analysis (decomposition) reaction, single-displacement reaction, isomerization reaction, and hydrolysis reaction.

23. A: van der Waals forces are the weak forces of attraction between two molecules. The van der Waals force is considered to be any of the attractive or repulsive forces between electrons that are not related to electrostatic interaction or covalent bonds. Compared to other chemical bonds, the strength of van der Waals forces is small. However, these forces have a great effect on a substance's solubility and other characteristics. The HESI exam may require you to demonstrate knowledge of all the major chemical forces.

24. D: Of the given gases, H_2 effuses the fastest. It has the smallest molecular weight, and it is therefore capable of moving faster than the molecules represented by the other answer choices. In chemistry, effusion is defined as the flow of a gas through a small opening. The rate of effusion of a substance is inversely proportional to the square root of the density of the substance. This means that the less dense a substance is, the faster it will effuse. This agrees with the common observation that thick smoke tends to linger in the same form for a longer period than thin smoke or steam.

25. B: Catalysts alter the activation energy during a chemical reaction and therefore control the rate of the reaction. The substrate is the actual surface that enzymes use during a chemical reaction (and there is no such term as *substrate energy*). Inhibitors and promoters participate in the chemical reaction, but it is the activation energy that catalysts alter to control the overall rate as the reaction occurs.

26. B: Carbon is not involved in many hydrogen bonds. A hydrogen bond occurs when an atom of hydrogen that has a covalent bond with an electronegative atom forms a bond with a third atom. The original covalent bond involving hydrogen gives away protons, and the third element receives them. One of the reasons that fluorine, oxygen, and nitrogen are frequently part of a hydrogen bond is that they have a strong electronegativity and are therefore able to form more durable bonds. Chlorine is another element frequently involved in hydrogen bonds.

27. D: The mass of 0.350 mol copper is 22.2 grams. This problem requires the use of the periodic table. There you will see that the molecular mass of copper is approximately 63.5. Take this figure and multiply it by the amount of copper given by the question: 0.350 mol. The resulting figure is 22.225, which, rounded to the nearest tenth, is 22.2 grams. In order to succeed on the HESI exam, you will need to be able to perform these simple calculations of mass.

28. A: There are five d orbitals in a d subshell (or sublevel). Each of these orbitals can hold two electrons, so sublevel d is capable of holding 10 electrons. The s subshell has one orbital, the p subshell has three orbitals, the d subshell has five orbitals, and the f subshell has seven orbitals. In chemistry, the electron configuration of an atom is expressed in the following form, using helium as an example: $1s^2$. In this notation, the 1 indicates that the electrons are found in the first energy level of the atom, the s indicates that the electrons are in a spherical orbit, and the superscript 2 indicates that there are 2 total electrons in the first energy level subshell.

29. D: The number of protons in an atom is the atomic number. Protons are the fundamental positive unit of an atom. They are located in the nucleus. In a neutral atom (an atom with neither positive nor negative charge), the number of protons in the nucleus is equal to the number of electrons orbiting the nucleus. When it needs to be expressed, atomic number is written as a subscript in front of the element's symbol, for example in $_{13}Al$. Atomic mass, meanwhile, is the average mass of the various isotopes of a given element. Atomic identity is not a concept in chemistry.

30. B: Rubidium is an alkali metal. The alkali metals are located in group 1 of the periodic table. These soft substances melt at a low temperature and are typically white in color. The alkali metals are lithium, sodium, potassium, rubidium, cesium, and francium. Rubidium, cesium, and francium are not commonly encountered in the natural world. The alkali metals are highly reactive, meaning that they easily engage in chemical reactions when combined with other elements. These metals have a low density and tend to react violently with water.

Anatomy and Physiology

1. A: The chromosomes separate during anaphase and move to the opposite ends of the cells.

2. D: The epiglottis covers the trachea during swallowing, thus preventing food from entering the airway. The trachea, also known as the windpipe, is a cylindrical portion of the respiratory tract that joins the larynx with the lungs. The esophagus connects the throat and the stomach. When a person swallows, the esophagus contracts to force the food down into the stomach. Like other structures in the respiratory system, the esophagus secretes mucus for lubrication.

3. B: The pads that support the vertebrae are made up of cartilage. Cartilage, a strong form of connective tissue, cushions and supports the joints. Cartilage also makes up the larynx and the outer ear. Bone is a form of connective tissue that comprises the better part of the skeleton. It includes both organic and inorganic substances. Tendons connect the muscles to other structures of the body, typically bones. Tendons can increase and decrease in length as the bones move. Fat is a combination of lipids; in humans, fat forms a layer beneath the skin and on the outside of the internal organs.

4. A: There are four different types of tissue in the human body: epithelial, connective, muscle, and nerve. Epithelial tissue lines the internal and external surfaces of the body. It is like a sheet, consisting of squamous, cuboidal, and columnar cells. They can expand and contract, like on the inner lining of the bladder. Connective tissue provides the structure of the body, as well as the links between various body parts. Tendons, ligaments, cartilage, and bone are all examples of connective tissue. Muscle tissue is composed of tiny fibers, which contract to move the skeleton. There are three types of muscle tissue: smooth, cardiac, and skeletal. Nerve tissue makes up the nervous system; it is composed of nerve cells, nerve fibers, neuroglia, and dendrites.

5. B: The epidermis is the outermost layer of skin. The thickness of this layer of skin varies over different parts of the body. For instance, the epidermis on the eyelids is very thin, while the epidermis over the soles of the feet is much thicker. The dermis lies directly beneath the epidermis. It is composed of collagen, elastic tissue, and reticular fibers. Beneath the dermis lies the subcutaneous tissue, which consists of fat, blood vessels, and nerves. The subcutaneous tissue contributes to the regulation of body temperature. The hypodermis is the layer of cells underneath the dermis; it is generally considered to be a part of the subcutaneous tissue.

6. C: Prolactin stimulates the production of breast milk during lactation. Norepinephrine is a hormone and neurotransmitter secreted by the adrenal gland that regulates heart rate, blood pressure, and blood sugar. Antidiuretic hormone is produced by the hypothalamus and secreted by the pituitary gland. It regulates the concentration of urine and triggers the contractions of the arteries and capillaries. Oxytocin is a hormone secreted by the pituitary gland that makes it easier to eject milk from the breast and manages the contractions of the uterus during labor.

7. D: Meiosis produces cells that are genetically different, having half the number of chromosomes of the parent cells. Mitosis produces cells that are genetically identical; daughter cells have the exact same number of chromosomes as parent cells. Mitosis is useful for repairing the body while meiosis is useful for sexual reproduction.

8. D: Of the given structures, veins have the lowest blood pressure. Veins carry oxygen-poor blood from the outlying parts of the body to the heart. An artery carries oxygen-rich blood from the heart to the peripheral parts of the body. An arteriole extends from an artery to a capillary. A venule is a tiny vein that extends from a capillary to a larger vein.

9. C: Of the four heart chambers, the left ventricle is the most muscular. When it contracts, it pushes blood out to the organs and extremities of the body. The right ventricle pushes blood into the lungs. The atria, on the other hand, receive blood from the outlying parts of the body and transport it into the ventricles. The basic process works as follows: Oxygen-poor blood fills the right atrium and is pumped into the right ventricle, from which it is pumped into the pulmonary artery and on to the lungs. In the lungs, this blood is oxygenated. The blood then reenters the heart at the left atrium, which when full pumps into the left ventricle. When the left ventricle is full, blood is pushed into the aorta and on to the organs and extremities of the body.

10. A: The cerebrum contains the parietal lobe, which is the part of the brain that interprets sensory information. The cerebrum is the largest part of the brain. The cerebrum is divided into two hemispheres, connected by a thin band of tissue called the corpus callosum. The cerebellum is positioned at the back of the head, between the brain stem and the cerebrum. It controls both voluntary and involuntary movements. The medulla oblongata forms the base of the brain. This part of the brain is responsible for blood flow and breathing, among other things. The hindbrain refers to a section of the brain including the medulla oblongata, pons, and cerebellum.

11. C: Collagen is the protein produced by cartilage. Bone, tendon, and cartilage are all mainly composed of collagen. Actin and myosin are the proteins responsible for muscle contractions. Actin makes up the thinner fibers in muscle tissue, while myosin makes up the thicker fibers. Myosin is the most numerous cell protein in human muscle. Estrogen is one of the steroid hormones produced mainly by the ovaries. Estrogen motivates the menstrual cycle and the development of female sex characteristics.

12. C: The parasympathetic nervous system is responsible for lowering the heart rate. It slows down the heart rate, dilates the blood vessels, and increases the secretions of the digestive system. The central nervous system is composed of the brain and the spinal cord. The sympathetic nervous system is a part of the autonomic nervous system; its role is to oppose the actions taken by the parasympathetic nervous system. So, the sympathetic nervous system accelerates the heart, contracts the blood vessels, and decreases the secretions of the digestive system.

13. C: As a haploid cell, normal human sperm must contain one chromosome of each of the 23 chromosome pairs. Twenty-two of these pairs are autosomal chromosomes, which do not play a role in determining gender. The remaining pair consists of either two X chromosomes in the case of a female, or of an X and a Y chromosome in the case of a male. Therefore, a normal sperm cell will contain 22 autosomal chromosomes and either an X or a Y chromosome—but not both—for a total of 23.

14. B: Urea is formed during the breakdown of proteins. It is a nitrogen-rich substance filtered out of the bloodstream by the kidneys and expelled from the body in the urine. Individuals with an elevated level of urea in their bloodstream may be suffering from kidney failure. In humans and most animals, urea is the primary component of urine. However, urine also contains uric acid and ammonia. Both of these substances can be toxic to humans if they are not expelled from the body. This is one of the dangers of kidney disease and kidney failure.

15. A: A hinge joint can only move in two directions. The elbow is a hinge joint. It can only bring the lower arm closer to the upper arm or move it away from the upper arm. In a ball-and-socket joint, the rounded top of one bone fits into a concave part of another bone, enabling the first bone to rotate around in this socket. This connection is slightly less stable than other types of joints in the human body and is therefore supported by a denser network of ligaments. The shoulder and hip are both examples of ball-and-socket joints.

16. B: Smooth muscle tissue is said to be arranged in a disorderly fashion because it is not striated like the other two types of muscle: cardiac and skeletal. Striations are lines that can only be seen with a microscope. Smooth muscle is typically found in the supporting tissues of hollow organs and blood vessels. Cardiac muscle is found exclusively in the heart; it is responsible for the contractions that pump blood throughout the body. Skeletal muscle, by far the most preponderant in the body, controls the movements of the skeleton. The contractions of skeletal muscle are responsible for all voluntary motion. There is no such thing as rough muscle.

17. A: An adult inhales 500 mL of air in an average breath. Interestingly, humans can inhale about eight times as much air in a single breath as they do in an average breath. People tend to take a larger breath after making a larger exhalation. This is one reason that many breathing therapies, for instance those incorporated into yoga practice, focus on making a complete exhalation. The process of respiration is managed by the autonomic nervous system. The body requires a constant replenishing of oxygen, so even brief interruptions in respiration can be damaging or fatal.

18. D: Plasma cells secrete antibodies. These cells, also known as plasmacytes, are located in lymphoid tissue. Antibodies are only secreted in response to a particular stimulus, usually the detection of an antigen in the body. Antigens include bacteria, viruses, and parasites. Once released, antibodies bind to the antigen and neutralize it. When faced with a new antigen, the body may require some time to develop appropriate antibodies. Once the body has learned about an antigen, however, it does not forget how to produce the correct antibodies.

19. B: The integumentary system includes skin, hair, and mucous membranes, all of which are responsible—in part, at least—for blocking disease-causing pathogens from entering the bloodstream. The circulatory system distributes vital substances through the body, and the lymphatic system sends leaked fluids from the cardiovascular system back to the blood vessels. The reproductive system stores bodily hormones that influence gender traits.

20. D: The force of blood pressure motivates filtration in the kidneys. Filtration is the process through which the kidneys remove waste products from the body. All of the water in the blood passes through the kidneys every 45 minutes. Waste products are diverted into ducts and excreted from the body, while the healthy components of the water in blood are reabsorbed into the bloodstream. Peristalsis is the set of involuntary muscle movements that move food through the digestive system.

21. A: Insulin decreases the concentration of blood glucose. It is produced by the pancreas. Glucagon is a hormone produced by the pancreas. Glucagon acts in opposition to insulin, motivating an increase in the levels of blood sugar. Growth hormone is secreted by the pituitary gland. It is responsible for the growth of the body, specifically by metabolizing proteins, carbohydrates, and lipids. The glucocorticoids are a group of steroid hormones that are produced by the adrenal cortex. The glucocorticoids contribute to the metabolism of carbohydrates, proteins, and fats.

22. A: The hypothalamus controls the hormones secreted by the pituitary gland. This part of the brain maintains the body temperature and helps to control metabolism. The adrenal glands, which lie above the kidneys, secrete steroidal hormones, epinephrine, and norepinephrine. The testes are the male reproductive glands, responsible for the production of sperm and testosterone. The pancreas secretes insulin and a fluid that aids in digestion.

23. C: Forty percent of female blood volume is composed of red blood cells. Red blood cells, otherwise known as erythrocytes, are large and do not have a nucleus. These cells are produced in the bone marrow and carry oxygen throughout the body. White blood cells, also known as leukocytes, make up about 1% of the blood volume. About 55% of the blood volume is made up of plasma, which itself is primarily composed of water. The plasma in blood supplies cells with nutrients and removes metabolic waste. Blood also contains platelets, otherwise known as thrombocytes, which are essential to effective blood clotting.

24. B: High-density lipoproteins (HDL) are considered to be the healthiest form of cholesterol. This type of cholesterol actually reduces the risk of heart disease. A lipoprotein is composed of both lipid and protein. These substances cannot move through the bloodstream by themselves; they must be carried along by some other substance. Although most people think of cholesterol as an unhealthy substance, it helps to maintain cell walls and produce hormones. Cholesterol is also important in the production of vitamin D and the bile acids that aid digestion. The other answer choices are low-density lipoproteins (LDL), very-low-density lipoproteins (VLDL), and very-high-density lipoproteins (VHDL).

25. A: The digestion of starch starts with its exposure to the enzyme amylase that is found in the saliva. Amylase attacks the glycosidic bonds in starch. This attack separates them to release sugars. This is the reason why some starchy foods may taste sweet if they are chewed for a long time. Another form of amylase is made by the pancreas. This amylase continues the digestion of starches in the upper intestine. The di- and tri-saccharides are the first products of this digestion. Later, they are converted to glucose. The glucose is a monosaccharide that is easily absorbed through the intestinal wall.

26. C: The vocal cords are located in the larynx. These elastic bands vibrate and produce sound when air passes through them. The larynx lies between the pharynx and the trachea. The pharynx is the section of the throat that extends from the mouth and the nasal cavities to the larynx, at which point it becomes the esophagus. The trachea is the tube running from the larynx down to the lungs, where it terminates in the bronchi. The epiglottis is the flap that blocks food from the lungs by descending over the trachea during a swallow.

27. A: Gas exchange occurs in the alveoli, the minute air sacs on the interior of the lungs. The bronchi are large cartilage-based tubes of air; they extend from the end of the trachea into the lungs, where they branch apart. The larynx, which houses the vocal cords, is positioned between the trachea and the pharynx; it is involved in swallowing, breathing, and speaking. The pharynx extends from the nose to the uppermost portions of the trachea and esophagus. In order to enter these two structures, air and other matter must pass through the pharynx.

28. B: Axons carry action potential in the direction of synapses. Axons are the long, fiberlike structures that carry information from neurons. Electrical impulses travel along the body of the axons, some of which are up to a foot long. A neuron is a type of cell that is responsible for sending information throughout the body. There are several types of neurons, including muscle neurons, which respond to instructions for movement; sensory neurons, which transmit information about the external world; and interneurons, which relay messages between neurons. Myelin is a fat that coats the nerves and ensures the accurate transmission of information in the nervous system.

29. A: The parathyroid gland is located in the neck, directly behind the thyroid gland. It is responsible for the metabolism of calcium. It is part of the endocrine system. When the supply of calcium in blood diminishes to unhealthy levels, the parathyroid gland motivates the secretion of a hormone that encourages the bones to release calcium into the bloodstream. The parathyroid gland also regulates the amount of phosphate in the blood by stimulating the excretion of phosphates in the urine.

30. B: In the lungs, oxygen is transported from the air to the blood through the process of diffusion. Specifically, the alveolar membranes withdraw the oxygen from the air in the lungs into the bloodstream. Osmosis is the movement of a solution from an area of low concentration to an area of higher concentration through a permeable membrane. Dissipation is any wasteful consumption or use. Reverse osmosis is a process for purifying a solution by forcing it through a membrane that blocks only certain pollutants.

Physics

1. B: Kinetic energy is the energy of motion and is defined as $KE = \frac{1}{2}mv^2$. Using this equation, if you double the mass and the velocity of an object, you find $KE = \frac{1}{2}(2m')(2v')^2$, or 8 times the original KE. Therefore, the motorcycle has 8 times as much kinetic energy as the bicycle.

2. C: The formula for velocity given constant acceleration is $v = v_0 + at$. Since the bicyclist starts from rest, $v_0 = 0$. So $v = (2\ \text{m/s}^2)(10\ \text{s}) = 20\ \text{m/s}$.

3. B: During one full rotation, the horse travels a distance of $\pi d \approx (3.14)(3\ \text{m}) = 9.42\ \text{m}$. The speed is then equal to distance divided by time, $(9.42\ \text{m})/20\ \text{s} = 0.47\ \text{m/s}$.

4. A: The temperature of a gas is related to the average kinetic energy of the component particles. If the molecule speed increases, the kinetic energy increases, and the temperature must also increase by definition. Any of the other choices *could* be true, depending on factors such as whether the gas is in a sealed and rigid container, but only choice A *must* be true.

5. D: The amplitude is in this case simply the maximum displacement from equilibrium (20 centimeters). The period is the time in which the point completes one full cycle (4 seconds), and the frequency is just the inverse of the period (0.25 Hz). To find the wavelength, however, information about a different point that corresponds to this one, or about the speed of the wave, is required and not given.

6. D: There are several different ways to approach this problem, but perhaps the simplest is by conservation of energy. On the flat stretch, we can take the car's gravitational potential energy as zero, so its mechanical energy is purely kinetic: $KE = \frac{1}{2}mv^2$. If the car just barely makes it to the top of the loop (like a projectile at the top of its arc), its velocity and therefore its kinetic energy are zero at that point, and its mechanical energy is purely gravitational potential energy: $PE = mgh$. Since energy is conserved, the energy at these two points must be equal: $\frac{1}{2}mv^2 = mgh$. The masses cancel, leaving $\frac{1}{2}v^2 = gh$, and solving for v yields

$$\begin{aligned} v &= \sqrt{2gh} \\ &= \sqrt{2(9.8\ \text{m/s}^2)(10\ \text{m})} \\ &= \sqrt{196\frac{\text{m}^2}{s^2}} \\ &= 14\ \text{m/s} \end{aligned}$$

7. A: The charge on the glass rod is positive and the charge on the cloth is negative when the glass rod is rubbed with a cloth made of polyester. This is an example of static electricity—the collection of electrically charged particles on the surface of a material. A static charge can be quickly discharged, commonly called a "spark," or discharged more slowly by dissipating to the ground. A static charge occurs because different materials have a capacity for giving up electrons and becoming positive (+), or for attracting electrons and becoming negative (−). The triboelectric series is a list of materials and their propensities for either giving up electrons to become positive or to gain the electrons to become negative. Polyester has a tendency to gain electrons to become negative and glass has a tendency to lose electrons to become positive.

8. C: Net work done is determined by the change in energy. Since the crate is not moving in the initial or final state, the relevant energy is gravitational potential energy. From the ground, the final change in altitude of the crate is 6 meters, which corresponds to a potential energy change of $mg\Delta h = (1{,}000\text{ N})(6\text{ m}) = 6{,}000\text{ J}$, and the net work done by the crane is 6,000 J. The fact that the crane first raised the crate to an altitude of 10 m before lowering it to 6 m is irrelevant for finding the net work.

9. D: The impulse is equal to the change in momentum. The initial momentum is $(0.4\text{ kg})(1\text{ m/s}) = 0.4\ (\text{kg}\cdot\text{m})/\text{s}$ towards the player. The final momentum is $(0.4\text{ kg})(8\text{ m/s}) = 3.2\ (\text{kg}\cdot\text{m})/\text{s}$ in the opposite direction. The change is then $(3.2\ (\text{kg}\cdot\text{m})/\text{s}) - (-0.4\ (\text{kg}\cdot\text{m})/\text{s})$, where the negative sign reflects the opposite directions), which equals $3.6\ (\text{kg}\cdot\text{m})/\text{s}$.

10. C: Since the ring isn't moving, the net force is zero. If we separate the force into perpendicular components, both components must be zero. If we consider the x direction to be to the right on the page, and the y direction to be upward, then one student is pulling completely in the $+x$ direction, and another is pulling completely in the $-y$ direction. Consider the y components first. One student is pulling with a force of 100 N in the $-y$ direction, while another is pulling at an angle with a force of 115 N. The y components of these forces must cancel, and the y component of the 115 N force must be 100 N. This means the Pythagorean theorem can find the x component of the force at an angle: $\sqrt{(115\text{ N})^2 - (100\text{ N})^2} = 57\text{ N}$ in the $-x$ direction. Since the x components of all the forces must also cancel, the unknown force must be 57 N in the $+x$ direction.

11. A: Heat between objects in contact with each other is transferred by conduction. Convection is transfer by currents within a body of fluid, and radiation is the transfer of heat between objects *not* in contact, through light rays emitted by the hotter object and absorbed by the cooler one.

12. D: Sound cannot travel through a vacuum, though it doesn't necessarily follow that it *can* travel through solids. Nor does the fact sound can travel through a solid follow from the fact that the atoms are packed tightly together. The fact that a sound is produced by knocking on a solid object also does not prove sound can pass through the object. However, if you hear a sound on the other side of a solid wall, the sound must have traveled through the wall.

13. A: The velocities of both the wind and the aircraft can be represented by vectors, with the length of the vector representing the speed, and the direction of the vector representing the direction of either the wind or the airplane. Since the wind speed opposes that of the plane, the pilot will measure the sum of the actual wind speed plus that of his aircraft:

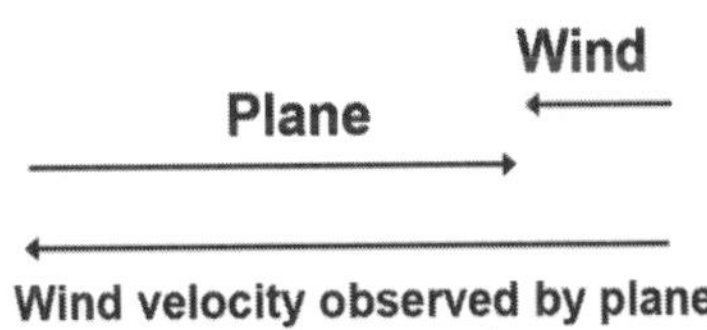

14. B: The effective resistance of two or more resistors in parallel is equal to the reciprocal of the sum of their reciprocal resistances. The two resistors in parallel therefore have an effective resistance of $((200\ \Omega)^{-1} + (500\ \Omega)^{-1})^{-1} = 142.9\ \Omega$. Resistances in series simply sum, so the total resistance of the parallel element plus the second 200 Ω resistor is $142.9\ \Omega + 200\ \Omega = 342.9\ \Omega$. Ohm's Law, $V = IR$, can be used to solve for current: $I = \frac{12\text{ V}}{342.9\ \Omega} = 0.035\text{ A} = 35\text{ mA}$.

15. C: If the 200 kg barrel has an acceleration of $0.13\ \text{m/s}^2$, the net force on the barrel is $\sum F = ma = (200\ \text{kg})(0.13\ \text{m/s}^2) = 26\ \text{N}$. Since Jim is exerting a force of 320 N, there must be a force working against him with a magnitude of $320\ \text{N} - 26\ \text{N} = 294\ \text{N}$.

16. B: Refraction is governed by Snell's law, $n_1 \sin\theta_1 = n_2 \sin\theta_2$. If n_1 is defined to be the index of refraction of air, and n_2 the index of refraction of amber, Snell's law yields $n_1 \sin 32° = n_2 \sin 20°$. Solving for n_2 using the fact the index of refraction of air is very close to 1 yields $n_2 = \frac{\sin 32°}{\sin 20°} = 1.55$. Note these calculations must be performed in degree mode rather than radian.

17. A: X-rays have a short wavelength (several orders of magnitude shorter than the wavelength of visible light), which rules out choices B and D. Choice C is true—photons with a shorter wavelength do have higher energies—but does not explain why x-rays are used in medical imaging. (If anything, the higher energy would seem to be a disadvantage for medical imaging since it would mean a greater chance of tissue damage.) Only choice A accurately explains why x-rays are used in medical imaging.

18. B: Choice D would violate the law of conservation of energy. If the chemicals heat up, their temperatures increase, and their kinetic energies therefore increase, so energy could not have been obtained from kinetic energy, so choice A is incorrect. Chemical reactions also do not typically involve absorption of heat from the environment as stated by choice C. Choice B correctly describes the situation: chemical bonds contain some amount of potential energy, which may be released in certain chemical reactions.

19. B: Ohm's Law states that voltage and current in an electrical circuit are directly proportional to one another. Ohm's Law can be expressed as $V = IR$, where V is voltage, I is current and R is resistance. Voltage is also known as electrical potential difference and is the force that moves electrons through a circuit. For a given amount of resistance, an increase in voltage will result in an increase in current. Resistance and current are inversely proportional to each other. For a given voltage, an increase in resistance will result in a decrease in current.

20. B: Since no information is given about how elastic the collision was, it is safest to avoid appealing to conservation of kinetic energy, but this problem can be solved using conservation of momentum. Before the collision, the total momentum is Before the collision, the total momentum is $(100\ \text{kg})(4.0\ \text{m/s}) = 400\ (\text{kg} \cdot \text{m})/\text{s}$. (The second sled's initial velocity is zero, so it has no momentum.) After the collision, the first sled's momentum is $(100\ \text{kg})(1.0\ \text{m/s}) = 100\ (\text{kg} \cdot \text{m})/\text{s}$. Since the total momentum is conserved, the second sled's momentum must then be $400\ (\text{kg} \cdot \text{m})/\text{s} - 100\ (\text{kg} \cdot \text{m})/\text{s} = 300\ (\text{kg} \cdot \text{m})/\text{s}$, and its speed must be $(300\ (\text{kg} \cdot \text{m})/\text{s}) \div (80\ \text{kg}) = 3.8\ \text{m/s}$.

21. B: The speed of sound, like the speed of other mechanical waves, depends on the density and the rigidity of the medium. The less dense and the more rigid a medium, the faster sound waves will travel through it. Aluminum is both less dense and more rigid than rubber or water, so we expect the speed of sound to be greater in aluminum than in either of these media. While aluminum is denser than air, it is much, much more rigid than air; in general, sound tends to travel faster through solids and liquids than through gases. We therefore expect the speed of sound to be greater in aluminum than in air as well, and B is the correct choice.

22. A: Acceleration is equal to the slope of the graph of velocity versus time. At points B and D, the slope of the graph is zero, so the acceleration is zero. The slope of the graph is steeper at point A than at point C, so the magnitude of the acceleration is greater at point A. Additionally, at point C the slope, and therefore the acceleration, is negative, less than any non-negative value. Therefore, of the four labeled points, the acceleration is greatest at point A.

23. D: Radiation therapy works because the high-energy photons or charged particles impact the DNA of the cancer cells, damaging it and harming the cells' ability to grow and reproduce. Of course, the radiation has the same effect on other cells, but healthy cells may have more resilient repair mechanisms for their DNA than cancer cells, making them somewhat less susceptible to radiation damage. Furthermore, the radiation is often applied in different beams that intersect at the site of the cancer cells, ensuring that the cancer cells get a much higher dosage than the surrounding healthy cells. Radiation therapy has nothing to do with destructively vibrating cancer cells or pulling them apart electromagnetically, nor does it have to do with destructive wave interference. While cancer cells, like other particles and objects, may have associated De Broglie wavelengths, these wavelengths are too small compared to those of the radiation used for interference to occur. The correct choice is D.

24. A: There are three different values for the current through different parts of this circuit: the current through the 6 V battery, the current through the 100 Ω resistor, and the current through the 9 V battery and 50 Ω resistor. Kirchhoff's circuit laws can calculate each of these currents: the junction rule gives one relation between the currents, and applications of the loop rule yield two more; three equations to solve for three unknowns. However, applying Kirchhoff's loop rule to the bottom loop yields an equation that can be solved directly for the current through the 100 Ω resistor. Specifically, a clockwise loop yields $6\text{ V} - (100\ \Omega)I = 0$, so that $I = \frac{6\text{ V}}{100\ \Omega} = 60\text{ mA}$, which is choice A. Determining which direction this current flows through the 100 Ω resistor, left or right, requires solving the system of Kirchhoff equations, but for this problem, the magnitude is sufficient.

25. D: Mario balances a book on his head. In this example, work is not applied to the book because the book is not moving. One definition of work is a force acting on an object to cause displacement. In this case, the book was not displaced by the force applied to it. Mario's head applied a vertical force to the book to keep it in the same position.

26. D: Convection is a process through which heat is transferred within a fluid by the movement of molecules, including large-scale internal flow of the fluid itself. Of the given choices, only the coastline heated by the warm ocean current fits this description. Food is cooked in a microwave through radiation, a pancake cooks primarily through conduction of heat from the burner to the pan to the pancake, and the sun heats planets through radiation of heat and energy through the intervening space. The correct answer is D.

27. C: The tension in the string is equal to the centripetal force keeping the ball in circular motion, given by $F = \frac{mv^2}{r}$. Since the circumference of the circle of motion is $2\pi r = 2\pi(0.75\text{ m}) = 4.71\text{ m}$, and the period of the motion is $\frac{1\text{ s}}{2\text{ period}} = 0.5\text{ s per period}$, the velocity is given by $\frac{4.71\text{ m}}{0.5\text{ s}} = 9.42\ \text{m/s}$. The centripetal force, the tension in the string, is therefore:

$$F = \frac{(0.080\text{ kg})(9.42\ \text{m/s})^2}{0.75\text{ m}} = 9.5\text{ N}$$

28. B: Stretching the spring gives it some elastic potential energy. The work done is equal to the total change in energy, so this (non-zero) potential energy must be taken into account to calculate the (non-zero) work, and D is incorrect. Knowing the mass of the weight and the displacement from equilibrium is enough to find the spring constant and therefore this energy, but that information is not given! What is given is the mass of the weight, and the displacement from the equilibrium position of the hanging mass; no information is given about how much the spring stretches when the mass is first hung. The information in choice A compounds the problem; it does not provide information about the "weighted" equilibrium position, and the time provided by choice C is irrelevant. Without knowing the additional potential energy in the stretched spring (or without knowing the spring constant, from which we could calculate the potential energy), it cannot be determined how much work was done on the spring. B is therefore correct.

29. A: This problem can be solved using conservation of energy. At the top of the swing, just before he steps off the platform, the boy's kinetic energy is zero. His potential energy is equal to $mgh = m(9.8\ \text{m/s}^2)(2.0\ \text{m}) = (19.6\ \text{m}^2/\text{s}^2)m$. (The answer must be expressed this way, since the boy's mass is not given.) At the bottom of the swing, $mgh = m(9.8\ \text{m/s}^2)(0.5\ \text{m}) = (4.9\ \text{m}^2/\text{s}^2)m$. Since the total energy is conserved, the kinetic energy he gains must be equal to the potential energy he loses, and the kinetic energy at the bottom of his swing must then be $(19.6\ \text{m}^2/\text{s}^2)m - (4.9\ \text{m}^2/\text{s}^2)m = (14.7\ \text{m}^2/\text{s}^2)m$. The undetermined mass cancels, and we can solve for v to get $v = \sqrt{2(14.7\ \text{m}^2/\text{s}^2)} = 5.4\ \text{m/s}$.

30. B: The amplitude is equal to the difference between the maximum displacement (for example, the height of the peak of the graph) and equilibrium. Here, equilibrium is at 0 cm, and the peak reaches 4 cm, so the amplitude is equal to (4 cm − 0 cm) = 4 cm. The x-axis (time) is irrelevant for finding the amplitude, and B is correct.

HESI Practice Tests #2 and #3

To take these additional HESI practice tests, visit our bonus page:
mometrix.com/bonus948/hesia2

How to Overcome Test Anxiety

Just the thought of taking a test is enough to make most people a little nervous. A test is an important event that can have a long-term impact on your future, so it's important to take it seriously and it's natural to feel anxious about performing well. But just because anxiety is normal, that doesn't mean that it's helpful in test taking, or that you should simply accept it as part of your life. Anxiety can have a variety of effects. These effects can be mild, like making you feel slightly nervous, or severe, like blocking your ability to focus or remember even a simple detail.

If you experience test anxiety—whether severe or mild—it's important to know how to beat it. To discover this, first you need to understand what causes test anxiety.

Causes of Test Anxiety

While we often think of anxiety as an uncontrollable emotional state, it can actually be caused by simple, practical things. One of the most common causes of test anxiety is that a person does not feel adequately prepared for their test. This feeling can be the result of many different issues such as poor study habits or lack of organization, but the most common culprit is time management. Starting to study too late, failing to organize your study time to cover all of the material, or being distracted while you study will mean that you're not well prepared for the test. This may lead to cramming the night before, which will cause you to be physically and mentally exhausted for the test. Poor time management also contributes to feelings of stress, fear, and hopelessness as you realize you are not well prepared but don't know what to do about it.

Other times, test anxiety is not related to your preparation for the test but comes from unresolved fear. This may be a past failure on a test, or poor performance on tests in general. It may come from comparing yourself to others who seem to be performing better or from the stress of living up to expectations. Anxiety may be driven by fears of the future—how failure on this test would affect your educational and career goals. These fears are often completely irrational, but they can still negatively impact your test performance.

Elements of Test Anxiety

As mentioned earlier, test anxiety is considered to be an emotional state, but it has physical and mental components as well. Sometimes you may not even realize that you are suffering from test anxiety until you notice the physical symptoms. These can include trembling hands, rapid heartbeat, sweating, nausea, and tense muscles. Extreme anxiety may lead to fainting or vomiting. Obviously, any of these symptoms can have a negative impact on testing. It is important to recognize them as soon as they begin to occur so that you can address the problem before it damages your performance.

The mental components of test anxiety include trouble focusing and inability to remember learned information. During a test, your mind is on high alert, which can help you recall information and stay focused for an extended period of time. However, anxiety interferes with your mind's natural processes, causing you to blank out, even on the questions you know well. The strain of testing during anxiety makes it difficult to stay focused, especially on a test that may take several hours. Extreme anxiety can take a huge mental toll, making it difficult not only to recall test information but even to understand the test questions or pull your thoughts together.

Effects of Test Anxiety

Test anxiety is like a disease—if left untreated, it will get progressively worse. Anxiety leads to poor performance, and this reinforces the feelings of fear and failure, which in turn lead to poor performances on subsequent tests. It can grow from a mild nervousness to a crippling condition. If allowed to progress, test anxiety can have a big impact on your schooling, and consequently on your future.

Test anxiety can spread to other parts of your life. Anxiety on tests can become anxiety in any stressful situation, and blanking on a test can turn into panicking in a job situation. But fortunately, you don't have to let anxiety rule your testing and determine your grades. There are a number of relatively simple steps you can take to move past anxiety and function normally on a test and in the rest of life.

Physical Steps for Beating Test Anxiety

While test anxiety is a serious problem, the good news is that it can be overcome. It doesn't have to control your ability to think and remember information. While it may take time, you can begin taking steps today to beat anxiety.

Just as your first hint that you may be struggling with anxiety comes from the physical symptoms, the first step to treating it is also physical. Rest is crucial for having a clear, strong mind. If you are tired, it is much easier to give in to anxiety. But if you establish good sleep habits, your body and mind will be ready to perform optimally, without the strain of exhaustion. Additionally, sleeping well helps you to retain information better, so you're more likely to recall the answers when you see the test questions.

Getting good sleep means more than going to bed on time. It's important to allow your brain time to relax. Take study breaks from time to time so it doesn't get overworked, and don't study right before bed. Take time to rest your mind before trying to rest your body, or you may find it difficult to fall asleep.

Along with sleep, other aspects of physical health are important in preparing for a test. Good nutrition is vital for good brain function. Sugary foods and drinks may give a burst of energy but this burst is followed by a crash, both physically and emotionally. Instead, fuel your body with protein and vitamin-rich foods.

Also, drink plenty of water. Dehydration can lead to headaches and exhaustion, especially if your brain is already under stress from the rigors of the test. Particularly if your test is a long one, drink water during the breaks. And if possible, take an energy-boosting snack to eat between sections.

Along with sleep and diet, a third important part of physical health is exercise. Maintaining a steady workout schedule is helpful, but even taking 5-minute study breaks to walk can help get your blood pumping faster and clear your head. Exercise also releases endorphins, which contribute to a positive feeling and can help combat test anxiety.

When you nurture your physical health, you are also contributing to your mental health. If your body is healthy, your mind is much more likely to be healthy as well. So take time to rest, nourish your body with healthy food and water, and get moving as much as possible. Taking these physical steps will make you stronger and more able to take the mental steps necessary to overcome test anxiety.

Mental Steps for Beating Test Anxiety

Working on the mental side of test anxiety can be more challenging, but as with the physical side, there are clear steps you can take to overcome it. As mentioned earlier, test anxiety often stems from lack of preparation, so the obvious solution is to prepare for the test. Effective studying may be the most important weapon you have for beating test anxiety, but you can and should employ several other mental tools to combat fear.

First, boost your confidence by reminding yourself of past success—tests or projects that you aced. If you're putting as much effort into preparing for this test as you did for those, there's no reason you should expect to fail here. Work hard to prepare; then trust your preparation.

Second, surround yourself with encouraging people. It can be helpful to find a study group, but be sure that the people you're around will encourage a positive attitude. If you spend time with others who are anxious or cynical, this will only contribute to your own anxiety. Look for others who are motivated to study hard from a desire to succeed, not from a fear of failure.

Third, reward yourself. A test is physically and mentally tiring, even without anxiety, and it can be helpful to have something to look forward to. Plan an activity following the test, regardless of the outcome, such as going to a movie or getting ice cream.

When you are taking the test, if you find yourself beginning to feel anxious, remind yourself that you know the material. Visualize successfully completing the test. Then take a few deep, relaxing breaths and return to it. Work through the questions carefully but with confidence, knowing that you are capable of succeeding.

Developing a healthy mental approach to test taking will also aid in other areas of life. Test anxiety affects more than just the actual test—it can be damaging to your mental health and even contribute to depression. It's important to beat test anxiety before it becomes a problem for more than testing.

Study Strategy

Being prepared for the test is necessary to combat anxiety, but what does being prepared look like? You may study for hours on end and still not feel prepared. What you need is a strategy for test prep. The next few pages outline our recommended steps to help you plan out and conquer the challenge of preparation.

Step 1: Scope Out the Test

Learn everything you can about the format (multiple choice, essay, etc.) and what will be on the test. Gather any study materials, course outlines, or sample exams that may be available. Not only will this help you to prepare, but knowing what to expect can help to alleviate test anxiety.

Step 2: Map Out the Material

Look through the textbook or study guide and make note of how many chapters or sections it has. Then divide these over the time you have. For example, if a book has 15 chapters and you have five days to study, you need to cover three chapters each day. Even better, if you have the time, leave an extra day at the end for overall review after you have gone through the material in depth.

If time is limited, you may need to prioritize the material. Look through it and make note of which sections you think you already have a good grasp on, and which need review. While you are studying, skim quickly through the familiar sections and take more time on the challenging parts.

Write out your plan so you don't get lost as you go. Having a written plan also helps you feel more in control of the study, so anxiety is less likely to arise from feeling overwhelmed at the amount to cover.

Step 3: Gather Your Tools

Decide what study method works best for you. Do you prefer to highlight in the book as you study and then go back over the highlighted portions? Or do you type out notes of the important information? Or is it helpful to make flashcards that you can carry with you? Assemble the pens, index cards, highlighters, post-it notes, and any other materials you may need so you won't be distracted by getting up to find things while you study.

If you're having a hard time retaining the information or organizing your notes, experiment with different methods. For example, try color-coding by subject with colored pens, highlighters, or post-it notes. If you learn better by hearing, try recording yourself reading your notes so you can listen while in the car, working out, or simply sitting at your desk. Ask a friend to quiz you from your flashcards, or try teaching someone the material to solidify it in your mind.

Step 4: Create Your Environment

It's important to avoid distractions while you study. This includes both the obvious distractions like visitors and the subtle distractions like an uncomfortable chair (or a too-comfortable couch that makes you want to fall asleep). Set up the best study environment possible: good lighting and a comfortable work area. If background music helps you focus, you may want to turn it on, but otherwise keep the room quiet. If you are using a computer to take notes, be sure you don't have any other windows open, especially applications like social media, games, or anything else that could distract you. Silence your phone and turn off notifications. Be sure to keep water close by so you stay hydrated while you study (but avoid unhealthy drinks and snacks).

Also, take into account the best time of day to study. Are you freshest first thing in the morning? Try to set aside some time then to work through the material. Is your mind clearer in the afternoon or evening? Schedule your study session then. Another method is to study at the same time of day that you will take the test, so that your brain gets used to working on the material at that time and will be ready to focus at test time.

Step 5: Study!

Once you have done all the study preparation, it's time to settle into the actual studying. Sit down, take a few moments to settle your mind so you can focus, and begin to follow your study plan. Don't give in to distractions or let yourself procrastinate. This is your time to prepare so you'll be ready to fearlessly approach the test. Make the most of the time and stay focused.

Of course, you don't want to burn out. If you study too long you may find that you're not retaining the information very well. Take regular study breaks. For example, taking five minutes out of every hour to walk briskly, breathing deeply and swinging your arms, can help your mind stay fresh.

As you get to the end of each chapter or section, it's a good idea to do a quick review. Remind yourself of what you learned and work on any difficult parts. When you feel that you've mastered the material, move on to the next part. At the end of your study session, briefly skim through your notes again.

But while review is helpful, cramming last minute is NOT. If at all possible, work ahead so that you won't need to fit all your study into the last day. Cramming overloads your brain with more information than it can process and retain, and your tired mind may struggle to recall even previously learned information when it is overwhelmed with last-minute study. Also, the urgent nature of cramming and the stress placed on your brain contribute to anxiety. You'll be more likely to go to the test feeling unprepared and having trouble thinking clearly.

So don't cram, and don't stay up late before the test, even just to review your notes at a leisurely pace. Your brain needs rest more than it needs to go over the information again. In fact, plan to finish your studies by noon or early afternoon the day before the test. Give your brain the rest of the day to relax or focus on other things, and get a good night's sleep. Then you will be fresh for the test and better able to recall what you've studied.

Step 6: Take a Practice Test

Many courses offer sample tests, either online or in the study materials. This is an excellent resource to check whether you have mastered the material, as well as to prepare for the test format and environment.

Check the test format ahead of time: the number of questions, the type (multiple choice, free response, etc.), and the time limit. Then create a plan for working through them. For example, if you have 30 minutes to take a 60-question test, your limit is 30 seconds per question. Spend less time on the questions you know well so that you can take more time on the difficult ones.

If you have time to take several practice tests, take the first one open book, with no time limit. Work through the questions at your own pace and make sure you fully understand them. Gradually work up to taking a test under test conditions: sit at a desk with all study materials put away and set a timer. Pace yourself to make sure you finish the test with time to spare and go back to check your answers if you have time.

After each test, check your answers. On the questions you missed, be sure you understand why you missed them. Did you misread the question (tests can use tricky wording)? Did you forget the information? Or was it something you hadn't learned? Go back and study any shaky areas that the practice tests reveal.

Taking these tests not only helps with your grade, but also aids in combating test anxiety. If you're already used to the test conditions, you're less likely to worry about it, and working through tests until you're scoring well gives you a confidence boost. Go through the practice tests until you feel comfortable, and then you can go into the test knowing that you're ready for it.

Test Tips

On test day, you should be confident, knowing that you've prepared well and are ready to answer the questions. But aside from preparation, there are several test day strategies you can employ to maximize your performance.

First, as stated before, get a good night's sleep the night before the test (and for several nights before that, if possible). Go into the test with a fresh, alert mind rather than staying up late to study.

Try not to change too much about your normal routine on the day of the test. It's important to eat a nutritious breakfast, but if you normally don't eat breakfast at all, consider eating just a protein bar. If you're a coffee drinker, go ahead and have your normal coffee. Just make sure you time it so that the caffeine doesn't wear off right in the middle of your test. Avoid sugary beverages, and drink enough water to stay hydrated but not so much that you need a restroom break 10 minutes into the test. If your test isn't first thing in the morning, consider going for a walk or doing a light workout before the test to get your blood flowing.

Allow yourself enough time to get ready, and leave for the test with plenty of time to spare so you won't have the anxiety of scrambling to arrive in time. Another reason to be early is to select a good seat. It's helpful to sit away from doors and windows, which can be distracting. Find a good seat, get out your supplies, and settle your mind before the test begins.

When the test begins, start by going over the instructions carefully, even if you already know what to expect. Make sure you avoid any careless mistakes by following the directions.

Then begin working through the questions, pacing yourself as you've practiced. If you're not sure on an answer, don't spend too much time on it, and don't let it shake your confidence. Either skip it and come back later, or eliminate as many wrong answers as possible and guess among the remaining ones. Don't dwell on these questions as you continue—put them out of your mind and focus on what lies ahead.

Be sure to read all of the answer choices, even if you're sure the first one is the right answer. Sometimes you'll find a better one if you keep reading. But don't second-guess yourself if you do immediately know the answer. Your gut instinct is usually right. Don't let test anxiety rob you of the information you know.

If you have time at the end of the test (and if the test format allows), go back and review your answers. Be cautious about changing any, since your first instinct tends to be correct, but make sure you didn't misread any of the questions or accidentally mark the wrong answer choice. Look over any you skipped and make an educated guess.

At the end, leave the test feeling confident. You've done your best, so don't waste time worrying about your performance or wishing you could change anything. Instead, celebrate the successful completion of this test. And finally, use this test to learn how to deal with anxiety even better next time.

Review Video: Test Anxiety
Visit mometrix.com/academy and enter code: 100340

Important Qualification

Not all anxiety is created equal. If your test anxiety is causing major issues in your life beyond the classroom or testing center, or if you are experiencing troubling physical symptoms related to your anxiety, it may be a sign of a serious physiological or psychological condition. If this sounds like your situation, we strongly encourage you to seek professional help.

Additional Bonus Material

Due to our efforts to try to keep this book to a manageable length, we've created a link that will give you access to all of your additional bonus material:

mometrix.com/bonus948/hesia2